Conducting and Reading Research in Health and Human Performance

Conducting and Reading Research in Health and Human Performance

Second Edition

Ted A. Baumgartner
University of Georgia

Clinton H. Strong
Indiana University (Retired)

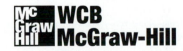

WCB
McGraw-Hill

Boston, Massachusetts   Burr Ridge, Illinois   Dubuque, Iowa
Madison, Wisconsin   New York, New York   San Francisco, California   St. Louis, Missouri

WCB/McGraw-Hill

A Division of The **McGraw·Hill** *Companies*

CONDUCTING AND READING RESEARCH IN HEALTH AND HUMAN PERFORMANCE

 This book is printed on recycled, acid-free paper containing 10% postconsumer waste.

1 2 3 4 5 7 8 9 0 KGP/KGP 9 0 9 8 7

ISBN 0-697-29509-5

Publisher: *Edward E. Bartell*
Associate Sponsoring Editor: *Theresa Grutz*
Project manager: *Donna Nemmers*
Production supervisor: *Laura Fuller*
Design freelance coordinator: *Mary L. Christianson*
Cover design: *Kay Fulton*
Cover image: *© David Bishop/PHOTOTAKE*
Compositor: *Electronic Publishing Services, Inc.*
Typeface: *10/12 Times Roman*
Printer: *Quebecor/Kingsport*

Library of Congress Cataloging-in Publication Data

Baumgartner, Ted A.
  Conducting and reading research in health and human performance /
Ted A. Baumgartner, Clinton H. Strong. — 2nd ed.
      p.   cm.
  Includes bibliographical references and index.
  ISBN 0-697-29509-5
  1. Medicine—Research—Methodology. 2. Health—Research—
Methodology. I. Strong, Clinton H.   II. Title.
R850.B365   1997
610'.72—dc21   97–8348

http://www.mhcollege.com

Defining the Problem   33
Developing the Research Proposal   37
   Proposal Title   38
   Writing Chapter 1: Introduction   39
   Statement of the Problem   39
   Purpose of the Study   40
   *Need for the Study (Significance of the Study, Justification for
     the Study)   41*
   Delimitations   42
   Limitations   43
   Assumptions   44
   Hypotheses   45
   Definition of Terms   45
   The Use of Literature in Research   46
   The Working Bibliography   47
   Research Reading   47
   Writing Chapter 2: Literature Review   49
   Sources of Literature   51
   Indexes   51
   Reviews   52
   Periodicals   53
   Computer Retrieval Systems   60
   Conducting a Computer Search   61
   Writing Chapter 3: Data Collection Procedures   62
   Example 2.1 An Opening Paragraph   64
   Example 2.2 Selection of Subjects   64
   Example 2.3 Selection of the Test Instruments   65
   Example 2.4 Design of the Study   66
   Example 2.5 Treatment of Data   66
Summary   67

3   Selected Elements of the Research Process   68

The Research Approach   69
   Time Frame of Interest   69
   Intent   70
Hypotheses   70
The Concept of Variables   71
   Quantitative and Qualitative Variables   71
   Discrete Variables   71
   Continuous Variables   72
   Independent and Dependent Variables   72
   Error-Producing Variables   73

Contents

Preface   xiii

PART I   THE RESEARCH PROCESS   2

---

1   The Nature and Purpose of Research   4

The Essence of a Profession: Knowledge   4
Research: The Knowledge Pipeline   5
The Search for Truth   5
The Scientific Method   7
   Example 1.1 Example of an Application of the Research Process   9
Research and Theory   11
Empiricism   12
Types of Research   12
   Pure, Fundamental, or Basic Research   12
   Applied Research   13
   Action Research   13
Research Classifications   14
Hypotheses and Research   17
The Significance of Research in HHP   20
Ethical Concerns   22
   Example 1.2 Protection of Human Subjects Form   24
   Example 1.3 Informed Consent Statement   26
Summary   27

2   The Research Problem   29

Steps in the Research Process   29
Selecting the Problem   31

Intervening Variables   73
Extraneous Variables   74
Attribute Variables   75
Control of Variables   75
Random Selection of Subjects   75
Equating or Matching by Some Criterion   75
Excluding the Variable   76
Data Collecting Methods and Techniques   76
  Observation Techniques   77
Direct   77
Indirect   77
Participant   77
  Measurement Techniques   78
Physical Measures   78
Cognitive Measures   78
Affective Measures   79
Measurement Techniques in HHP   79
  Questioning Techniques   85
Structured Questionnaire   85
Unstructured Questionnaire   86
Checklist   86
Structured Interview   86
Unstructured Interview   87
Delphi Technique   88
  Criteria for Selecting Methods and Techniques   88
The Data-Collecting Instruments   89
  Selecting the Instrument   90
  Revising the Instrument   91
  Instrument Development   92
Summary   93

4 Selection of Research Subjects: Sampling Procedures   95

Population and Sample   96
Sample Selection Methods   97
  Random Selection   97
  Stratified Random Sampling   99
  Systematic Sampling   100
  Cluster Sampling   101
  Multistage Sampling   101
  Deliberate Sampling   101
  Nonprobability Samples   102
Sample Size   103
Summary   105

PART II   TYPES OF RESEARCH   110

5   Experimental Research   110

Steps in Experimental Research   111
Internal and External Validity   114
Controlling Threats to Validity   115
   Threats to Internal Validity   115
   History   115
   Maturation   116
   Testing   116
   Instrumentation   116
   Statistical Regression   116
   Selection   117
   Experimental Mortality   117
   Interaction of Selection and Maturation or History   117
   Threats to External Validity   117
   Interaction Effect of Testing   117
   Interaction Effects of Selection Bias and Experimental Treatment   118
   Reactive Effects of Experimental Setting   118
   Multiple-Treatment Interference   118
Types of Designs   118
Validity in Summary   122
Methods of Control   122
Common Sources of Error   125
   Hawthorne Effect   125
   Placebo Effect   125
   "John Henry" Effect   126
   Rating Effect   126
   Experimenter Bias Effect   126
   Subject-Researcher Interaction Effect   127
   Post Hoc Error   127
Measurement in Experimental Research   128
Summary   128

6   Descriptive Research   130

Types of Descriptive Research   131
   Survey   131
   Developmental   131
   Case Study   132
   Correlational   132
   Normative   133
   Observational   134

Action   134
Ex Post Facto   134
Survey Research   135
Preliminary Considerations in Planning a Survey   135
Survey Methods   136
Phone Interview   136
Personal Interview   136
Administered Questionnaire   137
Distributed Questionnaire   138
Example 6.1 Example Questionnaire   146
Questionnaire Summary   149
Summary   150

7   Historical Research   151

The Nature of Historical Research   151
Data Control and Interpretation   152
Sources of Historical Data   153
Primary Sources   153
Secondary Sources   154
Evaluating Historical Data   155
External Criticism   155
Internal Criticism   156
Oral History   156
Biographical Research   157
Hypotheses in Historical Research   159
Historical Research in HHP   159
Format for Historical Research   161
Sample Format for Historical Research   161
Summary   164

8   Creative Activities   165

Introduction   165
Examples in HHP   166
Procedures and Evaluation   167
Fine Arts Departments   167
Other Departments   168
Standards and Documentation   169
Creative Activities for Graduate Students   170
Summary   171

9   Qualitative Research   172

Introduction   173
The Nature of Qualitative Research   174
Differences between Qualitative and Quantitative Studies   175

Theoretical Frameworks in Qualitative Research   176
  Symbolic Interaction   177
  Phenomenology   177
  Grounded Theory   178
  Critical Theory and Feminist Theory   179
Methods in Qualitative Research   179
  The Process of Qualitative Research   179
  Conceptualizing the Research   180
  Framing the Research Question(s)   180
  Collecting Data   180
  Analyzing Data   184
  Writing Up the Research   185
  Trustworthiness of Qualitative Data   185
Judging the Merit of a Qualitative Research Article   186
Uses and Applications of Qualitative Data   187
Summary   189

PART III   DATA ANALYSIS   192

10   Descriptive Data Analysis   194

Types of Scores   195
Common Units of Measure   196
Computer Analysis   196
Organizing and Graphing Test Scores   198
  Simple Frequency Distributions   198
  Grouping Scores for Graphing   200
Descriptive Values   202
  Measures of Central Tendency   203
  Mode   203
  Median   204
  Mean   204
  Measures of Variability   204
  Range   205
  Standard Deviation   205
  Variance   205
Measuring Group Position   206
  Percentile Ranks and Percentiles   206
  Standard Scores   207
Determining Relationships between Scores   207
  The Graphing Technique   209
  The Correlation Technique   210
  Interpreting the Correlation Coefficient   212

The Question of Accuracy   213
Summary   215

11   Inferential Data Analysis   217

Inference   218
Hypothesis-Testing Procedure   219
    Step 1: State the Hypotheses   219
    Step 2: Select the Probability Level   220
    Step 3: Consult the Statistical Table   220
    Step 4: Conduct the Statistical Test   220
    Step 5: Accept or Reject the Null Hypothesis   220
One-Group *t* Test   221
    Summary of Example   222
Two Independent Groups *t* Test   223
Two Dependent Groups *t* Test   224
Decision on Alternate Hypotheses and Alpha Level   227
Analysis of Variance   229
One-Way ANOVA   229
Repeated Measures ANOVA   232
Random Blocks ANOVA   234
Two-Way ANOVA, Multiple Scores per Cell   235
Other ANOVA Designs   241
Assumptions Underlying Statistical Tests   241
Overview of Two-Group Comparisons   243
Overview of Analysis of Covariance   244
Overview of Nonparametric Tests   244
    One-Way Chi-Square   245
    Two-Way Chi-Square   247
Overview of Multivariate Tests   249
Overview of Prediction-Regression Analysis   251
    Simple Prediction   252
    Multiple Prediction   252
    Nonlinear Regression   253
Overview of Testing Correlation Coefficients   253
Selecting the Statistical Test   254
Summary   254

PART IV   THE RESEARCH REPORT   258

12   The Research Report   260

Format of the Report   261
Divisions of a Thesis or Dissertation   261

Preliminary Items   261
The Text   261
Example 12.1A Title Page   262
Example 12.1B Acceptance Page   263
Example 12.1C Acknowledgments Page   264
Example 12.1D Table of Contents   265
Example 12.1E List of Tables   266
Example 12.1F List of Figures   267
Example 12.1G Abstract   268
Summary of Chapters 1–5   269
Example 12.2 An Opening Paragraph   270
Example 12.3 Sample Research Problem and Hypotheses   271
Example 12.4 Data Reporting Table for Response Rate Data   272
*Example 12.5 Data Reporting Table for Analysis: Chi-Square
    Analysis   273*
Example 12.6 Data Reporting Table for Analysis: F Test   274
Example 12.7 Discussion of Findings   276
References   278
Supplementary Items   278
Example 12.8 Sample of a Chapter 5   279
Example 12.9 References in APA Style   283
Abstract   284
Thesis Format versus Published Article Format   284
Preparing a Manuscript   286
Before Writing   286
During Writing   286
After Writing   287
*Example 12.10 Examples of Spelling and Writing Problems Not
    Easily Detected   288*
Critique of an Article   289
Criteria   289
Article Critique   289
Example 12.11 Checklist for Evaluating an Article   290
Example 12.12 Checklist for Evaluating a Research Paper   291
Summary   294

References   296

Appendix A Critical Values of *t*   310

Appendix B Critical Values of *F*   312

Appendix C Critical Values of Chi-Square   318

Index   319

Preface

This book was developed based on the methods its authors have used to teach the master's-level introduction to research course for many years. It is assumed that students come to this course with varied backgrounds in areas related to health and human performance, such as dance, exercise science, health, kinesiology, physical education, recreation, and sports management. The two major objectives of our courses are to teach the student how to conduct their own research and how to read with understanding the research that others have done. The book is comprehensive yet practical and understandable. Many examples of the application of various research methods and techniques are presented in an attempt to increase the students' grasp of the research process.

Many students begin the introduction to research course with little research background, little interest in research, and considerable fear about their ability to succeed in the course. These students typically do not write a master's thesis. However, it is still important that they develop an appreciation for research and an understanding of how different types of research are conducted so they will become good consumers and readers of the research of others. The book is certainly written with this type of student in mind.

Other students begin the introduction to research course knowing they will write a master's thesis or complete a master's project. These students need to be aware of the many possible research approaches and the procedures that are basic to many types of research. This book will also serve the needs of this type of student.

Doctoral students and beginning researchers who want an overview of the research process should find this book helpful. However, the procedures and techniques specific to a certain type of research in a specialized area are generally not covered in this book.

In chapter 2 we suggest that a research project begins with the identification of a research topic and progresses through a series of steps until the research is conducted and a report describing the research project is written. The book's chapters are organized in this manner. The first four chapters are essential to cover. Portions of chapters 5 through 9 may be covered quickly if only certain types of research are of interest to the student. Likewise, some of the content in chapters 10 through 12 could be omitted depending on the particular interests and needs of the students.

The two chapters on creative research and qualitative research are new and different. The two statistics chapters are inclusive but are presented with an orientation toward practical use and without emphasis on calculational ability. The computer programs accompanying the statistics chapters are presented with considerable explanation and use of examples. Even the emphasis on doing and understanding research is somewhat unique in this book.

The second edition of the book is not an extensive change from the first edition. Minor changes have occurred in each chapter to update the information presented, improve the presentation of the information, and eliminate a few problems identified in the first edition. The biggest changes are reference to a better computer program in the statistics chapters, the addition of key words and objectives at the beginning of each chapter, and the addition of formative evaluation of objectives at the end of each chapter.

This book is the product of the influence of many people and occurrences. First, the professors who trained and educated the authors must be recognized. Second, the research experiences of the authors have been influential. Third, the experience of teaching the introduction to research course and the feedback from the students in the course is reflected in the book. Finally, thanks must be expressed to people in the profession who reviewed the preliminary book manuscript and suggested improvements:

Stan Bassin
California State University, Pomona

Mary L. Dawson
Western Michigan University, Kalamazoo

Mark Huntington
Manchester College

Mark Kelley
Southeastern Louisiana University

Beverly Mitchell
Kennesaw State College

and to editors at McGraw-Hill Higher Education who improved the manuscript considerably.

Finally, the authors must thank their wives and families for allowing them to write the book. Adjustments and sacrifices were necessary by all in order for the book to be completed.

T.A.B.
C.H.S.

Conducting and Reading Research in Health and Human Performance

I

part

THE RESEARCH PROCESS

Research is exciting and challenging, and it makes an essential contribution to the development of those health and human performance (HHP) professionals who engage in it. Research accomplished by dance, exercise science, health, kinesiology, physical education, recreation, and sports management workers is exciting because the results frequently contribute to the pool of knowledge from which the fields of HHP can draw for purposes of application. It is challenging because the exploration of research ideas demands critical thinking and requires that judgment be exercised on procedural as well as conceptual questions. It contributes to the professional's development because the process builds a new set of skills that can be used to better comprehend the research literature and to recognize new questions that need to be researched.

Beginning graduate students in HHP frequently believe that research is foreign, abstract, and remote. They often feel totally incompetent, probably because they lack a basic understanding of the research process. A good course in research methods and statistics can lay the groundwork for attaining the high level of competency enjoyed by many of today's HHP professionals.

In Part I, the research process is introduced in four chapters. Chapter 1, "The Nature and Purpose of Research" details (1) the importance of research in the acquisition of knowledge by HHP professions, (2) how the scientific method of solving problems fits into the research process, (3) types of research, (4) the relationship of hypotheses to research, (5) the significance of research in HHP, and (6) ethical concerns in the research process. Chapter 2, "The Research Problem," discusses (1) how research problems are initiated, selected, and defined, (2) the importance of literature to the research process, and (3) the development of a research proposal.

Chapter 3, "Selected Elements in the Research Process," covers (1) the concepts underlying various approaches to research, (2) the way variables are used in research, (3) some of the more common HHP research methods and techniques, and (4) considerations in selecting or developing data collection instruments. Chapter 4, "Selection of Research Subjects: Sampling Procedures," addresses (1) the importance of procuring subjects appropriate for the research, (2) the concepts of population and sample, (3) subject selection methods, and (4) sample size.

1

The Nature and Purpose of Research

Key Words

Action research
Applied research
Basic research
Deductive reasoning (logic)
Directional hypothesis
Empiricism

Hypothesis
Imperfect induction
Induction
Nondirectional hypothesis
Perfect induction
Research classifications

Research hypothesis
Scientific method
Statistical (null) hypothesis
Syllogism
Theory

Objectives

Members of the HHP professions have a wealth of information upon which they make decisions. Quite frequently, this knowledge is passed down to us by other individuals, as opposed to our discovering knowledge through personal, direct observation types of experiences. Many times we don't bother to examine the source of the information prior to using it. However, when members of a profession engage in various aspects of the research process, current information can be checked out, along with the possibility of new knowledge being discovered.

After reading chapter 1, you should be able to:

1. Explain the relationship between research and a profession.
2. Know the various methods used in the way knowledge has been obtained in the past and how it is currently obtained.
3. Know the various types and classifications of research.
4. Distinguish between a hypothesis and a theory.

The Essence of a Profession: Knowledge

The professions of HHP produce a variety of monthly, quarterly, and annual publications. Articles, books, theses, and dissertations are a necessary part of the formal education and in-service education of the members of a profession, and the quality and quantity of such publications are an index of the vitality and soundness of a profession as a whole. The publications, and their use, also identify the professional stature of individual members. The information contained in the publications contributes greatly to the body of knowledge of a profession. A continuous flow of new facts and ideas must come from the laboratory and seminar, and this new information must be passed along. A profession's body of knowledge must not remain static and professional practices must be made applicable to new findings. If new knowledge suggests that an accepted practice is unsatisfactory, obsolete, or hazardous, then that practice must be modified or eliminated. The body of knowledge that characterizes a profession can and must be advanced for a profession to continue to contribute to the constituency it serves. The major vehicle by which a profession advances its knowledge base is the process of research.

Research: The Knowledge Pipeline

Research is a greatly misunderstood activity. Somehow, as soon as the word "research" is spoken, a barrier is raised. For many people, the term conjures up the image of a person in a white laboratory coat with a green visor pulled over his or her eyes. The perception is that this person, or researcher, is cold, shy, disinterested in people as individuals, interested in people only as subjects, and concerned primarily with figures, needles, stopwatches, and published articles.

Research is not like that. Nor is it a "mystical activity where the 'academic eggheads' go off to 'do their thing'" (Mobley 1980). In its simplest context, research is nothing more or less than finding solutions to problems in a logical, orderly, and systematic fashion. It is an organized attempt to obtain facts; it searches for the truth in human feelings, values, behaviors, activities, processes, elements, and relationships. Professional activity involves many problems that can be investigated through the research process. Solutions to research problems must be based on evidence that is as objective as possible. Objectivity is the key element, or the crux, of research, which is why researchers employ the scientific method of analysis in attacking research problems. The field of science offers researchers a structured means of finding the answers to research questions. Scientific solutions, in turn, can be used to help synthesize, validate, or change the philosophy, theoretical relationships, and, ultimately, the practices of a profession.

The Search for Truth

Men and women have been searching for truth since the beginning of time. In doing so they have relied, in general, upon five sources of evidence: (1) custom and tradition, (2) authority, (3) personal experience, (4) syllogistic or deductive reasoning, and (5) scientific inquiry (Good 1972). The earliest search for truth was characterized by the first three, and each provided a modicum of truth. While there is something valuable, secure, serene, and peaceful about customs and traditions, many were found to be erroneous. The truth is, there is no Santa Claus or Easter Bunny. Reliance on an authority served people well in the past, but fell short as a complete source of truth. Many authorities have been wrong. There was a time when the word of a coach, senator, or even the president was considered unimpeachable, but we now are reluctant to accept the assumptions of authorities merely because of the position they hold. There is also value in personal experience, but it, too, has limitations as a valid source of truth. Brothers and sisters in a family grow up differently because they have different experiences in the same situation. People may also need to know things that cannot be learned by experience. A group of graduate students cannot experience how to properly analyze physical fitness data until they know, at the very least, basic statistical techniques. As humans have thought about problems over the ages, each of these sources of evidence has played an important role. The obvious shortcomings of each, however, dictated gross inadequacies in the search for truth. Hence, arose the appeal to other sources for new knowledge, understanding, and insight.

Deductive reasoning (logic) was the first major contribution to the process of seeking truth systematically. In deductive reasoning, thinking proceeds from a general assumption to a specific application. Several pieces of rather general information, or facts, are woven together to produce a specific conclusion. Aristotle and other early philosophers ushered in the era of logic through statements referred to as a categorical **syllogism**. Following is such a statement:

> All philosophers are mortal. Socrates is a philosopher. Therefore, Socrates is mortal. (Sax 1979, 5)

Two ideas, or premises, form the basis for the conclusion. If the relationship between the two is true, then the conclusion is true. However, if either premise is false, the conclusion is also false. This represents the major weakness of deduction; that is, we have to accept the information contained in the premises as being true without really knowing that it is true.

> All heavy cigarette smokers die from cancer. John smokes six packages of cigarettes a day. John will die of cancer.

The ultimate truth or falsity of the conclusion concerning John's demise depends upon the truth of the first two statements. Do all heavy smokers die of cancer? Are six packs of cigarettes a day enough to cause cancer in John?

Sometimes rumors about someone are true, other times false. A teenager may observe that smoking marijuana is prevalent among his peers and conclude that such activity is okay for him. Peer pressure frequently leads to a deductive response. Phrases such as "It figures" or "That figures" also imply a conclusion based on deductive reasoning.

Deduction is valuable and is part and parcel of almost every research project. Reasoning of this kind enables the researcher to organize the information already known to exist concerning the research problem of current interest, to theorize about the relationship of this information to the problem, and then to deduce various hypotheses to be tested by the research. Despite the value of deductive reasoning in pointing up "new relationships as one goes from the general to specific, it is not sufficient as a source of new truth" (Ary, Jacobs, and Razaveih 1972).

The human thought process then turned to inductive reasoning, or scientific inquiry, in an attempt to get at the elusive truth. **Induction,** in which thinking proceeds from the specific to the general, is considered to be the basic principle of all science. Conclusions about events are based on information generated through many individual and direct observations. In the inductive process, the researcher observes an individual or group of individuals from a larger population of similar individuals. Then, based upon these observations of the smaller group, inferences, conclusions, or generalizations are made back to the larger population. Hence, thinking moves forward from the specific to the general. Deduction moves backward from the general to the specific. Ary, Jacobs, and Razaveih (1972) have clearly illustrated the difference between the deductive and inductive processes:

> *Deductive.* Every mammal has lungs. All rabbits are mammals. Therefore, every rabbit has lungs.
>
> *Inductive.* Every rabbit that has been observed has lungs. Therefore, every rabbit has lungs.

Induction, then, is based on seeking facts, which is the primary goal of science. There are two kinds of induction, **perfect** and **imperfect.** Perfect induction results in conclusions based on observations of selected characteristics of all members of a group or population. This is frequently not possible, especially when groups are large. Imperfect induction results in conclusions based on the observations of selected characteristics on a small, specific number of members of a population. Most research is based on imperfect induction. The information obtained may not be absolutely perfect, or true, but is sufficient to make fairly reliable generalizations. It is generally conceded that Darwin was responsible for integrating deduction and induction in his research in the nineteenth century. The integrated process became known as the **scientific method.**

The Scientific Method

The ultimate goal of science is the formulation of valid generalizations in the form of explanatory principles or laws. Researchers use accurate and important data in an attempt to explain some scientific phenomenon. However, this goal is rarely met, with researchers opting to use the data to make new hypotheses in the continual search for further insight into a problem area. Medical researchers have not yet solved the problems related to cancer cause and treatment, but data from countless cancer studies have been used to formulate hypotheses to be tested in subsequent investigations. With, perhaps, many additional studies the medical researchers hope to solve the problems associated with cancer. That is their ultimate, yet elusive, goal.

The scientific method of solving research problems has been delineated in many different ways in the past. It is an approach usually thought of as being accomplished in a series of logical steps.

1. Problem Identification
   Once the problem area of the research has been decided, then the specific problem should be spelled out or defined. When formulated, the problem statement

should provide direction for the research process. It should not be vague or too all-encompassing. A well-stated problem will imply a specific answer, or conclusion (Best 1981).

2. **Statement of Hypothesis**

   A **hypothesis** is a belief, hunch, or prediction of the eventual outcome of the research. It is a statement about the relationships between phenomena. It is a deductive idea from the theory concerning those relationships. Suppose a researcher wanted to study the effects of two different diets on selected health indices. Perhaps the theory is that a vegetarian diet provides a stronger and healthier person than does a nonvegetarian diet. If the theory is true, what observable consequences could be expected? The deduced hypotheses, in a series of separate statements, would predict that the individuals on the vegetarian diet would show (a) lower cholesterol levels, (b) lower blood pressure, (c) greater energy, (d) a higher strength index, (e) less body fat, (f) pinker cheeks, and so on, depending on the number of health indices observed.

3. **Collection and Analysis of Data**

   In this step the study is arranged in such a way as to test the hypotheses. The researcher will test, measure, weigh, experiment, or observe the phenomena in question and collect data to support or refute the hypothetical predicted outcome. In the diet study, the researcher might select two groups of people and place one group on a vegetarian diet and the other on a nonvegetarian diet. Initially, each group would be tested on the selected health indices, then proceed upon their respective diets for a preset period of time. At the end of the experimental period, data would again be obtained on the health indices.

4. **Confirming or Rejecting the Hypothesis**

   The collected data is now analyzed and an attempt is made to determine if the investigation confirms or refutes the hypothesis or hypotheses. In the case of the diet study, the data for each health index would be pitted against the stated hypothesis for that health indicator. Have the data supported the predicted outcome? Do the data refute it? A decision to accept or reject the hypothesis is made.

5. **Conclusion(s)**

   At this point the researcher puts an end to the study and summarizes, in one or more brief and definitive statements, what the investigation showed or did not show. The conclusions should not be restatements of the findings of the study. In general, the conclusions should be stated in concert with the acceptance or rejection of each stated hypothesis.

Example 1.1 provides a good illustration of the application of the scientific method using Seaman's (1970) abstract of a study by Robbins (1966). The problem is clearly and definitively stated, the hypotheses are appropriately deducted from theory and stated in a testable form, the procedures for collecting and analyzing the data are delineated, and the conclusions clearly reflect the data.

EXAMPLE 1.1
Example of an Application
of the Research Process

A Study of the Validity of Delacato's Theory of Neurological Organization

Robbins, Melvyn P., *Exceptional Children,* April, 1966, pp. 517–23

An Abstract
by
Janet A. Seaman

The problem of this study was to test the theoretical and practical implications of Delacato's theory of neurological organization. The central concept of the theory, that an individual's development of mobility, vision, audition, and language parallels his anatomical progress, was tested through the use of six null hypotheses.

Three classes of second-grade children were selected for participation in the study with no particular regard given to reading or other difficulties in the selection. Subjects were assigned to one of three groups on the basis of their intact classes. The first class ($n = 43$) was designated as a traditional control group and carried out its normal curriculum. The second class ($n = 38$), or experimental group, was subjected to a program consistent with Delacato's theory supplementary to their normal curriculum. The third or nonspecific group ($n = 45$) was supplemented with activities contrary to those deduced from the theory in addition to their normal curriculum. Although random selection techniques could not be used in assigning subjects to the three groups, the groups seemed to be reasonably matched and any differences across groups in the basic measures were partially controlled by using convariance analysis.

Standardized pretests were administered to all three groups for intelligence, reading, and arithmetic. An assessment was also made of creeping and laterality for each of the subjects. The experimental group underwent a three-month program of activities and postures prescribed by Delacato's theory. The nonspecific group participated in activities contraindicated by Delacato for the same period of time.

Analysis of pre- and posttest data was achieved by the testing of two sets of hypotheses. The first three hypotheses tested the influence on reading ability of laterality and creeping, both independently and conjointly. They were:

Hypothesis I: Creeping is not related to reading beyond chance expectancy.

Problem

Theory: The Basis for Hypotheses

Collection and Analysis of Data

Confirming or Rejecting the Hypotheses

EXAMPLE 1.1
Concluded

Hypothesis II: Mean reading differences between subjects who are lateralized and those who are nonlateralized do not exceed chance expectancy.

Hypothesis III: Mean differences in reading between subjects who are lateralized and those who are not lateralized do not exceed chance expectancy when controlled for differences in creeping.

These hypotheses were not rejected on the basis of analysis of data and therefore did not support the theory.

The second set of hypotheses compared pretest and posttest scores within the experimental group and between groups used in this study. These hypotheses were as follows:

Hypothesis IV: Mean posttest differences in reading between the group exposed to the experimental program and the other two groups are no greater than chance expectancy after pretest score differences have been controlled.

Hypothesis V: Mean posttest score differences between reading and arithmetic within the experimental class do not exceed chance expectancy when pretest score differences are controlled.

Hypothesis VI: The proportion of subjects lateralized after exposure to the experimental program does not exceed by greater than chance expectancy the proportion lateralized before the program was introduced.

These three hypotheses also were not rejected.

Conclusions   Within the limits of this study, the following conclusions were made:

1. The data did not support the postulated relationship between neurological organization and reading ability.
2. The prescribed program of activities effected with second graders did not in any way enhance the reading or lateral development of these children.

The essence of the scientific method is the marked control it can provide the researcher. For some research problems in HHP it is difficult to achieve a strict application of the scientific method. If all research problems were within the realm of natural science or always involved the use of animals and inert objects, perhaps maximum control could be attained. The use of human subjects diminishes the ability to handle them in a way that allows a highly controlled manner of experimentation. Performance-enhancing drugs may be harmful to the body. To truly determine their effect, a sample of athletes should be drawn from the population, these individuals should be given drugs over a period of time, and then the effects on various body organs should be observed. However, moral, ethical, and legal ramifications preclude studies designed in such a way. Research subjects have a right to expect researchers to prevent harm from coming to them and to pay attention to their safety and human dignity. Researchers cannot hope to know all potential risks and hazards to human subjects, but must inform them of all those that are known. There is much current evidence that performance-enhancing drugs are harmful. The use of drugs simply to see what happens to body organs five to ten years after they are ingested is a risk that should be avoided. Such a study would be difficult to justify from an ethical and moral standpoint. People cannot be treated in a harmful or dehumanizing way.

Also, many problems in HHP involve attitudes and are extremely subjective in nature. While science can discover potential health risks in smoking and drug use, it cannot prevent people from using those substances. Questions concerning whether or not abortion should or should not be legalized, whether participation in athletics is a right or a privilege, and at what grade level sex education should be introduced into school curricula are virtually impossible for science to answer.

Despite these limitations, respectable research on attitude and value types of problems is being done in a systematic manner. The major concern is that, whatever the problem, researchers try to be as scientific as possible in their attack. Control over the research situation will be more difficult to attain in studies done in gymnasia, swimming pools, camps, and playing fields.

Research and Theory

Through scientific research efforts, facts are discovered. Questions such as What do these facts mean? and What are the relationships among these facts? are asked. Theories must be postulated about the things inherent in the facts. The word "theory" is often misunderstood. Some believe that it is an esoteric term and that those who use it are "out in left field" or "in a world of their own." A **theory** is a belief or assumption about how things relate to each other. Basically, it is an explanation. According to Best (1981), "a theory establishes a cause and effect relationship between variables with the purpose of explaining and predicting phenomena" (p. 15). A theory is not a law, but the hypothesis deduced from a theory could become law through experimentation or observation.

Theory is a vehicle for obtaining new knowledge by providing hypotheses for additional research. Theories about the relationship between human beings and the environment abound. The good and bad features of that relationship are explained, and predictions are offered as to what will happen if certain human behaviors are not changed. Theories can lead to civil laws to control various behaviors. Gun control laws, for example, have been offered because of certain theories about the relationship between guns and crime. Today, children with disabilities are mainstreamed by law into the schools. This resulted from gathering sufficient facts through research that supported theory about the potential benefits to both disabled and nondisabled children from studying in the classroom together.

Theory, then, provides a structure for research. It can present guidelines for the procedures of research. A theory is general in nature and can lead to much practical application.

Empiricism

HHP has not always emphasized theory. In the past, many professionals in those fields have demonstrated greater interest in empiricism. Inductive reasoning is the major medium for establishing generalizations and principles. **Empiricism** is the idea that knowledge is obtained through experience, so it does not rely on theory or science. The empiricist utilizes facts, but has no interest in the when, how, or why of the facts. Empirical decisions are often based on pragmatic observations. Steroid and other performance-enhancing drug use by athletes is often the result of an empirical decision. These athletes may observe the total effect of steroid use in others without questioning its limitations. They do not solicit the deeper questions with regard to rapid strength and muscular gains steroid use provides. They are only interested in the end result. They tend to overgeneralize. The scientist digs deeper into all possible relationships of steroid use, seeking facts so as to theorize and explain such relationships. Empiricism may solve a problem in a quick and practical manner, but no new knowledge is discovered. Exclusive use of empiricism results in a knowledge status quo. It has been said that empiricism is "pseudo-scientific," which labels empiricism as being something other than scientific hypothesis testing.

Types of Research

Pure, Fundamental, or Basic Research

Generally, **basic research** aims to discover new knowledge. It is motivated by intellectual curiosity and interest in a specific problem area. Fundamental knowledge about such phenomena as the environment, space, human behavior, exercise, and human gene makeup is sought. Broad generalizations and principles, such as the overload and cross-transference principles and the laws of learning, frequently result from pure research. The results of this type of research may have no practical application. The majority of this research is done in highly controlled experimental laboratory settings, often with animal subjects. Selected variables have to be manipulated for maximum control. Some examples of what might be considered basic research studies are the following:

1. A study to determine the effect of lactic acid concentration on breast milk following different levels of exercise.
2. A study to determine the effect of various compounds on ventilation during normoxia and hypoxia.
3. A study to test the dynamic systems theory that infants learn motor skills through exploration and selection of adaptive responses.

Applied Research

Workers in the fields of HHP have seen real problems and are interested in solving them. They often engage in **applied research** in an effort to solve an immediate problem. A health educator may try out a new smoking cessation technique or a recreation practitioner may utilize a new method for improving the delivery of leisure services. A new motor learning theory may be applied by the physical education teacher. The idea is to improve products and processes and to test theoretical concepts. We are interested in improving our HHP practices and services. The results of this type of research are intended for universal population application. An adapted physical education researcher who finds that a particular motor activity is successful in improving the social skills of a sample of mentally retarded subjects, is likely to want to apply those results to all similar mentally retarded people. Seat belt studies and smoking and drug research are usually geared to producing results that will apply to the entire population. Some examples of what might be considered applied research studies are the following:

1. Application of the theory of self-efficacy to recreation supervisor's years of experience and number of employees supervised.
2. A study to determine if female children of divorce have more problems with trust and male children have more problems with intimacy when compared to children of a similar age from intact families.

Action Research

Action research is similar to applied research except that the interest is in local, not universal, applicability. This research can get very pragmatic and objective, but the problem exists in a local setting. A coach may experiment with his football punter, utilizing a new technique. His interest is in getting the punter to average ten yards further per kick. The coach is interested only in his local situation. This type of research has also been called "on the job" research. Methods, techniques, and practices are tried out which may promise better results and provide the basis for improved decisions. Behavioral modification, intervention, and in-service training skills are frequently employed in action research studies. To be successful, the researcher must adhere to sound research procedures. The approach should be as scientific as is possible given the lesser-controlled, local environment in which it takes place. Some examples of what might be considered action research studies are the following:

1. An investigation of various motivational techniques on the physical fitness test performance of sixth-grade children at McKinley Elementary School.
2. Citizen reaction to the environmental and recreational impact of a proposed highway in Indiana.

Research Classifications

There have been many attempts to classify research. The three basic **research classifications** are considered to be (1) historical, when the researcher is interested in the past; (2) descriptive, when the researcher is interested in the present; and (3) experimental, when the researcher is interested in the future. Experts in the field, however, differ in their classification criteria. How a given research problem is attacked depends largely on the nature of the problem and the purpose, or reason, for doing the research.

Isaac and Michael (1995, 46–47) have organized research into nine classifications based on differing problem characteristics:

Historical Approach: Reconstruct the past objectively and accurately, often in relation to the tenability of a hypothesis.

Examples:

1. Reconstruct the role of the media in women's sports since Title IX.
2. Trace the history of United States minorities' participation in the modern Olympic games.
3. Test the hypothesis that Charles H. McCloy is the "Father of Biomechanics."

Descriptive Approach: Describe systematically, factually, and accurately a situation or area of interest.

Examples:

1. Population census studies
2. Public opinion surveys
3. Fact-finding surveys
4. Status studies
5. Task analysis studies
6. Job description
7. Surveys of the literature
8. Documentary analyses
9. Anecdotal records
10. Critical incident reports
11. Test score analysis
12. Normative data

Developmental Approach: Investigate patterns and sequences of growth and/or change as a function of time.

Examples:

1. A longitudinal study of the overhand ball-throwing patterns of children from age 6 to 18.
2. A cross-sectional study of the overhand ball-throwing patterns by sampling groups of children at five different age levels.
3. A trend study projecting the educational need for comprehensive health education programs in the schools from past health education curricular patterns.

Case and Field Approach: Study intensively the background, current status, and environmental interactions of a given social unit (e.g., individual, group, institution, or community).

Examples:

1. The case history of a skilled athlete who exhibits bizarre social behavior.
2. An intensive study of a violent teenage gang.
3. An intensive study of the personality characteristics of a group of high-level women gymnasts.

Correlational Approach: Investigate the extent to which variations in one factor correspond with variations in one or more other factors based on correlation coefficients.

Examples:

1. A factor-analytic study of the factor-pattern differences in tests of physical fitness, motor ability, and skill among men and women physical education majors.
2. A factor analysis of selected tests for speed of body movement.
3. An investigation of the relationships of selected variables to exercise adherence and nonadherence.
4. A study of the relationship of whole body movement response time and the fielding average of baseball players.

Causal Comparative or Ex Post Facto Approach: Investigate possible cause-and-effect relationships by observing some existing consequence and searching back through the data for plausible causal factors.

Examples:

1. Identify factors common to Indiana University dropout students during the period from 1990 to 1992 using student personnel data.
2. Determine similarities and differences in teenage drug users and nonusers, recreationally active and inactive senior citizens, and Little League players who continue in sports through high school and those who do not, based on data already on file.

True Experimental Approach: Investigate possible cause-and-effect relationships by exposing one or more experimental groups to one or more treatment conditions and comparing the results to one or more control groups not receiving the treatment (random assignment being essential).

Examples:

1. Study range of motion as a method of teaching the overhand throwing pattern of children.
2. Investigate the effect of plasma and erythrocyte magnesium concentrations on the VO_2 max in male cyclists.
3. Investigate two different methods of improving self-esteem in adolescent children.

Quasi-Experimental Approach: Approximate the conditions of the true experiment in a setting that does not allow the control and/or manipulation of all relevant variables.

Example:

A cause-and-effect study where only one group is observed, random assignment of subjects is not possible, and maximum control of the variables is lacking.

Action Approach: Develop new skills or approaches in order to solve problems or improve performance in the classroom or other applied setting.

Examples:

1. An in-service training program to help camp counselors develop skill in stress challenge techniques.
2. Experimentation with a new intervention program designed to decrease teenage drug use.

No attempt should be made to assign these classifications to a hierarchy of importance; one is not better than another. The researcher's interest and the nature of the problem to be investigated usually determine the category of research. The most important consideration should be that, whatever research is attempted, it be done in a careful and systematic manner. The classifications simply imply that different types of problems will necessitate a different plan of attack in seeking solutions.

Hypotheses and Research

Statements of hypothesis are important to almost all research projects. Most researchers proceed in their studies with the idea that a certain outcome will result. This idea is then stated as a "tentative explanation of the relationship between two or more variables" (Best 1981). The predicted outcome is referred to as a **research hypothesis.** It has been hypothesized that extensive use of anabolic steroids by athletes leads to the deterioration of certain body parts and to disease. Many research studies have been done on the relationship between steroid use and serious illness, and the results have generally supported that the relationship is as the hypothesis suggests.

In general, research hypotheses possess these characteristics:

1. They are based on theory or previous research findings.
2. They state a relationship between at least two variables.
3. They are simple and clear statements with no vague terms clouding the relationships.
4. They are testable; that is, the stated variables can be measured, and theoretical or previous research knowledge exists to permit a clear and testable hypothesis.
5. They have the capability of being refuted; the prediction can be evaluated in terms of "yes, it occurred" or "no, it did not occur."
6. They are related to available techniques of design, procedure, and statistical analysis.

Research hypotheses can be stated in a **directional** or a **nondirectional** manner. If the researcher believes that a particular relationship or difference exists between groups of subjects, the hypothesis is stated directionally, or in the direction of the expected result.

Example:

Children with a high IQ are more easily motivated than children with a low IQ.

The researcher is predicting that there is a difference between children in how easily they are motivated and that this difference favors or is in the direction of those with high IQs. A nondirectional hypothesis is stated when the researcher has no reason to believe that a difference or relationship exists in any direction.

Example:

There is a difference in the motivational level of children with a high IQ and those children with a low IQ.

In this case the researcher expects a difference but does not indicate the direction it will take. The topic of the directional versus the nondirectional hypothesis is related to a statistical analysis procedure that will be described in a later chapter.

The number of research hypotheses in a given study will depend upon the number of variables being investigated. The more variables, the greater the number of relationships; hence, the greater the number of hypotheses. This point is related to the scope of the study, which increases as the number of hypotheses increases. All research hypotheses are stated in the present tense and before collecting data on the variables.

The research hypothesis is not tested directly by the data. Rather, the **statistical (null) hypothesis** is tested by the data. It states that there is no difference between the groups being studied. For example:

Research hypothesis: Students exposed to an experimental leisure counseling program show greater improvement in the organization of their lives than do students who have not been exposed to this program.

Statistical or null hypothesis: There is no difference in the organization of the lives of students who have been exposed to an experimental counseling program and students who have not been exposed to the program.

The statistical procedures used for analyzing research data can only test hypotheses stated in the form of a null hypothesis. If the data support the null hypothesis it will be accepted; if the data refute the null hypothesis it will be rejected. Usually the research and null hypotheses are stated in opposite terms; the research hypothesis is a positive statement of expected outcome, while the null hypothesis simply states that no difference will be found.

Research hypothesis: Children who perform on physical fitness tests under team competition obtain higher test scores than children who perform on physical fitness tests under competition against someone of nearly equal ability.

Statistical or null hypothesis: There is no difference in the test scores of children who perform on physical fitness tests under team competition and those children who perform on physical fitness tests under competition against someone of nearly equal ability.

If the null hypothesis is accepted, then the researcher rejects the research hypothesis and concludes that there really is no difference between the two motivating conditions. If the data showed that team competition was the superior condition, the null hypothesis is rejected and the research hypothesis is accepted. Of course, the research hypothesis would also be rejected if, in fact, competition against someone of nearly equal ability was found to be associated with superior performance on the physical fitness test.

Sometimes the research hypothesis is stated the same way as the statistical hypothesis. A researcher may go into an investigation expecting no difference. In this case whatever action is taken on the statistical hypothesis, as dictated by the data, will also be taken on the research hypothesis.

Stating hypotheses helps to make a researcher's thought process about the research situation more concrete. If a prediction of a specific outcome is made, this forces more thorough consideration of which research techniques, methods, test instruments, and data collecting procedures should be employed. Hypotheses also help set up the way the data will be analyzed and how the final report will be organized and written.

All experimental studies and those descriptive investigations in which comparisons are made will have hypotheses. Readers of those studies deserve to know what the researcher expected would be revealed by the experiment or the descriptive comparison. Simple descriptive and historical studies can also include hypotheses, but sometimes do not. Occasionally, the researcher may not have any reason, by virtue of his or her experience or based on the literature, to make a prediction of outcome.

What happens if the hypotheses are not supported by the results of the study? A frequent misconception is that the research was faulty and is of no value. Perfectly well-conducted research can reveal data that do not support what was expected. In such a situation the researcher should review the assumptions that served as the basis for the hypotheses, the theoretical relationships involved, and the design of the study. On the other hand, the truth may be that the research hypotheses should have been rejected. There really may be no relationship between the groups.

The Significance of Research in HHP

The body of knowledge in each of the fields of health and human performance (HHP) is currently expanding at a rapid rate. Tremendous progress has been made because scholars in these fields have focused on all aspects of the human being—the physical, mental, and emotional. The whole person is studied in relation to movement, attitude, and lifestyle. The research has been both theoretical and practical and has reflected a sharp increase in quality, range, and depth.

Health education has produced a variety of conceptual and methodological approaches for dealing with problems in health promotion and disease prevention. Important attitudes, beliefs, intentions, and norms for people of all ages with regard to human sexuality, alcohol and drug use, smoking, family relationships, obesity, and nutrition have been identified. The thrust of Health Education research has been on promotion and prevention as opposed to researching ways to eliminate or treat existing health problems. Torabi, Seffrin, and Yarber, along with various colleagues, have done excellent studies with regard to these variables (Torabi, et al., six studies dealing with attitude, tobacco, alcohol, cancer, and HIV). In addition, Torabi has published several articles on the statistical evaluation of research studies in applied health science. Many epidemiological studies have recently produced an abundance of scientific knowledge concerning the relationship between exercise and longevity, controlling chronic illness, retarding the aging process, and the important roles of nutrition, sleep, exercise, and lifestyle in providing good health.

Physical education research continues to make essential contributions to the better understanding of the various physiological responses to exercise and stress through biochemical and histochemical studies. Research in motor learning and motor control has added a great deal to the understanding of the acquisition and retention of motor skills, motor response processing, and the varied roles of the nervous system in movement. Adapted physical education has produced significant information as a result of biomechanical and energy cost studies of the activity performance of disabled individuals. The area of measurement and evaluation has developed increasingly more reliable and valid measures of physical fitness, motor skill, and mental ability and has contributed excellent theoretical work concerning reliability and validity, measurement scales, probability and sampling theory, and statistical design. Biomechanics, sport psychology, sport sociology, sport history, and motor development have generated research data which have been indispensable to the understanding of how people behave as they interact with the environments of physical education, exercise, and sport.

Recreation and Park Administration has long provided exceptional services to people so they may improve the quality of their lives. Research has been a major tool for obtaining the knowledge that has led to better delivery of these services, such as physical and mental health, administrative behavior, leadership evaluation, facility design, outdoor recreation, and leisure counseling (Pelegrino 1979, 5). Studies relating life-span development to the effects of recreation on people, the cultural impact of increased leisure time on society, the improvement of playground surfaces and equipment, the impact of recreation on the environment, the effect of tourism on society, and the spiritual and moral aspects of recreation have led to better recreation programs, practices, and services.

Dance is a unique and dynamic field of study whose research is best characterized as a creative activity. Choreography, the act of forming and performing dances, is a method of research unique to dance. Movement notation research has provided, for movement, a complete and accurate language and vocabulary. Rhythm has been studied as a language which transmits ideas and meaning through the "signs, symbols, sounds, and motions of the human body" (Cooper and Andrews 1975, 61). The biomechanics of dance, physiological responses resulting from dance, and injuries peculiar to dance performers are other popular dance research topics.

The rapid progress in HHP research has resulted, at least in part, from improved instrumentation and the development of new methods, techniques, and procedures. These developments have led to better research designs, a more objective research approach, and more reliable and valid data. Better data has enabled HHP researchers to increase the quality of their generalizations.

The volume of research emerging from the fields of HHP has increased in the past five to ten years. The HHP professional journals are facing an increasing backlog of both basic and applied research articles waiting to be published, and not all of these studies are being done by professional researchers. The HHP practitioner has become more active in research, while the focus of the professional researcher appears to have become more fixed on research having utilitarian value. The so-called gap between the researcher and the practitioner appears to be narrowing. A stronger feeling of cooperation seems to be growing in both camps as it relates to both theoretical and applied problems. Theoretical applications can help solve practical kinds of problems, while basic research frequently needs the results from the applied research to round out its theoretical concepts.

In its simplest form, research is just another way of looking at the problems which permeate the fields of HHP. Research is for everyone, and everyone can and should engage that process. Deep knowledge of statistics and research design is not necessary to carry out creditable research. All that is needed is someone who is interested and willing to undertake the activity and who has some background knowledge of the problem to be studied. Research should not be relegated to just a few "name" people in the profession, but rather it is the responsibility of many people. In the past, a few HHP "names" gave those fields good leadership and direction in research circles. This impetus was needed but resulted in research narrowly focused in just a few interest areas. Larger numbers of people engaging in research are needed to guarantee that the problems, questions, and interests of all fields of HHP are represented in research investigations. Research can help broaden the knowledge and improve the practices that have long been associated with HHP. It is, and should continue to be, an active and continuing ingredient of the scholarly efforts of those fields. It is a tool that HHP cannot do without. It is the lifeblood of a profession and must be pursued vigorously.

Ethical Concerns

Human subjects have been used to generate research data since ancient times. Only in the past fifty years, however, has a concerted effort been made to protect the rights and welfare of research subjects. The impetus for such protective measures came from studies that brought some form of harm (injury, death, disrepute) to people who served as subjects. A classic example of such studies is the long list of atrocities committed by the Nazi Germans when they experimented on prisoners of war during World War II (Rubinson and Neutens 1987). The quest for knowledge is important to a profession and how such knowledge can improve society is of paramount importance. We now work into the equation the element of subject rights and document any possible harm or risk that could come to people who supply the data for the knowledge we seek from research.

Most agencies and collegiate institutions require all researchers, from graduate students to full professors, to submit a Protection of Human Subjects Form to a Human Subjects Review Committee. The form includes a checklist regarding the types of data to be collected and the methods to be used which the researcher must complete. The checklist in example 1.2 is used at Indiana University. In addition to the checklist, the researcher must provide information concerning these items:

1. The nature and purpose of the proposed research and where it will take place.
2. A description of how the subjects will be recruited, how many subjects will be recruited, how many subjects will be involved, and how much time will be

required of them. Eligibility requirements, including those criteria that would exclude otherwise acceptable subjects, are also to be identified.

3. If minors under age 18, fetuses, abortuses, pregnant women, persons with mental disabilities, prisoners, and economically or educationally disadvantaged people are to be used as subjects, the necessity for doing so needs to be stated.

4. All procedures to be used on the subjects must be listed.

5. Potential risks (physical, psychological, financial, social, legal) connected with the proposed procedures must be indicated.

6. Procedures (including methods to assure confidentiality) for protecting against, or minimizing, potential risks must be indicated, as well as some assessment of their likely effectiveness.

7. Any benefit to the subject is to be stated. In the event of monetary gain, all payment arrangements (amounts of payment and the proposed method of disbursement), including reimbursement of expenses, are to be identified. Partial payment if the subject withdraws prior to completion of the study needs to be included. If class credit is awarded, the amount should be indicated.

8. An indication of what information will accrue to science or to society in general as a result of the research should be included.

9. A description on how risks to subjects are reasonable in relation to anticipated benefits should be presented.

10. The investigator, co-investigator, cooperating departments, and institutions should be noted. Investigator signatures are required, along with a letter from any cooperating institution.

The researcher must also prepare an Informed Consent Statement for the subject to read and sign. It is prepared from a checklist of items pertaining to the conduct of the study. The Informed Consent Statement used at Indiana University is presented in example 1.3. Depending on the ages of the subjects, the physical and mental status of selected groups, and various conditions of other vulnerable groups, different guidelines are followed for obtaining consent. All forms regarding human subjects must be completed before an investigation is begun.

All subjects in human research are entitled to the right of privacy and confidentiality. They have the right to request that their individual identities remain anonymous, to know who will see the data derived from them, and to be given a thorough understanding of the data's importance. In many survey studies, questions about sensitive issues (e.g., drugs, sex) are frequently asked. Subjects may feel that these questions are an invasion of their privacy. They will answer the questions if they can be convinced that the information is crucial to the purpose of the research project and if they can be assured that the information they provide will in no way harm them physically, mentally, or emotionally. The researcher must be truthful in detailing the nature and purpose of the research to the subjects. Subjects should in no way be deceived by being told one particular procedure will be conducted when another one will be used. Subjects should be given an honest and fair explanation of the procedure, including the type of experimental or survey methods that will be utilized. There should be no misconception in the subjects' minds as to how the data will be collected, interpreted, or applied. The Informed Consent Statement, which must be signed by the subject, should reflect the subject's right to privacy and confidentiality. It should also assure the subject that information is not being concealed from them.

Protection of human subjects is perhaps the major ethical responsibility facing researchers. Other ethical concerns include the proper establishment of authorship, the use of nonsexist language, ethnic bias designations, the care and use of animals, and the reproduction of copyrighted material. All of these concerns are delineated in detail in the *Ethical Principles of Psychologists,* American Psychological Association, 1981. The reader is encouraged to become familiar with those guidelines if any concerns of this type may apply to contemplated research studies.

EXAMPLE 1.2
Protection of Human
Subjects Form

Protection of Human Subjects Form

DIRECTIONS: This form is to be completed and submitted to the Committee when the investigator plans a research project which, in the investigator's judgment, requires expedited or full Committee review. Items 1–13 are the categories which may qualify for expedited review. *If "yes" is the response to any of items 14–17, the study does not qualify for expedited review (full Committee review will be required).*

STUDIES INVOLVING MINORS AND ECONOMICALLY OR EDUCATIONALLY DISADVANTAGED PERSONS MAY, IN THE DISCRETION OF THE CHAIR, REQUIRE FULL COMMITTEE REVIEW.

STUDIES INVOLVING PREGNANT WOMEN, FETUSES, ABORTUSES, PRISONERS, OR PERSONS WITH MENTAL DISABILITIES WILL REQUIRE FULL COMMITTEE REVIEW.

Yes No

___ ___ 1. Collection of hair and nail clippings in a nondisfiguring manner; collection of deciduous teeth and permanent teeth if patient care indicates a need for extraction.

___ ___ 2. Collection of excreta and external secretions including sweat and uncannulated saliva; collection of placenta at delivery; collection of amniotic fluid at the time of rupture of the membrane before or during labor.

___ ___ 3. Recording of data from subjects 18 years old or older using noninvasive techniques such as measurements, weighing,

EXAMPLE 1.2
Concluded

Yes No

electrocardiography, echocardiography, or thermography. Research involving radiation outside the visible range, i.e., x-ray, must receive full Committee review.

___ ___ 4. Collection of blood samples by venipuncture, in amounts not exceeding 450 milliliters in an eight-week period and no more than two times per week from subjects who are 18 years of age or older and who are in good health and not pregnant.

___ ___ 5. Collection of both supra- and subgingival dental plaque and calculus, provided the procedure is not more invasive than routine prophylactic scaling of the teeth, and the process is accomplished in accordance with accepted prophylactic techniques.

___ ___ 6. Voice recordings made for research purposes such as investigations of speech defects.

___ ___ 7. Moderate exercise by healthy volunteers.

___ ___ 8. The study of existing data, documents, records, pathological specimens, or diagnostic specimens.

___ ___ 9. Research on individual or group behavior or characteristics of individuals, such as studies of perception, cognition, game theory, or test development, where the investigator does not manipulate subjects' behavior and the research will not involve stress to subjects.

___ ___ 10. Research on drugs or devices for which an investigational new drugs (IND) exemption or an investigational device exemption (IDE) is not required.

___ ___ 11. Videotaping, filming, or audio taping (other than 6 above).

___ ___ 12. Use of minors under age 18, or economically or educationally disadvantaged persons.

___ ___ 13. Use of deception.

___ ___ 14. Use of prisoners, pregnant women, fetuses or abortuses, the seriously ill, or persons with mental disabilities, or incompetent individuals.

___ ___ 15. Collection of information or recording of behavior which, if known outside of the research, could reasonably place the subject at risk of civil or criminal liability or damage the subject's social standing, financial standing, or employability.

___ ___ 16. Collection of information regarding sensitive aspects of the subject's behavior such as: drug and alcohol use, illegal conduct, or sexual behavior.

___ ___ 17. This project includes procedures that present more than minimal risk to the subject.

___ ___ 18. The subjects are free to withdraw from the study at any time without prejudice.

EXAMPLE 1.3
Informed Consent
Statement

Information

You are invited to participate in a research study, titled

_____.

The purpose of this study is _____

_____.

List in detail:

1.   All procedures, preferably in chronological order, which will be employed in the study. Point out any that are considered experimental and explain technical and medical terminology.

2.   The amount of time required of the subject per session and for the total duration of the study.

3.   The risks, if any, of each of the procedures to be used in the study and any measures that will be used to minimize the risks.

4.   The benefits you anticipate will be achieved from this research, either to the subjects, others, or the body of knowledge.

If applicable to your study, list:

1.   Alternative procedures or courses of treatment [when experimental procedures are being used].

2.   The number of subjects that will be participating in the research.

3.   Information concerning taping or filming.

4.   A disclaimer for the use of deception.

Confidentiality (Item 5)

The information in the study records will be kept confidential. Data will be stored in a locked cabinet and will be made available only to persons conducting the study unless you specifically give permission in writing to do otherwise. No reference will be made in verbal or written reports which could link you to the study.

If applicable to your study, add the following information on Compensation and Emergency Medical Treatment here.

Compensation

For participating in this study you will receive _____.
If you withdraw from the study prior to its completion, you will receive

_____.

_____
Subject's initials

EXAMPLE 1.3
Concluded

Emergency Medical Treatment

In the unlikely event of physical injury resulting from your participation in this research, emergency medical treatment will be provided at no cost to you. Be certain that you immediately notify the researcher if you are injured. If you require additional medical treatment you will be responsible for the cost. No other compensation will be provided if you are injured in this research.

Contact

If you have questions at any time about the study or the procedures, or you experience adverse effects as a result of participating in this study, you may contact the researcher, [name], at [address], and [phone number].

Participation

Your participation in this study is voluntary, you may decline to participate. If you decide to participate, you may withdraw from the study at any time without penalty and without loss of benefits. If you withdraw from the study prior to its completion your data will be returned to you or destroyed.

Consent

I have read and understand the above information. I have received a copy of this form. I agree to participate in this study.

Subject's signature _____ Date _____

Investigator's signature _____ Date _____

Summary

Research is the lifeblood of a profession because it produces information that adds to the profession's body of knowledge. The research process is a formal, systematic, and logical attack on a problem using the scientific method of analysis. An organized endeavor to obtain facts about some subject, research attempts to discover truth. Properly conducted research requires a clear understanding of the functions research performs. Different problems need different approaches in seeking their solutions. Within the three major types of research (basic, applied, and action), Health and Human Performance (HHP) scholars have produced a variety of conceptual and methodological approaches for dealing with all aspects of the human being (physical, mental, and emotional). Research productivity in the fields undergirding HHP has expanded at a rapid rate and reflects much quality, range, and depth.

Formative Evaluation of Objectives

Objective 1   Explain the relationship between research and a profession.

1. Select a piece of information that you have always assumed to be true (Examples: An aspirin a day prevents a stroke; there is only one sure way to make a free throw) and indicate how you would attack the study (research) of such information.

Objective 2   Know the various methods used in the way knowledge has been obtained in the past and how it is currently obtained.

1. Construct a categorical syllogism that makes sense and one that does not (also indicate why it doesn't make sense).

2. Select a problem in which you are interested and apply the scientific method to researching it.

Objective 3   Know the various types and classifications of research.

1. Provide examples for each of the following: pure or basic research, applied research, action research.

2. Provide a research problem example for each of the research classifications.

Objective 4   Distinguish between a hypothesis and a theory.

1. Explain the difference between a theory and a hypothesis.

The Research Problem

2

Key Words

Assumptions
Computer search
Conceptual literature
Critical reading
Data collection plan

Definition of terms
Delimitations
Hypotheses
Limitations
Problem statement

Purpose statement
Related research literature
Working bibliography

Objectives

Beginners in the realm of research frequently have difficulty in selecting an appropriate problem. The inability of students to recognize the many problems that exist in a profession is the result of inexperience. They simply do not understand, through no fault of their own, the nature of research and problem-solving elements. The emphasis of this chapter is on the learning process of students faced with the necessity of selecting a researchable problem for the first time.

After reading chapter 2, you should be able to:

1. Select a suitable research problem.
2. Know the various sources of research problems.
3. Understand the various steps of the research process.
4. Systematically review literature relevant to the selected problem.
5. Plan and develop an attack on the problem.

Steps in the Research Process

The research process operates in several steps. Each step is undergirded by certain necessary elements, and from each step definite results can be expected. Many of these steps combine mental activity, such as reflective thinking, and the physical activities of searching, evaluating, interpreting, and writing. In reality, there is no universally applicable order in which these steps are incorporated in a given research project. The order and importance of these steps will vary according to the type of research being conducted, the purpose for doing the study, and the whims of the researcher. In many instances, various steps will be combined or accomplished concurrently. For example, the steps of initiation selection, and definition of the problem for a research investigation involve, simultaneously, a literature search, an estimation of the success potential of the study, consideration of the way in which the research will be approached, and a statement of hypothesis. It is believed by the authors of this text that the following steps, originally proposed in a model presented by Fox (1969),[1] apply to most experimental and descriptive research projects. The content embodied in these steps is discussed in appropriate sections of the book. The steps are as follows:

1. **Initiating the idea, need, or problem area:** Becoming aware of research problems, where to look for them, and how to select and define problems.

2. **Initial review of the literature:** Reading sources which will provide an understanding of a basic body of facts to help round out the problem.

3. **Defining the specific research problem:** Providing a specific statement of the problem along with statements of why the problem is important and how it is delimited.

4. **Estimating the success potential of the proposed research:** Reflective thinking regarding whether or not the study will meet the goals and objectives of the researcher. Should the project go forward, be revised, or be abandoned?

5. **The second review of the literature:** Becoming thoroughly knowledgeable in the problem area and obtaining ideas about methods, techniques, and instrumentation needed to attack the problem.

6. **Selecting the research approach:** Depending on the researcher's interest in the past, present, or future time frames, determining whether the problem will be attacked historically, descriptively, or experimentally.

7. **Stating the hypothesis(es) of the research:** Based upon the literature and the researcher's experience, establishing the expected outcomes of the research.

8. **Selecting the data-collecting method(s) and technique(s):** Determining what methods and techniques will specify the instrumentation to provide the needed research data. Considering cost, demands made on the research subjects, and the level of skill possessed by the researcher.

9. **Selecting and developing data-collecting instrument(s):** Considering the availability and adequacy of the instrument(s), deciding what instrument(s) will procure the needed research data.

10. **Developing the data-analysis plan:** Depending upon the nature of the research variables and types of data produced by the research, identifying what statistical procedure(s) will be applied.

11. **Designing the data-collecting plan:** Planning how the experimental or descriptive study will be conducted and how the study will be designed so as to properly test the hypothesis(es).

---

1. From *The Research Process in Education,* by David J. Fox, 1969, Holt, Rinehart & Winston, Inc. Reprinted with permission.

12. **Identifying the population and sample:** Determining the type of subjects who will produce the needed research data. Are the subjects appropriate? How many subjects are needed? How will they be selected?

13. **Conducting pilot studies of the approach, method(s), instrument(s), and data-analysis plan:** Performing a trial run of the research procedures to determine if the needed data will be obtained according to plan, to try out the statistical design, and to be sure that everything works. If problems develop, what revisions need to be made?

14. **Implementing the data-collection plan:** Conducting the research as designed.

15. **Implementing the data-analysis plan:** Analyzing the collected data and testing the hypothesis(es).

16. **Preparing the research report:** Writing the report according to appropriate research writing criteria.

17. **Disseminating the findings:** Publishing the research report or presenting the findings at a professional conference.

Selecting the Problem

A researcher necessarily begins any study with a problem. The source of research problems will vary according to the experience of the person contemplating an investigation, but it is generally agreed that the process begins with an idea or need. Wherever the process starts, it will always end in a problem area (Fox 1969). In HHP there are many problem areas within which exist many potential research problems. Basketball is a problem area. Someone interested in basketball may have the *idea* that basketball officials can be classified as inferior, superior, or average, based on a measure of their personality characteristics, knowledge of the game, previous playing experience, and previous officiating experience. This *idea* might then be translated to a specific problem to be studied (Fratzke 1973). On the other hand, another basketball enthusiast may believe that there is a definite *need* to determine the physiological fitness of officials in relation to the demand placed on them during game situations. This *need* could then be translated into a researchable problem (Holland 1970). Gaunt, in 1979, saw a *need* to study basketball skills in an attempt to compile a battery of tests that might predict basketball playing ability. Henry, in 1974, studied the shooting accuracy of third graders when the basketball goal was less than ten feet high.

The beginner in research, most frequently graduate students with no previous research experience, oftentimes confuses a problem with the problem area. If asked, "In what area are you particularly interested?" they may reply, "Well, I am interested mostly in administration." Or, they may mention health promotion, outdoor education, exercise science, or some other problem area, but are vague as to a specific problem. Each of those areas contain innumerable research problems.

There are many reasons why people engage in research, as delineated by Fox in 1969. Curiosity is as good a motivational factor as any. A recent graduate student was interested in the broad problem area of dietary disorders and illnesses, specifically, anorexia nervosa and bulimia. This student was curious about where the attitude began that led to the development of these disorders in teenagers and young adults. Is it possible that the dietary problems are rooted in childhood? Such curiosity led to an excellent study in which an attempt was made to determine and compare body figure perception and preferences among male and female preadolescent children, in grades 1 through 3 in Georgia and Indiana (Collins 1989). So, from a problem area, a definitive problem was identified.

Many methods for finding worthwhile research problems have been suggested to graduate students by their professors over the years. The following list represents some of the methods which have been helpful in the past:

1. Write out your philosophy of the field of HHP in which you are studying. Divide the field into its several parts and study them. When you come to something you would like to know, but do not know, write it down for your research "hope chest."

2. In reading, in discussions, at lectures, and at all times, write down at once any hunches or ideas that come to you. Many times reading or philosophizing will reveal gaps in your present field of knowledge. Write these down. Read the best studies in your interest area. Think about a problem, and note the questions which arise. Criticize and challenge statements made in current professional periodicals, in books and research studies, and in your own and allied fields. Hundreds of research problems exist in those sources.

3. Prepare a paper on some subject that interests you and extend it into unknown realms. When you meet an obstacle in your thinking, analyze it for the problem it suggests.

4. With what in your field are you dissatisfied? What problems does it suggest? Investigate these.

5. Analyze, challenge, and criticize the popular beliefs and practices in your field of interest. You will be appalled by their unquestioned acceptance. Again, note your hunches.

6. What procedures or practices in your field interest you? Observe the problems inherent in those procedures and practices that could be researched.

7. Browse reference and bibliographical lists in books, journals, magazines, and theses. Just running down a list of titles frequently sparks a viable idea for a research problem. Examine the lists of master's and doctoral studies done at your institution. Then, move on to the lists from other institutions or research centers.

Several of the suggestions listed above involve the utilization of hunches. Becoming sensitive to such ideas can become a valuable mental habit. Upon inspection, most of them will not be viable research problems or will already have been studied. Occasionally, though, a hunch will lead to an important research problem that, when solved, will make a major contribution.

Defining the Problem

Once the idea for a problem has been decided upon, the student should then begin a literature search in an attempt to obtain additional background information to assist in rounding out or fully defining the problem. Fox (1969) delineated two kinds of literature that should be consulted. **Conceptual literature** includes books and articles written by experts or authorities in a problem area. Through their writing they have passed on their ideas, opinions, and theories about what is good, bad, desirable, and undesirable in the problem area. Most of the time conceptual literature is not to be considered research literature as such, but the information disseminated frequently is based on research. An article by Mull (1991) in the *Journal of Health Education* provides a good example of conceptual literature that discusses the role of the health educator in the development of self-esteem in children. Mull gave full support to the idea that self-esteem is an important part of the makeup of healthy people and used previous research to support her argument. Several concepts are presented for health educators assisting children in the development of their self-esteem.

A second type of literature is **related research.** This category includes previous studies in the problem area. Similar or related studies are reviewed to determine what is already known about the main issues inherent in the problem. Using the self-esteem example, examining previous research in that problem area would uncover what earlier work has shown about that characteristic as it relates to children.

In reality, the literature should be consulted throughout the research project. However, the majority of the review should be accomplished before the final plans for conducting the research have been completed. The first plunge into the literature will provide the neophyte researcher with a broader and deeper understanding of what facts are already known in the problem area. If a decision is made to actually investigate the problem, the second review of the literature will provide helpful information on methods, techniques, instrumentation, and procedures for conducting the study.

In making the final determination as to whether or not the problem should be studied, certain common criteria should be considered:

1. **Is the problem in the realm of research? Will it add to the store of knowledge?**
   A researchable topic is one that can be attacked. If there is no way to get at a problem, it is considered to be unresearchable and one that would not increase knowledge.

2. **Does it interest you?**
   It may be a splendid problem, but you should pass it by if you are not interested in it. People tend to do a better job with a problem that was their own idea or something that they created. Faculty advisors frequently are reluctant to "give" a research topic to a graduate student.

3. **Does the problem possess unity?**
   It is important that all components of a problem work together toward the desired objective. Each aspect should be an integral part of the problem. The situation

where several elements exist that should be attacked separately should be avoided. Very frequently one selects too large a problem. If the problem contains experimental, historical, and descriptive elements, these should be separated to clear the way for the main problem.

4. **Is it worth studying? Will it unify knowledge? Does it have real substance? Will it make a real contribution?**

   This criterion can be difficult to satisfy. Most individuals believe that the problem they are studying is important and worthwhile. This criterion is related to a researcher's goal. If a graduate student engages just any problem simply to fulfill a degree requirement, the problem may be of questionable worth. Likewise, if a college professor is pressured into research in order to be promoted and tenured, the selection of the problem may lack the necessary quality to meet this criterion.

5. **Is it feasible from the standpoint of difficulty, time, expense, and availability of data?**

   A student may have a deep interest in history but will forego studying a historical problem because of the extended period of time this type of research entails. Historical studies can also be expensive and frequently involve extensive travel. Sometimes an excellent research problem is conceived and developed only to find that the subjects needed to produce the relevant data are unavailable. No subjects, no data, no study!

6. **Is it timely?**

   There have been times when a research problem has been proposed but not carried out because there was no great demand for its solution. At other times, no effective measurement instrument was available to obtain the needed research data. Until the last fifteen years there was no great demand for the solution of the world's AIDS problem. When the disease reached epidemic proportions, researchers immediately began investigating it, trying to understand it, and attempting to develop a cure. Suddenly AIDS research became timely.

7. **Is it a problem that you can attack without prejudice?**

   If the answer to this question is no, then it is better to pass the problem on to someone else. All researchers, beginners and veterans alike, need to be objective. It is desirable to have a firm conviction and be emotionally charged by a problem, but bias is out of place in research. Bias can creep into a study through the way subjects are selected, instrumentation is developed, and procedures are conducted. A prejudicial viewpoint on how one's hypothesis should turn out can become a reality.

8. **Do you have sufficient formal training and experience in the problem area to conduct the study?**

   This is a common deficiency in beginning researchers, but most students could answer "yes" to this question. It is an obstacle, but one that can be overcome. Research skill and understanding can be achieved, given necessary intellectual qualities, interest, and an in-depth study in one's chosen field. Beginning researchers have often profited by engaging in low-keyed, or modest, studies as a way to learn about research. Research methodology, then, is something one can learn by doing, rather than just reading about it.

Another helpful exercise in defining one's problem, especially for the beginner in research, is to prepare an outline of the problem. Such an outline is usually created after the first review of the literature has been completed. The outline task will enable the student to think through the research problem from beginning to end. The process involves determining what research questions need to be answered as a result of investigating the problem. The questions, in turn, imply what data need to be collected, what methods need to be employed to collect it, and what statistical techniques need to be used to analyze it. The following is an example of such an outline of the problem as prepared for an ex post facto study.

Outline of the Problem

I.   *Topic:* **Student Attrition at the College Level**

II.   *Statement of the Problem.* **The problem was to determine the extent to which students in teacher education programs drop out of college, the reasons for their dropping out, and the relationship of various facts to loss of enrollment.**

III. *Results of Previous Studies*

IV.   *Questions to be Answered*

    A. What is the extent of the attrition?

    B. What is the nature of the attrition? (That is, among various groups of students?)

    C. What are the causes of the attrition?

    D. What is the relationship of the cause of attrition to each type of attrition?

    E. Are there any factors that explain the causes of attrition?

V.   *Collection of Data*

    A. What specific questions need to be answered?

        1. What is the extent of the attrition?

            (a) In each semester or year?

            (b) Among students matriculated for each degree?

            (c) Among majors in each of various areas?

Outline of the Problem—*Continued*

2. What is the nature of the attrition among what groups?
   (a) Students entering at different ages?
   (b) Boys and girls?
   (c) Students in the different types of high school programs offering different patterns of entrance units?
   (d) Students at different scholarship levels?
   (e) Students of different intelligence levels?
   (f) Veterans and nonveterans?
   (g) Students with deficiencies in college entrance requirements?
   (h) Combinations of the above?

3. To what extent is attrition due to:
   (a) Poor scholarship?
   (b) Economic reasons?
   (c) Personal (other than economic) reasons?
   (d) Personality (emotional) difficulties?

4. What is the relationship of the causes of attrition to each of the categories under VA?

5. Are there any particular causes for attrition due to:
   (a) Poor scholarship?
   (b) Economic reasons?
   (c) Other personal reasons?
   (d) Personality difficulties?
   (e) Other reasons?

B. What data need to be obtained? and

C. What methods should be employed to obtain these data?
   1. Obtain the official college record for each student who was dropped or resigned during the last five years.
   2. Select record cards of all students who entered in August of the years 1992–1996.
   3. Prepare a code for the following:
      (a) Reason for being dropped or resigning
      (b) Class
      (c) Level at which student left college (lower freshman, etc.)

> ### Outline of the Problem—*Concluded*
>
>   (d) Achievement record at time of separation
>
>   (e) Age at entrance
>
>   (f) Sex
>
>   (g) Type of high school program completed
>
>   (h) High school achievement
>
>   (i) Degree for which matriculated
>
>   (j) College major
>
>   (k) Entrance deficiencies
>
>   (l) Veteran or nonveteran
>
> **VI.** *Statistical Treatment to Which Data Need to Be Subjected*
>
>   A. Tabulation of number of cases of separation for each of the five class groups by:
>
>   1. Class level at time of separation
>
>   2. Degree for which matriculated
>
>   3. Major
>
>   4. Other traits listed under VA
>
>   B. Computation of appropriate means, percents, and other measures needed for interpretation of data.
>
>   C. Preparation of a table for each item or group of items listed in VA.
>
> **VII.** *Interpretation of Data*
>
> **VIII.** *Conclusions*

The outline process helps solidify thinking about the problem. Many important details are less apt to be forgotten if this task is carried out conscientiously.

Developing the Research Proposal

The final definition of the problem occurs when the graduate student develops a research proposal for the thesis or dissertation that is being planned. In most instances the proposal consists of three chapters: introduction, review of related literature, and procedures for collecting data. Those three chapters ultimately become the first three chapters of a thesis. It is in the first chapter that the final definition of the problem is noted. Before discussing the content in chapter 1 in detail, a few words about the title of the research project are appropriate.

Proposal Title

Quite frequently, the title of the research project is the last decision made by the researcher. All proposals will be titled, but the name given to the project at this time is considered only temporary. It may be changed several times before being finalized. The title is important in that it is the first thing the reader sees. Based on the title, the reader will continue reading or lose interest. A brief title, one that is streamlined, is currently preferred. This title is too long:

> An Analysis of the Specific Curriculum Content for the Preparation of Recreation Majors and the Relationship between the Details of the Curriculum and the Details of the Majors' On-the-Job Duties

Not only is this title overly long, it also includes some redundancy and is confusing. The title should be long enough to cover the subject of the research, but short enough to be interesting. Usually, twelve to fourteen words is sufficient. The beginning researcher should ask these questions when contemplating a project title:

1. Does the title precisely identify the area of the problem?
2. Is the title clear, concise, and adequately descriptive to permit indexing the study in its proper category?
3. Are unnecessary words avoided, such as "an analysis of," "a comparison of," "a study of," "the effect of," and "the relationship between"? (*Note:* These words and other catchy, misleading, and vague phrases unnecessarily lengthen titles and do nothing to add substance. They are superfluous.)
4. Do nouns, as opposed to adjectives, serve as the key words in the title?
5. Are the most important words placed at the beginning of the title?

Following are some examples of appropriate titles:

1. Self-Consciousness and Physical Self-Efficacy in Relationship to Exercise Adherence (Visker 1986)
2. Group Cohesiveness and Team Success Among Women's Intercollegiate Basketball Teams (Cotter 1978)
3. Body Figure Perceptions and Preferences Among Preadolescent Children (Collins 1989)
4. Needs Assessment of Indiana Convention and Visitor Bureaus (Peña 1990)
5. A Health Knowledge Test for Male College Freshmen in Saudi Arabia (Hashim 1988)

All of these titles meet the criteria for a streamlined, yet complete, title. Each accurately reflects the research problem.

Writing Chapter 1: Introduction

Chapter 1 of the proposal usually begins with a brief introduction. Customarily, the researcher includes a paragraph or two (perhaps more depending on the nature of the problem) to help lead the reader into the problem. The researcher specifies the problem being investigated and establishes why it is important. How the researcher became interested in the problem is usually indicated. Some references to the literature can be made, but it is more desirable if the content of this section represents the researcher's own thoughts. If too much literature is used to stimulate interest, the introduction begins to look like a review of the literature, which is more properly done in chapter 2. Again, it is not necessary that this section be long. Following are two examples of good introductory sections:

1. The three major points of emphasis in the field hockey drive according to most coaches and authors are: (1) quickness, (2) power, and (3) accuracy. In particular game situations, a player may desire to sacrifice some accuracy to execute the drive as quickly as possible, or he/she may choose to sacrifice some power to achieve a more accurate pass. What differences, if any, exist in the mechanics of the field hockey drive under various conditions? It was the nature of this question that prompted this investigation (Hendrick 1981).

2. Obesity is prevalent in our society and its treatment is constantly being explored. All proper weight loss programs for the moderately obese include aerobic exercise as well as dietary restriction. Obese individuals are often told to exercise two or three times a day for short periods in order to burn more calories. The goal of exercise is to mobilize fats from adipose tissue stores for energy production. It is, however, not known if this is the most effective method of achieving weight loss. The optimal exercise prescription for the moderately obese has not been determined. This study, then, examined the duration of exercise in an attempt to determine the most effective exercise prescription for moderately obese women (Sun 1988).

Statement of the Problem.   Immediately after the introductory comments, the **problem statement** should appear. This will always be a declarative statement that indicates what question or issue was addressed in the research project. The problem should be stated clearly, concisely, and definitively. All of the problem elements, including the variables to be studied, should be expressed in an orderly system of relationships. The statement results from the researcher's analysis of all of the facts and explanations that might possibly be related to the problem. Typically, the statement of the problem begins in a manner similar to one of the following:

1. "The problem of the study was to . . ."
2. "The study was concerned with . . ."
3. "The focus of the research was on the . . ."

Although it is sometimes seen, the phrase "The study investigated . . ." is not a good choice. Inanimate objects cannot take action; hence, a study cannot investigate.

Following are a few examples of problem statements that meet the criteria for clarity and conciseness.

1. The problem was to investigate the influence of cohesiveness on the team success of women's intercollegiate basketball teams (Cotter 1978).

2. The problem was to apply the Feldt (1975) and Kristof formulas (1974) to motor performance tests consisting of several trials in order to compare the resulting estimates of reliability with those obtained by currently recommended methods (Frye 1977).

3. The problem of the study was to determine if the psychological facts of self-consciousness and physical self-efficacy discriminate between female adults who adhere to exercise programs and female adults who do not adhere to exercise programs (Visker 1986).

Purpose of the Study. The **purpose statement** must indicate *why* the study was done. Again, brevity is stressed. The researcher spells out the reason(s) or objective(s) for doing the study and answers the question, "What potential impact will the results of the study have on the current body of knowledge?" The problem and purpose are often confused by research neophytes and veterans alike. Consider the following:

1. The problem tells *what* was done in the study (i.e., what was tested, determined, effected, compared, analyzed, evaluated, etc.).

   The purpose tells *why* the study was done. What good could possibly come out of the study? How will the findings be used or applied?

2. It is incorrect under the problem statement to say, "The purpose of the study was to . . ." It is also incorrect in a purpose statement to say that the purpose of the study was to test, to determine, to analyze, or to compare something. Such a statement is a problem statement. Just remember that the purpose tells why you want to test, determine, analyze, or compare.

This example illustrates the difference between the two statements:

Statement of the Problem: The problem of the study was to evaluate five options of coping with smoking in the workplace: (1) improvement of ventilation, (2) installation of air cleaning devices, (3) segregation of smokers and nonsmokers, (4) smoking only in designated areas, and (5) a total smoking ban. Included in the study was an attempt to identify the effects of these options on the economical and productivity aspects while an acceptable indoor air quality was maintained. (Padilla 1986)

Purpose of the Study: The purpose of the study was to provide employers with guidelines to initiate or improve smoking policies in the workplace. (Padilla 1986)

Following is the purpose statement for the cohesiveness problem previously mentioned:

> If cohesiveness is a significant factor in predicting team success, coaches should devote greater time, effort, and personnel to the development and cultivation of group cohesion. If low cohesiveness is a better predictor of success, coaches may seek to increase success by generating conflict among players. Cohesiveness may not show any prediction ability for team success, in which case the time and energy of the coach would be better spent on other aspects of coaching. (Cotter 1978)

In the body perception and preference study discussed earlier, the reason or purpose for doing the study was given as follows:

> If concerns for thinness and weight loss are occurring among children of normal weight, health education intervention and prevention strategies must be addressed at earlier ages than has been believed previously. It was believed that the information provided in the study would assist in targeting the age at which health education for counteracting an unrealistic standard of attractiveness should begin. (Collins 1989)

Need for the Study (Significance of the Study, Justification for the Study).   This section of chapter 1 follows the purpose statement, and its function is to elaborate on the purpose. One of the three section heads listed above should be selected. Which of the three is most appropriate will depend upon: (1) the nature of the study, (2) the reasons the study was undertaken, and (3) the researcher's preference. Use the literature to help show why the study is needed, to explain why it is significant, or to justify its content. This is the place to present examples of how the problem has manifested itself in society. The development of this section will attempt to show that one or more of the following is true:

1. Knowledge gaps exist between the theoretical and practical aspects of the problem.
2. More and better knowledge is needed in the problem areas.
3. Present knowledge in the problem area needs validation.
4. Current practices concerning the problem need to be clarified.
5. A solution to the problem needs to be found.

The following example of a need for the study section appeared in a research proposal in which the problem was to determine the impact of rotation from day shift to periodic night shift work on nurses' performance and frequency of medication errors during the night shift sessions:

Medical accident and error statistics continue to reflect significant numbers of accidental injury, fatalities, and inadequate care related to improper dosage and/or route of administration of medicines in medical care facilities (Smith 1990). Further evidence indicates that nurses rotating to night shift work from other shifts are likely to encounter biorhythm interference that adversely affects performance (Klein and Bruce 1989). Management knowledge of hazards has been recognized as a key element in the prevention of various industrial accidents (Accident Prevention Manual for Industrial Operation 1981). This includes work environments such as nursing. Medication error rates will continue to be a major problem in health care settings until proper countermeasures are identified and controls are instituted to reduce occurrence. Therefore, management action through knowledge is essential to correct the situation. The focus of this study was to provide an accurate assessment of the relationship between night shift rotation and medication errors which should lead to a more informed management. This information could provide new insight into shift workers' performance and contribute toward better decisions on shift rotation assignments in the future. (Welcher 1991)

Delimitations. In research circles, **delimitations** refers to the scope of the study. It is in this section of chapter 1 that the researcher draws a line around the study and, in effect, "fences it in." This segment identifies what is included in the research. Delimitations spell out the population studied and include those things the researcher can control. It establishes the parameters on such characteristics of the study as (1) number and kinds of subjects, (2) number and kinds of variables, (3) tests, measures, or instruments utilized in the study, (4) special equipment, (5) type of training program, (6) the time and duration of the study (e.g., date, number of weeks, time of year), and (7) analytical procedures. These are the ingredients that the researcher uses to attack the problem. If an item does not appear in the list of delimitations, then it is of no concern in the research. A particular population is targeted on which selected variables will be studied. The variables will be measured by specific test instruments. A certain training program may be involved and the study will be conducted over a specified period of time. Following is an example of the delimitations that appeared in a proposal for studying an obesity problem (Sun 1988):

The study was delimited to:

1. Thirty moderately obese and previously sedentary women subjects, aged 25–55, who had been obese for at least five years and were free of any diagnosed metabolic or cardiovascular disease.

2. The subjects were randomly assigned to one of three groups as follows: Exercise Group One; Exercise Group Two; Control Group.

3. All subjects followed a daily diet of 500 calories less than their current weight maintenance diet using dietary exchanges. The diets were well balanced and nutritionally adequate with the contribution of nutrients as follows: 12–15 percent protein, 50–55 percent carbohydrate, and 30–35 percent fat. Three-day food diaries and 24-hour recalls were used for diet analyses.

4. Exercise groups walked at 50–60 percent of maximal heart rate reserve, four days per week for six months.

5. Exercise Group One walked 30 minutes twice a day and Exercise Group Two walked 60 minutes a day. The Control Group did not participate in any formal exercise program.

6. Three of the exercise sessions per week were under the supervision of the Indiana University Adult Fitness Program. The other exercise sessions were supervised by the investigator.

7. Percent body fat was determined by skinfold measurements, circumferences, and hydrostatic weighing. All measurements were performed by the investigator.

8. Pretraining and posttraining concentrations of plasma FFA, glycerol, and lipolytic hormones (epinephrine, norepinephrine, adrenocorticotropin, triiodothyronine, tetraiodothyronine, growth hormone, glucagon, and insulin) concentrations were obtained from blood samples taken at 0, 10, 20, 30, 40, 50, 60, and 90 minutes of exercise or rest.

9. The study was conducted for a period of six months between February and August, 1988.

Limitations.   In research terminology **limitations** refer to weaknesses of the study. All studies have them because compromises frequently have to be made in order to conform to the realities of a situation. Limitations are those things the researcher could not control, but that may have influenced the results of the study. The reader of a research report should always know at the outset those conditions of the study that could reflect negatively on the work in some way. Only those things that might affect the acceptability of the research data should be presented. The researcher will, of course, try to eliminate extremely serious weaknesses before the study is commenced. Among the items that typically involve statements of limitation are the following:

1. The research approach, design, method(s), and techniques

2. Sampling problems

3. Uncontrolled variables

4. Faulty administration of tests or training programs

5. Generalizability of the data

6. Representativeness of subjects

7. Compromises to internal and external validity

8. Reliability and validity of the research instruments

It is important that all statements of limitation sound like, or imply, weakness. The statement, "The sample size was small," is not sufficient, because a small sample does not necessarily assume a weakness of the study. However, the statement, "The sample size of the study ($N = 30$) is small, necessitating caution in extrapolation of the data to a larger obese population," implies a possible weakness of the study.

The limitations of the obesity study were presented as follows.

The study was limited by:

1. The sample size of this study is small ($N = 30$) necessitating caution in extrapolation of the data to a larger obese population.

2. Daily activities of the subjects other than the exercise program were not controlled.

3. Although subjects were requested to stay on a diet that was well balanced and restricted by 500 calories a day, occasional variance from this could not be controlled. In addition, due to the nature of the diet analyses performed, changes in caloric intake may not have been detected.

4. The investigator was unable to personally conduct all of the maximal graded exercise tests in pretraining and posttraining as well as the exercise sessions. To insure standardization in testing and training, she met with the staff of the Indiana University Adult Fitness Program in order to discuss the testing and training procedures.

5. Resting metabolic rate was not measured following the exercise sessions and lipolytic changes during this time could not be determined.

6. Since plasma FFA, glycerol, and lipolytic hormones can be affected by conditions other than exercise, it is possible that such conditions did exist.

7. Plasma FFA do not reflect FFA flux in adipose or skeletal muscle tissue and, therefore, conclusions concerning fat metabolism must be interpreted with caution. (Sun 1988)

Assumptions.   **Assumptions** are derived primarily from the literature. Assumptions then become the basis for the hypotheses, or predictions of eventual outcome, of the study. In other words, what does the literature tell the researcher that can be assumed to be true for purposes of planning the study? The information gleaned from the literature frequently serves as the basis for much of the development of the research project. The literature provides information about a particular behavior being investigated and the various conditions influencing that behavior, and sometimes contains factual evidence explaining the behavior. The researcher undertakes a study with certain assumptions about this information. Assumptions are also made about the way the instrumentation, procedures, methods, and techniques will contribute to the study. In a study that involved teaching the overhand throwing pattern to children, the following assumptions were made:

1. The maturational and environmental influences are unique to each child.

2. The throwing force of children increases with age due primarily to improved coordination.

3. A mature throwing pattern conforms to mechanically correct execution patterns.

4. Distributed practice is essential in the proper learning of motor skills.

5. Elementary school children have delimited information and are able to handle only a few items at a time.

6. A child's information processing abilities improve with age, experience, and training. (Luedke 1980)

The researcher may also assume that certain things that could not be controlled or documented may have happened in the study. The following are examples of this type of assumption:

1. All subjects completed the questionnaire honestly and correctly.

2. The subjects complied with the researcher's request to perform maximally on all trials of the test.

3. The test instrument was a reliable and valid measure of self-esteem.

Hypotheses.   A detailed discussion about the nature of hypotheses was presented in chapter 1. The assumptions made by the researcher provide the launching pad for hypotheses. The **hypotheses** permit the researcher to predict the outcome of the study in advance, and they present tentative explanations for the solution of the problem. It is extremely important that the hypotheses be testable. In a therapeutic recreation study (Pate 1987) to determine the effect of sea kayak touring on the self-concept of patients with low-level spinal cord injuries (SCI), the following hypotheses were stated:

1. Patients with a low level of SCI of at least one year duration exhibit an increased self-concept after participation in a two-week sea kayak tour.

2. Increased self-concept changes are significantly greater for those patients participating in the sea kayak tour than for patients participating in a two-week camping experience or in a regular rehabilitation center program.

3. Self-concept does not change for those patients participating in a two-week camping experience or in a regular rehabilitation program.

4. Self-concept remains elevated for those patients participating in the sea kayak tour for six months after completion of the tour.

Definition of Terms.   **Definition of terms** is a necessity since many terms and concepts have multiple meanings. The researcher should define terms as they will be interpreted and used throughout the study. Always define operational and behavioral terms and concepts, and check special terms in technical dictionaries or have them reviewed by experts in the field. An operational definition gives meaning to a concept or term by indicating what operation has to be accomplished so as to be able to measure the concept. In experimental studies a researcher will cause a particular result to occur by using a certain procedure or operation. An operational definition of personality might refer to the "scores on the Cattell 16 Personality Factor Inventory" or some other personality test selected by the researcher. Directly quoted or accurately paraphrased time-honored definitions, if they fit the research situation, are considered superior to definitions made up or "coined" by the researcher. Once defined, a term should be applied consistently throughout the study so as not to confuse the reader. It is customary to alphabetize the terms in a list of operational definitions. Following is an example of a partial list of terms defined in a study of women victims of sexual coercion (Ogletree 1991):

> For consistency of interpretation the following terms are defined:
>
> *Acquaintance Rape.* "A forced sexual intercourse that occurs either on a date or between individuals who are acquaintances or romantically involved" (Meyer 1984, 2). This term excludes incest, authority rapes, spousal rape, and rape of children under age 14. This phenomenon is also called "date rape."
>
> *Assertiveness.* "A response, direct and specific, to an aggressive act" (Bakker and Bakker-Rabdau 1973, 59).
>
> *Self-esteem.* "A positive or negative attitude toward a particular object, namely the self" (Rosenberg 1965).
>
> *Sexual Coercion.* "Sexual intercourse subsequent to the use of menacing verbal pressure or misuse of authority" (Koss et al. 1987, 163) or attempted rape or rape.

The Use of Literature in Research

As discussed earlier, the literature is a big help in providing the beginning researcher with an initial understanding of the facts in the problem area. The information gained from the preliminary excursion into the literature helps to round out the problem. As the problem planning continues, the literature search becomes increasingly more pointed and specific. Related research becomes critical. Studies related to the proposed study are sought out in terms of problem, variable, and population similarity. The researcher will attempt to find out just how far human inquiry into the problem has progressed. What is known and what is not known concerning the problem? Are there any gaps in the literature with respect to the relevant information surrounding the problem? These questions can be answered by a thorough literature search.

The researcher will also become knowledgeable about methodology and procedures for attacking the problem, as well as ideas on instrumentation and design. Conceptual and theoretical relationships among the essential variables will be found. A major outcome of the search is that the researcher will develop a theoretical basis for the study and justification for its conduct. It has often been said that the more sound and thorough knowledge of the previous research, the better will be the planning of subsequent study in the problem area. "Knowledge of the literature in the field and critical insight into the research in the student's major field of interest is considered evidence of high scholarship" (Bookwalter and Bookwalter 1959).

It is recommended that the literature be searched by looking at the most current literature first, then working backward in time. This will familiarize the researcher with the newer methods, techniques, procedures, instrumentation, and data analysis designs that have been developed in the problem area. Chances are better that mistakes made in previous studies will have been corrected, old theories revised, new ones postulated, and more sophisticated designs developed. Again, all background reading should be completed before final plans for conducting the study are made.

Searching the literature is hard and demanding work. It is absolutely essential that graduate students contemplating a research project for the first time build plenty of library time into their schedules. The literature search can be a frustrating and not particularly romantic task. However, it can be exciting to increase the knowledge base on the topic to be researched. One of the more frustrating occurrences for the beginner is to discover that the proposed study, or closely related study, has already been done. In this situation the researcher must weigh the merits of replicating the previous study or of revising the proposed study to attack a different part of the overall problem.

The Working Bibliography

Once the literature search has identified promising sources, the researcher creates a **working bibliography;** this list should include all sources that are pertinent to the problem. People differ in their methods for developing a bibliography, but a very common and helpful approach is to record the information on 3" × 5" or 4" × 6" index cards. Take care to accurately note all of the bibliographic information for each source. Typically, this information includes the author's last name and initials; title of the journal article, book, report, or review; volume or issue number, year, and month of the journal; publisher of the book; edition and date of when the book was published; page numbers of the article or book reference; and library call number.

Research Reading

After the working bibliography has been completed, the sources have to be located. This is usually accomplished through the use of the card catalog in the library, which is divided into a subject list and an author list. The student will learn the two library classification systems used in the United States, namely, the Dewey decimal and Library of Congress systems. Other available resources for seeking out specific topics are the dictionary, encyclopedias, abstracts, and indexes to various periodicals and reviews. (*Note:* With increasing computer technology, the card catalog retrieval system may soon become obsolete. Most college and university libraries have developed computerized catalogs that list information about books, magazines, journals, newspapers, and other regularly published periodicals and serials that these libraries hold. Through the Internet, the globally-distributed collections of computer networks that exchange information, researchers can access all of these catalogs.

Because computer-generated source location systems may not contain the volume included in the card catalog medium, it might be wise to use both systems.)

After identifying each source in the working bibliography, the next task is to quickly evaluate the potential value of the book, article, report, or abstract, to the proposed research. This is done by scanning the table of contents, book indexes, chapter summaries, and article abstracts. Even though a title may seem to indicate that the content will be useful, frequently it is misleading. As the scanning process continues, the working bibliography will change. Some references will be thrown out because they hold no promise of being helpful, while new ones may well be discovered that will be of use. The research focus may even change as the study develops which would, in turn, render changes in the working bibliography.

When it has been determined which sources will be valuable to the proposed study, each one must be read in depth. Bookwalter and Bookwalter (1959) referred to this process as **critical reading** or gleaning. This means reading a large amount of material while at the same time thinking about, reflecting upon, and analyzing what is being said. While doing critical reading it is essential that the researcher take notes. This has been referred to as developing an annotated bibliography. Again, it is recommended that index cards be used for this process. The first card for each source will contain all of the relevant bibliographic information. Each additional card will contain source notes pertaining to the items that have a close relationship to the proposed research. Figure 2.1 is an example of a note card containing the type of information usually recorded.

Notes should be taken only from the sources most pertinent to the current problem of interest. In transcribing notes from the source to the cards, use extreme care to ensure accuracy. If any of the information will be quoted directly when it appears in the research paper, use quotation marks to identify those items on the cards. Note page numbers accurately.

After the notes have been taken from all relevant and pertinent sources, they should be sorted and classified. The researcher should gain insight into agreements, differences, relationships, and trends as a result of this process. When two or more literary sources do not agree, both sides of the issue should be noted. Beginning researchers sometimes have the mistaken idea that they should seek out only those hypotheses, findings, and conclusions with which they agree.

While notes gathered from reading usually will be the most profitable, notes from speeches, lectures, class discussions, interviews, letters, and taped television programs can also represent related literature sources. The point is that no stone should be left unturned during the literature search. The annotated bibliography is an excellent mechanism for establishing control over a large amount of material. It is recognized that in this age of the Xerox machine and the highlighter pen, many graduate students will be tempted to duplicate book chapters and journal articles and highlight appropriate information. With the increasing popularity of the Internet, temptation exists to simply print out relevant information. This is a common way of "taking notes" today. However, cards are much easier to handle and the information is easier to organize in that form than are several hundred $8\frac{1}{2}$" × 11" sheets of paper.

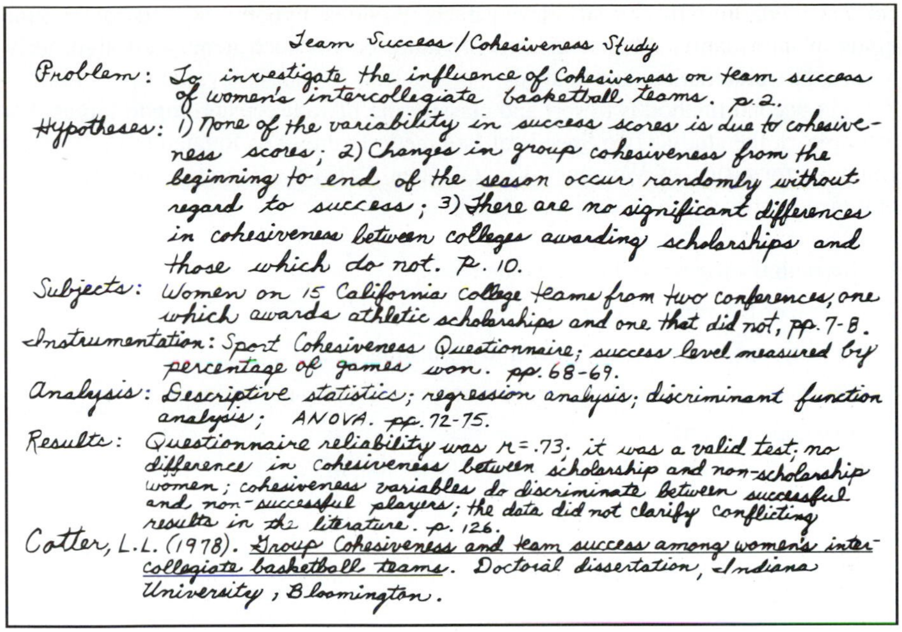

Team Success/Cohesiveness Study

Problem: To investigate the influence of Cohesiveness on team success of women's intercollegiate basketball teams. p. 2.

Hypotheses: 1) None of the variability in success scores is due to cohesiveness scores; 2) Changes in group cohesiveness from the beginning to end of the season occur randomly without regard to success; 3) There are no significant differences in cohesiveness between colleges awarding scholarships and those which do not. P. 10.

Subjects: Women on 15 California college teams from two conferences; one which awards athletic scholarships and one that did not. pp. 7-8.

Instrumentation: Sport Cohesiveness Questionnaire; success level measured by percentage of games won. pp. 68-69.

Analysis: Descriptive statistics; regression analysis; discriminant function analysis; ANOVA. pp. 72-75.

Results: Questionnaire reliability was r = .73; it was a valid test; no difference in cohesiveness between scholarship and non-scholarship women; cohesiveness variables do discriminate between successful and non-successful players; the data did not clarify conflicting results in the literature. p. 126.

Cotter, L.L. (1978). Group Cohesiveness and team success among women's intercollegiate basketball teams. Doctoral dissertation, Indiana University, Bloomington.

FIGURE 2.1
Sample research note card.

Writing Chapter 2: Literature Review

After the literature has been thoroughly reviewed, the researcher will then organize the notes and transpose them into a chapter 2, which is usually called the "Review of Related Literature," "Related Literature," or "Literature." This section should be a well-organized chapter that consists of an insightful analysis and evaluation of each research source as it relates to the objectives of the current study. The literature review helps to justify the study. This is not automatically or arbitrarily determined; it must be shown. A careful analysis of related studies is important in verifying the worth of the study and in helping to establish the overall justification. Only those studies that have a significant relationship to the current problem should be included. It is also important to note that all references located will not be included in this chapter. Some will not be used at all or will be used in other chapters.

The review of literature should not merely present previous studies in chronological order, leaving it to the reader to assimilate the facts and to draw relationships between the cited research and the problem. Above all, the literature review should not be presented as a series of abstracts of various studies. Facts and theories should be presented and their relationships shown. Gaps in the existing knowledge in the problem area should surface.

Researchers vary in the way they organize the literature, but two methods are more common than others. In one, the sources are divided into literature related to the present study in content, and literature related in method. Discussion of the content literature will present relevant facts, theories, hypotheses, and background kinds of information. Method-related literature covers such items as design, techniques, instrumentation, and analysis.

A second method is to sort and classify the literature according to topics. For example, in the study "Two Speeds of Isokinetic Exercise as Related to the Vertical Jump Performance of Women" (Van Oteghen 1973) the literature reviewed was organized under the following topic headings:

1. Strength testing reliability of women
2. Nature of the vertical jump
3. Validity and reliability of vertical jump testing
4. Effects of weight training programs on vertical jump performance
5. Isokinetic training
6. Isokinetic training related to strength development
7. Summary

Chapter 2 should always begin with an opening paragraph that relates the literature to the problem and explains how the chapter is organized. Following is an example from Collins's (1989) study:

> The literature related to perception of bodily attractiveness in American culture is reported in this chapter. For organizational purposes, the literature is presented under the following topics: (1) Body Image and Self-Esteem, (2) Attractiveness in American Culture, (3) Influence of the Mass Media, (4) The Thin Standard of Bodily Attractiveness for Women, (5) Impact of the Thin Standard, (6) Body Dissatisfaction in Non-Clinical Populations, (7) Measurement of Body Image, and (8) Summary.

Chapter 2 is the only one in the proposal that may need a summary. It appears as the last section of the chapter and should be relatively brief. An attempt should be made to, in sum, indicate what the literature has told us. What is it that we know? Don't know? What gaps need to be filled? The summary should not be used to report or present any more specific references to the literature; this should already have been done in detail. Instead, the summary should be a series of statements that tie all of the previous reporting together. The following example (Hendrick 1981) illustrates the function of a summary.

> The majority of publications reviewed on the field hockey drive were considered conceptual. In addition, much of the information obtained from these sources was contradictory and inconclusive. Phrases like, the hands are to be placed 'close together,' the stick is to be held 'firm,' 'a strong forward foot,' and wrists should be 'cocked slightly,' but remain 'firm,' are just a few examples of the ambiguity that existed. How close is close? How firm is firm? Does 'cocked' mean flexed or extended? What is a 'strong foot?'

Pubic Affairs Information Service (PAIS), 1915–date. A monthly index to books, current periodicals, government documents, and pamphlets pertaining to economics and public affairs.

Psychological Abstracts, 1927–date. A monthly bibliography listing new books and articles grouped by subjects, with a signed abstract of each item.

Applied Science and Technology Index, 1958–date. A cumulative subject index to periodicals in the fields of aeronautics, automation, chemistry, construction, electricity and electrical communications, engineering, geology and metallurgy, industrial and mechanical arts, machinery, physics, transportation, and related subjects.

Business Periodicals Index, 1958–date. A cumulative subject index to periodicals in the fields of accounting, advertising, banking and finance, general business, insurance, labor and management, marketing and purchasing, office management, public administration, taxations, specific businesses, industries, and trades.

Wall Street Journal Index, 1958–date. A monthly index with annual cumulation.

Biological and Agricultural Index, 1964–date. A cumulative subject index to periodicals in the fields of biology, agriculture, and related sciences. (Formerly the *Agricultural Index.*)

Social Sciences and Humanities Index, 1965–date. A quarterly guide to periodical literature in the social sciences and humanities. (Formerly the *International Index.*)

Current Index to Journals in Education. (CIJE) 1969–date. Monthly.

Dissertation Abstracts. University Microfilms, Inc. Monthly.

Research Quarterly Index. References in physical education, exercise, and sport. Yearly.

Reviews. Another excellent means by which to begin a literature search is to utilize the many reviews that are available. There are several in the areas of health and human performance (HHP) and others exist in the fields of education, psychology, physiology, and sociology. The following is a representative list of such reviews:

Exercise and Sport Reviews
Physical Fitness Digest
What Research Tells the Coach
Encyclopedia of Physical Education, Fitness and Sport
Science and Medicine of Exercise and Sport
Annual Review of Physiology
Annual Review of Psychology
Athletic Performance Review
Review of Educational Research

Each author seemed to have his or her own viewpoint on the execution of the field hockey drive. There were no two descriptions that were completely alike. The two research studies available also led to inconclusive generalizations. There is definitely a large gap in the literature as to the components of the optimal field hockey drive. Cohen (1969) summed up the information well when she concluded that more research must be done in order to formulate any generalizations regarding the execution of the field hockey drive.

Sources of Literature

The first step in acquiring literature resource materials is to determine if they exist. It is necessary that students become familiar with the large range of references that are frequently housed in both public and academic libraries. Invariably, students will benefit from the assistance that can be provided by the reference librarians who are only too willing to help. These people are professionals who possess a sound knowledge of what sources are available and how to locate them.

Indexes. Indexes provide a valuable resource for locating related literature. The *Education Index* includes comprehensive author and subject guides to educational literature from most significant American sources. The *Reader's Guide to Periodical Literature* leads to content in the mainstream popular magazines and journals. The *Physical Education Index* contains subject entries for nearly two hundred journals, including some foreign publications. Articles from journals representing almost all of the areas comprising HHP can be found in this index. The *Bibliographic Index of Health Education Periodicals (BIHEP)* is a comprehensive index to the professional literature through 1983 in the areas of Health Education, Health Business, Health Promotion, and the Social Aspects of Health. Other indexes frequently used by HHP researchers include the following:

Indices Medicus. Subject-author index of over two thousand biomedical journals.

Palmer's Index to the Times (London), 1790–1941. Indexes early period of the *Times*.

Engineering Index, 1884–date. Guide to engineering literature of the world.

U.S. Superintendent of Documents. United States government publications: Monthly Catalog 1895–date.

Book Review Digest, 1905–date. Excerpts from reviews of current books published in the United States.

Dramatic Index, 1909–1949. Index to articles on drama.

New York Times Index, 1912–date. Master key to news.

Industrial Arts Index, 1914–1957. A subject index to periodicals in the fields of business, finance, applied science, and technology.

Encyclopedia of Educational Research
Annual Review of Public Health

Periodicals.   As the fields of HHP have become specialized by several subdisciplines, the number of periodicals has increased dramatically. Added to those available in HHP are the many relevant journals from fields outside of HHP. It is not possible to mention all of them here, but the following list is representative of what is at the disposal of HHP researchers. The sources have been arranged by subject.

APPLIED HEALTH SCIENCE

Addictions

Alcohol Health and Research World
Bibliography on Smoking and Health
Bottom Line on Alcohol in Society
British Journal of Addictions
Changes
Prevention Pipeline
Smoking and Health Bulletin
Tobacco-free Young America Reporter

Diseases/Dying

Ca-A Cancer Journal for Clinicians
Journal of Cancer Education
Omega Journal of Death and Dying

Family Studies

American Journal of Family Therapy
Family Life Educator
Family Perspective
Family Process
Family Relations
Journal of Divorce
Journal of Family Issues
Journal of Family Violence
Journal of Marital and Family Therapy
Parenting Studies
Sage Family Studies Abstracts
Single Parent

Health Education

Health Education (AAHPERD)
Health Education Quarterly
Health Education Research

Health Values
International Quarterly of Community Health Education

Human Sexuality

Current Research Updates in Human Sexuality
Journal of Sex Education and Therapy

Nutrition

American Journal of Clinical Nutrition
Annual Review of Nutrition
Clinical Nutrition
Food and Nutrition News
International Journal of Obesity
Journal of Nutrition
Journal of Nutrition Education
Journal of the American Dietetic Association
Nutrition Abstracts
Nutrition Action Newsletter
Nutrition & Cancer
Nutrition Reviews
Sports Nutrition News

Preventive Medicine

American Journal of Preventive Medicine
Behavioral Medicine
Indiana Medicine
Optimal Health
University of California, Berkeley Wellness Letter

Public Health

Accident Analysis and Prevention
Accident Facts
AIDS Education and Prevention
American Journal of Health Promotion
American Journal of Public Health
Canadian Center for Occupational Health and Safety
Canadian Journal of Public Health
Indiana State Board of Health Bulletin
Journal of American College Health
Journal of School Health
Public Health Reports

Youth and Adolescence

Adolescence
Adolescent Psychiatry
International Journal of Adolescence and Youth

Journal of Adolescent Research
Journal of Youth and Adolescence

Unclassified

American Health
Health

EXERCISE AND SPORT SCIENCES

Advances in Pediatric Sport Sciences
Canadian Journal of Sport Sciences
Exercise and Sport Sciences Review
Journal of Sport Sciences
Medicine and Science in Sports and Exercise
Research Quarterly for Exercise and Sport
Scandinavian Journal of Sport Sciences
SPORTS - Science
American Journal of Human Biology
Pediatric Exercise Science

PHYSICAL EDUCATION/KINESIOLOGY

Adapted Physical Education

Adapted Physical Activity Quarterly
Paleastra

Athletic Training

Athletic Training
NATA News
National Strength and Conditioning Association Journal

Biomechanics, Kinesiology, Physiology

Clinical Kinesiology
European Journal of Applied Physiology and Occupational Physiology
International Journal of Sport Biomechanics
Journal of Applied Physiology
Journal of Biomechanics
Journal of Motor Behavior
Journal of Sport and Exercise Physiology

Coaching/Referee

Coaching Clinic
Journal of Applied Research in Coaching & Athletics
Referee
Scholastic Coach
Spotlight on Youth Sports

Dance

American Journal of Dance Therapy
Dance Teacher Now
IDEA Today
Kinesiology and Medicine for Dance

History, Psychology, Philosophy, and Sociology of Sport

Arena Review
International Journal of Sport Psychology
International Journal of the History of Sport
Journal of Sport and Exercise Psychology
Journal of Sport and Social Issues
Journal of Sport Behavior
Journal of Sport History
Journal of Personality and Social Psychology
Journal of the Philosophy of Sport
North American Society for Sport History Newsletter
Personality and Individual Differences
Psychology and Sociology of Sport
Sociology of Sport Journal
Sport Psychologist

Individual Sports

International Gymnast
Journal of Swimming Research
Sports 'n Spokes
Swimming Technique
Swimming World and Junior Swimmer
Track and Field News

Physical Therapy/Rehabilitation

International Journal of Rehabilitation Research
Journal of Cardiopulmonary Rehabilitation
Journal of Orthopaedic & Sports Physical Therapy
Physical Therapy

Sport Medicine

American Journal of Sports Medicine
Annals of Sports Medicine
Archives of Physical Medicine and Rehabilitation
British Journal of Sports Medicine
Clinics in Sports Medicine
Electromyography & Clinical Neurophysiology

International Journal of Sports Cardiology
International Journal of Sports Medicine
Journal of Sports Medicine and Physical Fitness
Medicine & Science in Sports & Exercise
Physical Fitness/Sports Medicine (Index)
Physician and Sportsmedicine
Sports Medicine
Sports Medicine Digest
Yearbook of Sports Medicine

Sports Administration/Marketing

Athletic Administration
Athletic Business
Club Business International
College Athletic Management
Corporate Fitness
Employee Health and Fitness
Executive Edge
Fitness Management
Journal of Sport Management
Sports Careers
Team Marketing Report

Sports Law

Exercise Standards and Malpractice Reporter
Sports and the Courts

Teaching Physical Education

Great Activities Newspaper
Gym Dandies Series
Journal of Teaching in Physical Education
Physical Educator
Quest
Strategies

Unclassified

American Academy of Physical Education: Academy Papers
Athletic Performance Review
Human Movement Science
International Journal of Physical Education
Journal of the International Council for Health, Physical Education and Recreation
NCAA News
Olympic Message

Olympic Panorama
Physical Education Index
Soviet Sports Review
Sport Bulletin/International Union of Students
Sportsearch (Index)
Women's Sports and Fitness

RECREATIONAL SPORTS

National Intramural Recreational Sports Association
NIRSA Journal
NIRSA Proceedings
Rec Sports Report

GENERAL

AAHPERD: Abstracts of Research Papers
Alliance Update
Completed Research in Health, Physical Education, Recreation and Dance
Computers in Human Behavior
Ergonomics
ERIC on CD-ROM
Futurist
IAHPERD Journal
Journal of Physical Education, Recreation & Dance
Medline on CD-ROM
Sociology of Leisure Sports Abstracts
Sports, Parks and Recreation Law Reporter
SPRE Annual on Education
The Kappan

RECREATION AND PARK ADMINISTRATION

Gerontology

Aging Research and Training News
Gerontologist
Journal of Aging and Health
Journal of Applied Gerontology
Journal of Gerontology
Research on Aging
Topics in Geriatric Rehabilitation

Leisure Studies

Journal of Leisurability
Journal of Leisure Research

Leisure Information Quarterly
Leisure Sciences
Leisure Studies
Loisir & Societe (Society and Leisure)
Newsletter, World Recreation and Leisure Association
Play and Culture
World Leisure and Recreation Association Journal

Outdoor/Environmental Education

Camping Magazine
Conservation Directory
Journal of Experiential Education
Journal of Outdoor Education
North American Environment
Outdoor Communicator
Outdoor Indiana
Restoration and Management Notes

Recreation and Parks

Design
Grist
Journal of Park and Recreation Administration
Marking Recreation Classes
Park Maintenance & Grounds Management
Park Practice Program Index
Parks and Recreation
Recreation and Park Education Curriculum Catalog
Recreation and Parks Law Reporter
Trends

Therapeutic Recreation

Programming Trends in Therapeutic Recreation
Therapeutic Recreation Journal

Travel and Tourism

Annals of Tourism Research
Cornell Hotel and Restaurant Administration Quarterly
Journal of Travel Research
Leisure, Recreation and Tourism Abstracts
Travel and Tourism Executive Report

Unclassified

Employee Services Management
Recreation Canada

Recreation Executive Report
Recreation Research Review
Recreation, Sports & Leisure

Computer Retrieval Systems. The advent of the computer has added great speed to the process of searching the literature. Many reference sources are now available in the compact disk (CD-ROM) format, enabling complex searches to be performed that would be much more difficult, if not impossible, using paper resources. These reference sources include indexes to journals and other publications (sometimes accompanied by the full text of the cited article), abstracts, statistical reference materials, and compilations of useful data (Indiana University Libraries Bulletin 1992).

Learning to do a **computer search** for literature is a relatively simple matter. Select the key words, or descriptors, from the title or problem statement of the proposed research topic. These key words are entered into the computer, which uses them to search for related information from the databases upon which a particular system operates. The computer generates a printout with the titles of studies, reports, reviews, conference papers and proceedings, and other sources. Some systems include a brief abstract describing the content of each reference. These printouts may be available in a few hours; others may take up to a week to appear. There are many computer retrieval systems. Those that seem to be of the most value to HHP are the following:

Education Resources Information Center (ERIC). This very useful database contains thousands of materials from education and allied areas, including HHP, and houses information from the printed indexes, *Current Index to Journals in Education and Resources in Education,* from 1966 to the present.

Sport Discus. This is the primary research database for sport, physical fitness, sport science, and recreation. It is international in scope and covers such subjects as exercise physiology, leisure, biomechanics, coaching, sport psychology, and motor development.

Medline. This is an enlarged version of the printed *Index Medicus.* It contains references to journal articles in all areas of clinical and research medicine, including biomedical research, health administration, nursing, veterinary science, and others. It is of potential use for students and researchers in fields ranging from anatomy to zoology.

PsycLIT. This database provides users with information about articles in psychology-related journals. PsycLIT is a computerized version of *Psychological Abstracts.* It includes articles published from 1974 to the present.

Direct Access to Reference Information (DATRIX). This database focuses on the dissertation references at University Microfilms, Ann Arbor, Michigan and is the computerized version of the printed *Dissertation Abstracts.*

Conducting a Computer Search.   Many computer reference sources are now available in most college and university libraries that subscribe to a variety of databases. The reference sources include indexes to journals and other publications, and may include the full text of the cited article, statistical reference materials, and compiled data. Most libraries utilize an on-line computerized information system that permits the researcher to gain immediate access to the needed literary citations.

Graduate students typically learn to do a computer search in one of two ways—through a seminar-type course sponsored by the institution or a HHP department, or with the help of a librarian highly skilled in using the various methods for retrieving information. In conducting the search, the following five steps must be performed:

1. **State the research problem precisely.** If the statement is too long and rather general, there will be too many descriptors. This will result in an unwieldy list of references, most of which will be irrelevant to the research problem. A brief and specific statement like "physical fitness status related to improved self-esteem of elementary school students" is definitive and gives focus to the search. The descriptors (physical fitness, self-esteem, and elementary school students) will generate a limited number of references, yet provide the needed information.

2. **Determine what database(s) should be used.** In this step the researcher decides which database will provide the most information about articles pertinent to the research problem. One database, ERIC, may be sufficient; but, in some cases, two or more will need to be searched. In the physical fitness/self-esteem example, it may be necessary to use ERIC, Sport Discus, and PsycLIT to generate a helpful list of literature sources.

3. **Determine what descriptors will be used.** Select key words (descriptors) from the research problem statement. This tells the computer what direction the search should take. From the problem of fitness related to self-esteem, logical descriptors are physical fitness, self-esteem, and elementary school students. The computer will also want to know the year the search is to commence. If 1990 is selected, the resultant list of references will contain only those articles published from that year on. It is also necessary to indicate in what language the literature source should be written. This is usually English.

4. **Do the search.** The selected database software is inserted into the computer and the descriptors are entered. After a few minutes it is prudent to ask the computer to print out a small list of references to be sure the descriptors are providing helpful sources. If relevant sources are being obtained, the computer can then be asked to provide a printout containing all available references.

5. **Study the list of references.** The researcher obtains and reads, in detail, the articles that are determined to be the most pertinent to the research problem. Frequently, the bibliographic information in these articles provides other helpful sources and may prompt another computer investigation of the literature.

Writing Chapter 3: Data Collection Procedures

The third chapter of a research proposal deals with the procedures for collecting data. Alternative titles for chapter 3 are "Procedures," "Methodology," "Experimental Procedures," and "Survey Procedures." All proposals must include a detailed and appropriate **data collection plan** for attacking the problem. Earlier in the proposal (primarily in chapter 1), the rationale for selecting certain methods, techniques, and procedures was presented as background information for the problem. However, a more detailed rationale is needed in chapter 3. The entire research proposal is like a contract between the student researcher and a faculty committee. If the research study is conducted as proposed, the committee cannot seriously complain about the procedures at the final defense meeting. Hence, the procedures section becomes extremely critical. The soundness of the study will depend on the appropriateness of the planned attack on the research problem. The reader will analyze this section closely and relate the methods, techniques, and procedures to the relative quality of the research data to be obtained.

The procedures chapter is considered to be the "cookbook" or "recipe" portion of the proposal or research report. Its presentation requires much attention to detail as the researcher illuminates the reader about where the data come from (sources), how the data were gathered (collection methods), and how the data were analyzed (treatment). This step-by-step set of instructions for conducting the investigation should be so detailed that if another researcher wanted to replicate the study, there would be no trouble in doing so. The reader should not have to make any assumptions about what or how something was done in the research situation.

The first paragraph of chapter 3 always includes a restatement of the problem (stated exactly as it was in chapter 1) and indicates how the chapter is organized. In general, most studies will include these items:

1. A discussion of the subjects used in the study and the sampling techniques used for obtaining them
2. A discussion of the tests, instruments, or measures that were used to collect the data
3. A discussion of the design of the study within which the data were collected
4. A discussion of the administrative procedures used to collect the data
5. A discussion on how the data were treated or analyzed

Depending on the nature of the study and the whims of the researcher, these five items are translated into a variety of section topics. Following are some of the topic headings typically found in this section:

1. Arrangements for Conducting the Study
2. Selection of Subjects

3. Selection of the Test Instrument(s)

4. Development of the Test Instrument(s)

5. Procedures for Testing and Gathering Data

6. Instrumentation

7. Jury of Experts

8. Selection of the Jury

9. Design of the Study

10. Training Program

11. Preliminary Investigation

12. Pilot Study

13. Administration of Tests

14. Treatment of Data

Whatever choices the researcher makes for organizing this chapter, all topic headings will be centered and underlined. Only the first letter of the important words are capitalized. Variations will depend upon the style manual used at the various institutions. Typically, the Treatment of Data section does not have to be unduly long, but must clearly indicate the researcher's plan for treating, or statistically analyzing, the data. The following questions can be used as a guide to providing the appropriate information in chapter 3:

1. Was the population clearly specified?

2. Is the design appropriate to the problem?

3. Were the sampling procedures clearly specified and the total sample adequate?

4. If a control group was involved, was it selected from the same population?

5. Were the various treatments (including control) assigned at random?

6. Were appropriate statistical treatment procedures selected and the level of significance selected in advance?

7. Were the reliability and validity of the data-gathering instruments and procedures established and reported?

8. Were the treatments and/or methods of the collection of data described so clearly and completely that an independent investigator could replicate the study?

9. Are the characteristics of the subjects clearly representative of the population?

10. Were extraneous sources of error either held constant or randomized among subjects of all groups?

Examples 2.1 through 2.5 demonstrate the various content areas of chapter 3 of a research report.

EXAMPLE 2.1
An Opening Paragraph
(Luedke 1980)

> The problem of the study was to determine if an instructional emphasis on increasing the range of motion in the overhand throwing pattern of second and fourth graders results in improved throwing form and velocity. The conduct of the study included the following procedural steps: (1) arrangements for conducting the study, (2) selection of subjects, (3) development of instructional approaches, (4) selection of measurement tools, and (5) treatment of data.

EXAMPLE 2.2
Selection of Subjects
(Wasilak 1988)

> All of the subjects were volunteers and were enrolled at Indiana University during the course of the investigation. The main criteria for participation included: (a) all subjects were males, (b) all subjects had previous high school competitive swimming experience with no collegiate experience (age-group swimming experience was considered to be an adequate substitute), (c) all subjects had a minimum of four years of competitive swimming background, (d) each subject had a personal best 50-yard time of 28.6 seconds or better, and (e) subjects had a minimum and maximum age of 18 and 22 years, respectively.
>
> These criteria were selected to give the study an external validity factor that would allow the results to be generalized to a population of high school, or age-group swimmers. This population was selected because it has the largest number of participants relative to the total swimming population, and has the greatest potential for improvement. The number of years of competitive swimming experience, and the emphasis on minimum and maximum age added power to the analysis of the experimental data by reducing the intersubject variance in scores.

EXAMPLE 2.3
Selection of the Test
Instruments
(Umansky 1976)

Three measures were selected to assess perceptual-motor abilities of the subjects: the Perceptual Quotient score of the Frostig Developmental Test of Visual Perception (1966), and the developmental age scores from the Perceptual-Motor and Pre-Academic scales of the Assessment-Programming Guide for Infants and Preschoolers (Umansky 1973).

The Frostig DTVP is a five-part test that purportedly assesses five distinct perceptual functions: eye-hand coordination, figure-ground perception, form constancy, position in space, and spatial relationships. Standardized on a group of 2,116 children between three and nine years of age, the sample largely consisted of middle-class white children from southern California. The test yields raw scores from each subtest which are converted to scale scores, and then summed up to produce a Perceptual Quotient. Test-retest reliability for the Perceptual Quotient for first and second graders tested two weeks apart was .80, as reported by the authors of the test. Subtest scale score test-retest correlations were reported from .42 to .80 by the authors (Frostig 1964).

The Assessment-Programming Guide for Infants and Preschoolers (Umansky 1973) is an eclectic tool compiled by the investigator a number of years ago as a developmental evaluation instrument for young children. A list of sources upon which the Guide was based is presented in Appendix F. It is a criterion-referenced checklist composed of six developmental subscales. The Perceptual-Motor and Pre-Academic subscales were used for this investigation (Appendix B). The subscales consist of specific skills divided into appropriate age groups. A perceptual-motor age score and pre-academic age score were derived for the subscales.

EXAMPLE 2.4
Design of the Study
(Miller 1990)

The subjects were randomly assigned to either the Adventure Group or the Control Group. Both groups completed the pretest one day prior to the involvement of the Adventure Group in the Challenge Education Program. The Adventure Group participated in a six-hour sequentially based Challenge Education program conducted at Bradford Woods. The Control Group participated in the normal daily activities of the psychiatric hospital, which included various therapies, counseling sessions, and unstructured leisure time. One day following the Adventure Group's Challenge Education experience, both groups were administered the posttest.

Both the pretest and the posttest were administered by the investigator, in the company of a recreation therapist familiar to the subjects. The investigator also facilitates the Challenge Education experience for the Adventure Group. The Adventure Group was also accompanied by the same recreation therapist that assisted with the test administration. Additionally, a nurse accompanied the Adventure Group to monitor the health of the subjects, many of whom were under various forms of medication.

EXAMPLE 2.5
Treatment of Data
(Van Oteghen 1973)

To test the hypothesis that there is no significant increase in vertical jump performance, a t-test for correlated samples, repeated measures design, was conducted utilizing pretraining and posttraining scores. The sum of a subject's three trials was used as his criterion score for a testing period. The null hypothesis was tested using a one-tailed test at the .05 level of significance.

The sum of the trials was also used as the criterion score for strength test measurements for testing the hypothesis of no significant increase in leg strength development. Again, pretraining performance was compared to posttraining performance by utilizing a t-test for correlated samples repeated measures design. The null hypothesis was tested using a one-tailed test and a .05 level of significance.

The difference between the pretraining and posttraining scores on each variable was determined for each subject. The relationship between muscle strength and vertical jump performance was tested by correlating the change in scores on the vertical jump with the change in scores on the cable-tensiometer using a Pearson product-moment r. The correlation coefficient which was obtained was tested for significance at the .05 level.

Summary

The research problem is perceived, developed, and attacked in several steps as discussed in detail in this chapter. Crucial to the success of any research endeavor is a complete review of the related literature determined to be pertinent to the problem being investigated. This chapter has provided a compiled list of many sources of information useful to HHP research efforts. The usual procedures for conducting a research project have been delineated in some detail and have been illustrated using several examples extracted from successful graduate student research projects.

Formative Evaluation of Objectives

Objective 1   Select a suitable research problem.

1. Select an area of HHP of major interest to you, and list five problems requiring investigation that have been published in the literature in the past year.

Objective 2   Know the various sources of research problems.

1. Identify the more effective ways to find an appropriate research problem.

Objective 3   Understand the various steps of the research process.

1. Select a research problem and:
   a) state the problem.
   b) indicate the purpose of the study.
   c) delimit the study.

Objective 4   Systematically review literature relevant to the selected problem.

1. List the various sources of literature you would use in developing a background for the proposed problem in Objective 3.

Objective 5   Plan and develop an attack on the problem.

1. State the hypothesis for the problem, indicating how it will be tested, what data need to be obtained, and what data-gathering instruments or procedures will be employed.

3

Selected Elements of the Research Process

Key Words

Attribute variables
Comparison
Continuous variables
Data collecting instrument
Dependent variables
Description
Descriptive approach
Discrete variables
Evaluation
Experimental approach

Extraneous variables
Halo effect
Historical approach
Hypotheses
Independent variables
Internal consistency reliability
Intervening variables
Measurement techniques
Objectivity
Observation techniques

Qualitative variables
Quantitative variables
Questioning techniques
Reliability
Stability reliability
Time frame of interest
Validity
Variable

Objectives

The process of developing a research project involves many interrelated elements. In the previous chapter various research procedures were discussed. The nature of problems, the importance of the problem, and the related literature were also addressed. Now it is important to consider the details of a research plan which include the research approach, methodological steps, instruments to be used, and how the instruments will be administered to capture the needed data obtained on the selected variables for study.

After reading chapter 3, you should be able to:

1. Suggest one study that could be researched under each of the three research approaches.
2. Group the significance of the terms used to describe (define) a variable.
3. Know when it is appropriate to apply the different methods of collecting data.
4. Know the various techniques available for each data-collection method.
5. State the criteria for selecting the appropriate research instrument.

The Research Approach

Once a definitive research problem has been identified and a thorough search of the literature has been accomplished, the researcher decides on the best approach to take in systematically collecting the data, or information, needed to solve the research problem. The three generally accepted approaches available to the researcher are historical, descriptive, and experimental. The choice of approach will be made on the basis of an interaction between two dimensions: (1) the time frame in which the researcher is interested and (2) the intent the researcher has for the research (Fox 1969).

Time Frame of Interest

If the **time frame of interest** is the past, the **historical approach** is used. In this case the researcher will be concerned with conditions and occurrences that have already taken place that may provide insight and understanding of a current situation or condition. For example, the National Athletic Training Association (NATA) is a highly respected and formidable force in the area of sports medicine today. It is largely responsible for the rise of athletic training to a position of high stature. Why did this happen and how did it occur? What were the events and who were the key people in the growth and expansion of the concept of athletic training? What past successes and failures have enabled those who practice the art of athletic training today to benefit from the experiences of those who labored years before? An in-depth study of the history of the NATA might help us to better understand and appreciate the present situation in which athletic training finds itself.

If the research interest lies in the present, then the **descriptive approach** is used. Here the researcher studies a current issue or problem of current status, one which now exists, and seeks to describe in detail that which is presently happening. Exploratory, fact-finding, attitude-opinion, and evaluation studies provide up-to-date information concerning prevailing conditions, practices, interests, thoughts, and judgments. The question "To what extent has the computer influenced the administrative, management, and programming practices of recreation and park districts in the United States?" might be answered by an extensive descriptive study.

Researchers are often interested in comparing several methods, techniques, substances, or programs to determine the best one to use in the future; this calls for the **experimental approach.** The concepts associated with skeletal muscular contractions can be learned in a variety of ways. This phenomenon could be studied by looking at three different teaching strategies (for example, the lecture approach, the programmed approach, and the classical textbook, abstract, and journal approach) to compare their effectiveness in promoting the learning of the concepts of skeletal muscular contraction among undergraduate exercise science majors. The objective of such an experiment is the desire to generalize which teaching strategy should be applied on a larger scale in the future.

Intent

The second important dimension when considering the research approach is that of the researcher's intention for the study when it is finished. There are three aspects to the intent dimension: **description, comparison,** and **evaluation** (Fox 1969). One might conduct a study of the salaries of women in sport management positions with the intention simply to describe the salary situation as it presently exists, nothing more. On the other hand, the researcher may collect data on both men and women who occupy sport management positions with the intention of comparing the salary condition of the two groups. Comparative judgments are made about the similarities and differences between salaries. The researcher could also intend to evaluate by judging the quality, good or bad, of the salary situation as indicated by the information obtained. In making such judgments, a criterion should be established. In the sport management situation, for example, if one group's salary was 25 percent higher than the other for the same type of work, the prevailing salary discrepancy could be judged as bad. The figure of 25 percent serves as the criterion measure, or standard, for making the evaluation judgment.

The interaction between the time frame of interest and intent dimensions then guides the selection of the research approach and results in a variety of different kinds of studies. Table 3.1, developed by Fox (1969, 46), provides an excellent illustration of this interaction.

Hypotheses

A detailed discussion of the role of hypotheses in the research process was presented in chapter 1; a few additional comments here are warranted because of the intimacy of the relationships between the research problem, the approach used to attack it, and the need to predict what outcome might result from the study. Once the research topic has been reduced to a specific and manageable problem and the type of approach needed to study it has been determined, the researcher then states the **hypotheses** or, more specifically, the predicted outcome(s) of the study. Any research project can include hypotheses, and they are mandatory for experimental and comparative descriptive studies. Occasionally, historical studies and simple descriptive studies may not have them. This will be true when the researcher has no basis for believing a particular outcome will result from the historical or descriptive research. A hypothesis is warranted whenever a reasonable expectation of outcome is anticipated. Usually the hypothesis will indicate an expected relationship between the variables (e.g., characteristics, traits, attributes) being investigated. The researcher may have several objectives for a research project, and a hypothesis should be stated for each one. The usual intent of a research study is to predict a series of outcomes based on the objectives of the research problem. Once the research data have been collected, the hypotheses are tested to determine their truth or falsity.

DIMENSION 2 **INTENT OF RESEARCH**	**DIMENSION 1** **TIME IN WHICH INTEREST LIES**		
	Past: Historical	**Present: Descriptive**	**Future: Experimental**
Description	Simple Historical	Simple Survey Case Study	Single Group Experiment
Comparison	Parallel Historical	Multiple Group Survey Correlational Survey	Multiple Group Experiment
Evaluation	Historical and Criterion Measure	Single Group or Multiple Group Survey and Criterion Measure	

TABLE 3.1 Interaction of Time and Intent Dimensions to Consider in Selecting the Research Approach

Note: From *The Research Process in Education,* by David J. Fox, 1969, Holt, Rinehart & Winston, Inc. Reprinted with permission.

The Concept of Variables

The focus of the researcher's effort is always on the **variable.** A variable is a characteristic, trait, or attribute of a person or thing that can be classified or measured. Eye color, sex, and church preference are classifications. Skill, self-concept, strength, heart rate, and intelligence are variables that can be measured. The term *variable* indicates that a characteristic can have more than one value. There are two genders in the human race, male and female, and if both appear in a research project then gender becomes a variable. When a characteristic does not vary, it is referred to as a *constant.* In a study of the manual dexterity of second-year nursing students, the characteristic, second-year, is a constant; it does not vary among the student nurses.

Quantitative and Qualitative Variables

Variables can be **qualitative** if they are classified by some characteristic, attribute, or property. People are categorized as to sex (male, female), eye color (blue, brown, green), church preference (Catholic, Protestant, Jew), and political affiliation (Republican, Democrat, Independent). Qualitative variables are usually unmeasurable. Variables are called **quantitative** if they can be measured in a numerical sense. The heights of five starters on a basketball team may be 5'10", 6'2", 6'5", 6'8", and 7', respectively. Their ages range from 18 years, 6 months to 22 years, 3 months. There are two basic types of quantitative variables, **discrete** and **continuous.**

Discrete Variables. This type of variable is usually thought of as being a whole unit, one that cannot be fractionated or divided up into smaller parts. Examples of discrete variables are football scores, and the number of correct answers on a test. Football scores are recorded in whole numbers (e.g., 3, 7, 10, 14) and cannot be divided into smaller parts like 7.5 or 11.75.

Continuous Variables.　This type of variable can be divided into fractional amounts in large or small degrees. Strength and endurance scores, track and field times, height, weight, and girth measures are considered to be continuous variables. Time in a 100-yard dash is sometimes to the nearest tenth of a second, but in high level competition it could be one one-hundredth of a second. The height of a person could be measured in feet and inches, in half-inches, or in quarter-inches, depending on the precision desired and the ability to measure height accurately.

Independent and Dependent Variables

In research, particularly experimental research, the terms **independent** and **dependent** variable are used. The experimental approach involves observing what effect different amounts of one variable (independent) have on a second variable (dependent). The independent variable is referred to as the *experimental treatment.* The researcher controls what treatment will be selected and how much will be applied. The treatment, or independent, variable will not change during the research or as a result of the research. The dependent variable is the one that is expected to change as a result of the treatment. It is not under the control of the researcher. Said another way, the independent variable is expected to *cause* some *effect* on the dependent variable. The changed, or affected, variable is referred to as dependent because its value depends on the value of the independent variable (Tuckman 1978). Actually, the independent variable forms or defines groups; the dependent variable generates data.

Following are some examples of independent and dependent variables:

1. *Hypothesis:* Fourth-grade orienteering students score higher on a map reading skills test when taught by the direct practice method than by the conventional practice method.

   Independent variable: Type of practice method (qualitative; discrete).

   Dependent variable: Score on the map reading skills test (quantitative; continuous).

2. *Hypothesis:* There is a difference in the self-confidence of female adults who adhere to exercise programs and the female adults who drop out of exercise programs.

   Independent variable: Exercise program adherence or nonadherence (qualitative; discrete).

   Dependent variable: Self-confidence score (quantitative, continuous).

3. *Hypothesis:* An HIV (AIDS) education unit taught in a health class is more effective in changing ninth- and tenth-grade students' HIV-related attitude and knowledge than when the HIV (AIDS) education unit is taught in a biology class.

   Independent variable: Curriculum unit (qualitative, discrete).

   Dependent variable: HIV-related attitude and knowledge score (quantitative, continuous).

4. *Hypothesis:* A vegetarian diet produces stronger and healthier people than does a nonvegetarian diet.

   Independent variable: Type of diet (qualitative; discrete).

   Dependent variable: Strength and health score (quantitative; continuous).

5. *Hypothesis:* Physically disabled children who participate in a two-week stress challenge course develop a higher self-concept than do physically disabled children who participate in a conventional two-week camping experience.

   Independent variable: Type of program (qualitative; discrete).

   Dependent variable: Self-concept score (quantitative; continuous).

Some of the most common independent variables in HHP are exercise, diet, medicines, drugs, motivation, programs, procedures, methods, techniques, sex, social class, attitude, and intelligence. Some of the most common dependent variables are performance, fitness, learning, health, knowledge, achievement, and behavior.

Variables can be used as independent in one study and dependent in another study. In one experiment, the effect of losing (independent) on motivation (dependent) might be studied, while in a second study the effect of motivation (independent) on physical performance (dependent) might be the research objective.

Error-Producing Variables

While the independent variable is to serve as a stimulus to evoke a response from the dependent variable, there are usually other factors (variables) that could possibly cause the same response. To conclude that one type of physical fitness training is more effective than another, the researcher must be able to show that all factors that conceivably could have caused the difference were the same for the subjects in each group, and that only the two types of training were permitted to vary. Perhaps the most frequent and most serious mistake made by the beginning researcher is the failure to either control or account for the variables that could contribute error in an experiment. These variables are commonly known as **intervening, extraneous,** and **attribute variables.**

Intervening Variables.   Also referred to in the literature as *modifying variables,* this type of variable intervenes between the independent and dependent variables, that is, between the cause and the effect. The desired effect of the independent variable is blocked.

For example, a coach may experiment with a different method of practice in an attempt to get the players to perform better. If no improvement takes place, the coach may think that some other factor or variable, which cannot be controlled, is influencing the relationship. An intervening variable, such as fear, anxiety, motivation, learning, fatigue, drive, or frustration, is probably operating to prevent the independent variable (practice method) from having the desired effect. These variables are difficult to control because they cannot be measured or manipulated. They are assumed to affect the research situation, but cannot be used as an explanation for the results. For the most part, the impetus for an intervening variable to become operative comes from within an individual.

Extraneous Variables. Also referred to as *confounding variables,* extraneous variables come from outside of the research situation and interact with the dependent variable to make the independent variable extremely effective or ineffective. They correlate with, and affect, the dependent variable in a way that can invalidate the research conclusions.

A researcher studied the effect of motivation (independent) on the physical fitness test scores (dependent) of sixth-grade boys and girls. The two motivating conditions were team competition and level of aspiration (goal-seeking). The subsequent finding that the group receiving level of aspiration was significantly better than the group receiving team competition was surprising because the literature contains much information proclaiming the superiority of team competition as a motivational vehicle.

A detailed check into the composition of the groups participating under each condition revealed that they came from classes that were divided into high, average, and low academic achievement. The sixth graders who performed under the level of aspiration condition came from the high achievement category and possessed a mean intelligence quotient (IQ) of 132. The literature clearly indicates that, in general, the more intelligent an individual is, the easier it is to get that person "up," or motivated. So, IQ, a variable that was not included in the design of the study, served as an extraneous variable that slipped into the research situation, interacting with the dependent variable (fitness score) to make the condition (level of aspiration) look extremely potent and effective. The researcher presumed that IQ, while not a planned part of the study, was a substantive contributor to its results. That variable, like all extraneous variables, was not manipulated by the researcher.

There are many extraneous variables that can have a significant influence on the dependent variable and can invalidate research conclusions. Other such extraneous variables besides IQ, and depending on the specific type of experiment, are sex, socioeconomic level, teacher competence, personality, enthusiasm, physical health, emotional health, age, and the use of volunteers and intact groups as subjects. If a researcher conducted a study on the effect of three different methods of teaching outdoor education concepts on elementary students' appreciation and knowledge of the outdoors, with one recreation instructor assigned to each method, instructor personality could play an important role in the ultimate results of the study. Extraneous variables are difficult, if not impossible, to control. A good design of a study can help to play down the effect of such variables. In the teacher personality example above, the outdoor education teachers could be screened for personality characteristics; the one with the best personality would then be assigned to teach the outdoor education concepts under the three different methods. Teacher personality would be the same for all three groups of subjects and so, in this case, the teacher personality variable would be controlled, or neutralized. However, it is assumed here that the teacher is equally effective in teaching with each method.

Attribute Variables.   Also referred to as *organismic variables,* attribute variables are characteristics that are already determined and are unchangeable. Examples are sex, race, and age. If more than one sex, race, or age are included in an experiment, the researcher cannot manipulate the particular variable because it is already determined and already varies within the group to be studied. Thus, attribute variables either define the groups to be compared or must be equally distributed across all treatment groups.

The question of whether nine-year-old girls show greater tumbling achievement than nine-year-old boys presents a situation in which gender is an attribute or organismic variable that forms the groups being studied. The methods of teaching the tumbling stunts will be the same for each group. Because sex, or gender, has already been determined, it will not be manipulated by the researcher; it is already varying in the study. A second example: Each of three groups is taught by a different method. To equate the groups, twenty-five boys and twenty-five girls are placed into each group. If a researcher does not want race, sex, or age to vary in an experiment, then it should be designed to include only the desired gender, race, or age group.

Control of Variables

Many experiments in the fields of HHP are conducted outside of the laboratory using human subjects, and many variables surround the research situation which could alter the results in some substantive way. It becomes imperative that the researcher maintain as much control over these variables as possible so as to prevent or reduce their effect. At the same time it must be recognized that not every variable that could make a difference can be controlled. Following are some of the procedures that are frequently used in an attempt to control extraneous variables:

Random Selection of Subjects.   When the laws of probability are permitted to operate in the selection of two or more experimental groups of subjects, systematic bias is removed and the effect of extraneous variables is minimized. It is assumed that the groups are equal and that if any difference does exist, it is due to probability or chance factors (Best 1981).

Equating or Matching by Some Criterion.   The subjects are paired on some characteristic, such as age, sex, height, weight, ability, or the results of preliminary testing. After the pairing is completed, the members of each pair are assigned at random, one to the experimental group and the other to the control group. If a researcher wanted to use 15-, 16-, and 17-year-old boys and girls to study methods of developing flexibility, it might be desirable to match on age and gender so that the experimental and control groups would be comparable on those two variables at the beginning of the experiment. Each boy and girl in each age group would be randomly assigned to either the experimental or control group.

By matching subjects it is also possible to reduce the variation among them because of chance differences in initial ability. It is a relatively simple matter to match on one or two characteristics. As the number of traits to match increases, so does the difficulty in obtaining accurate pairs.

Excluding the Variable. A researcher may simply choose to not include a particular trait in the study. Only one age group, or one gender, may be studied so as to remove them as variables. This is sometimes referred to as controlling for the variable. If a researcher's presence might change subjects' behavior, such distraction could be a source of bias in an experimental study. To obviate such bias, a one-way mirror could be used to shield the researcher from subject view (Best 1981).

Data Collecting Methods and Techniques

The research process includes three different methods of procuring information, or data. They are **observation, measurement,** and **questioning.** The researcher may watch subjects perform and record relevant data about them; he/she may test subjects or apply a device to subjects to measure certain qualities; or he/she may ask subjects questions to obtain information that cannot be obtained in any other way.

Fox (1969) has delineated the relationship of each method to each of the three research approaches in the following way:

1. *Observation*

   a. This is accomplished retroactively in the historical approach by viewing museum artifacts, antiques, photographs, and printed material.
   b. In the descriptive approach, a subject can be watched in the research situation, although it is recognized that subjects' awareness of being observed could change their response and generate invalid data.
   c. Observations in the experimental approach represent only a small portion of some future reality.

2. *Measurement*

   a. With the descriptive and experimental approaches, the researcher can directly measure a large variety of variables (e.g., attitude, knowledge, physiological qualities, and personality traits).
   b. Direct measurement of cognitive and affective variables is not possible in the historical approach. The personality of a deceased famous person can only be determined by inference from other existing data. Physical remains (e.g., buildings, bridges, toys) can be measured directly.

3. *Questioning*

    a. In the historical approach, questioning has to be retroactive and must rely on the memory of those who were there at the time.

    b. The descriptive and experimental approaches permit questioning about past, present, and future activities.

A variety of techniques may be used to carry out each of these methods. Depending on the scope and objectives of the study, a research project may incorporate several methods and techniques.

Observation Techniques (Fox 1969)

Direct. Under the direct technique, subjects are cognizant of being observed and they usually know why they are being observed. *Example:* Subjects being observed exercising in different training programs using the biokinetics swim bench to determine front crawl stroke hand-speed patterns.

In many cases, it is important to the study that subjects be directly observed, but unaware they are being watched. *Example:* Any situation in which the researcher's presence might cause a change in the subjects that would inhibit them from reacting in a natural way. Elementary school subjects, knowing they were going to be observed performing a series of motor skill activities, might get nervous and feel intimidated, or become hyperactive in their behavior and not perform to their true ability. In this case, direct observation could be accomplished through the use of a one-way mirror so the youngsters would not know they were being watched.

Indirect. Indirect observation is a technique accomplished when a group of subjects are filmed or videotaped. *Example:* A group of physically disabled youngsters serve as subjects in a stress-challenge study. They are told that their performances will be videotaped first, and then they and the researchers will view the tapes to evaluate the various rope techniques, both good and bad. Observing the tape is indirect observation. The alternative to letting the subjects know they are being filmed is to use a hidden camera. In this situation, the term "bugging" could be applied. Whether or not the subjects know they are being taped, the direct observer is always the camera.

Participant. In the technique of participant observation, the observer participates in the research situation. *Example:* The researcher is studying the attitude and behavior of teenage campers and participates in a two-week camp experience, engaging in all activities, attending meetings, and so forth. The subjects know that the researcher is an outside person who wants to learn as much as possible about teenage camper attitude and behavior. In certain instances it may be appropriate that the outside participant's motives be unknown to the subjects, as in the case of an undercover agent infiltrating an agency, association, or group to collect data on its activities.

Measurement Techniques (Fox 1969; Best 1981)

Almost anything can be measured, evaluated and assessed. Physical measures, cognitive measures, and affective measures are presented here. Although these three categories of measures by no means exhaust the possibilities, they are ones frequently applied in research.

Physical Measures. The very nature of the activity inherent in the fields of HHP provides countless opportunities for physical measure. Physical education and the various areas of exercise science have produced a large variety of tests to measure physiological fitness, motor behavior and learning skills, sport skills, anthropometric attributes, and biomechanics variables. Following are a few examples of the thousands of research topics dealing with physical parameters.

1. Factor pattern differences in tests of physical fitness, motor ability, and skill in selected populations of men and women.
2. Static and dynamic strength tests for both sexes in various age groups.
3. Kinematic and kinetic factors involved in pole vaulting.
4. Task complexity effects on reaction times, movement time, and accuracy.
5. Sodium-calcium ratios and central body temperature in men during exercise and recovery.
6. Physiological responses to training.
7. Physical activity related to health promotion programs.
8. Distance, interval, and mixed methods of training for competitive swimming.

Cognitive Measures. The HHP literature is profuse with tests developed to measure the acquisition of health, fitness, sport, and leisure knowledge. Typical examples include:

1. Oral and dental knowledge assessment of college students.
2. Health knowledge test for elementary school teachers.
3. A gymnastics apparatus knowledge test for college men in professional physical education.
4. Knowledge and practice of women physical education teachers regarding negligence.
5. Developing environmental knowledge and perceptivity in early childhood.
6. Cognitive learning related to motor performance in school orientation.
7. Leisure-time knowledge, activities, and interests of older Americans.

Affective Measures. Factors such as opinion, attitude, personality, motivation, interest, personal problems, mood, drive, and frustration are more difficult to capture quantitatively than are physical and cognitive variables. They are less objective and more unstable. Many change rapidly over time. The instruments developed to measure these variables have typically been paper-and-pencil self-report scales. If people are unwilling to provide information accurately and objectively, however, these measures may lack considerable validity. Nonetheless, there has been a considerable amount of research done on affective variables in the fields of HHP and better instruments have been developed to measure them. A few typical examples include the following:

1. Self-motivation and adherence to therapeutic exercise.
2. Leisure attitudes of selected populations.
3. Leisure-time activities and interests of aged residents.
4. Personality related to the sport of gymnastics.
5. Personality traits of highly skilled basketball and softball women athletes.
6. Attributes of nationally rated intercollegiate basketball officials.
7. Personality and attitude of selected traffic violators and nonviolators.
8. Attitudes toward and beliefs about AIDS among adolescents.
9. Self-concept related to lifestyle attitude and practice.

The measurement method utilizes more techniques than either of the other two methods.

Measurement Techniques in HHP.   Following are descriptions of some of the techniques frequently used in HHP studies.

Inventory.   With the use of this technique the researcher tries to measure interests, attitudes, personality, personal problems, likes and dislikes, and motivation. Most inventories are self-report instruments on which subjects "take stock" of themselves. Questions are asked or statements are presented to which the research subjects are asked to respond. The total amount of information obtained represents a measure of the variable being studied. Following is an excerpt of ten statements from the Athletic Motivation Inventory developed by Tutko, Lyon, and Ogilvie in 1969.[1] The original instrument contained some two hundred statements. "The purpose of the test is to provide information that can be personally beneficial to an athlete" (Tutko, Lyon, and Ogilvie 1969, 1).

I believe that the coach is not always right . . . . (A) sometimes (B) seldom (C) never
I seldom stay after practice to work out . . . . (A) true (B) somewhat true (C) false
I lose my temper during competition . . . . (A) sometimes (B) seldom (C) never
There is absolutely no excuse for being
late for practice . . . . (A) true (B) uncertain (C) false

---

1. From *Athletic Motivation Inventory,* by T. A. Tutko, L. P. Lyon, and B. C. Ogilvie, 1969, Institute for the Study of Athletic Motivation at California State University, San Jose. Reprinted with permission.

There are usually one or two fellow athletes
with whom I can't get along . . . . (A) sometimes (B) seldom (C) never
When the team loses it is usually my fault . . . . (A) true (B) uncertain (C) false
I would like the responsibility of being a coach . . . . (A) very true (B) true (C) uncertain
I perform poorly after being harshly criticized . . . . (A) sometimes (B) seldom (C) never
Most athletes do not wear uniforms . . . . (A) true (B) seldom (C) never
When new athletes join the team or competition I . . . (A) try to show them up (B) hope they
compete well (C) try to help them

Sociometric Technique.   This technique attempts to measure social relationships
by having members of a group indicate individual preferences based on some social
criterion (Fox 1969). Though not applied on as large a scale in HHP as are some of the
other measurement techniques, there appears to be a growing body of HHP research
using sociometric analysis. The following question was used in a cohesiveness/
cooperation study of a football team: "What member of the team would you select,
regardless of the amount of playing time, as being the most inspirational leader on
the team?" In a larger sense, it is well known that the sociometric technique is used
when youngsters "choose up" sides for a playground or gymnasium game and when
members of a team select a captain or most valuable player.

Projective Technique.   The use of this technique attempts to measure the real feelings, values, attitudes, and needs of an individual (Best 1981). A stimulus is present
and the subject's response is recorded in some psychological dynamic (Fox 1969).
The Rorschach Inkblot Test is a good example of the projective technique. A spot of
ink is dropped on a piece of paper, which is then folded. When the paper is unfolded,
the subject is asked to indicate what the resultant inked figure looks like. Associations and perceptions can also be stimulated in subjects by having them view car-
toons and pictures or having them listen to particular words. A scream or the use of a
whistle often evokes a variety of responses which tend to reveal the "real person."

Scaling Techniques.   Scales are devices used by researchers to attempt to quantify responses to various concepts and variables. Subjects are asked to rate or order
concepts along a continuum (Fox 1969). Scales can be used to obtain data on almost
any topic, object, or subject. Attitude, opinion, behavior, performance, and perception are frequently measured by some scaling device. Evaluation and assessment are
often accomplished through the use of various scaling techniques. Several of the
most popular types of scales are presented below.

Rating Scales. These scales can be numerical or verbal. Observers rate each
item by selecting a verbal or numerical point on the scale that corresponds to
their impression of the item. Table 3.2 represents a verbal rating scale administered to selected sport managers. The researcher's objective is to obtain data
indicating how the importance of various administrative concepts relates to the
successful operation of a sport management program.

TABLE 3.2 Administrative Concept Scale

CONCEPTS	NO IMPORTANCE	MODERATE IMPORTANCE	GREATEST IMPORTANCE
Staff Discipline			
Communication			
Personnel Management			
Objectives and Goals			
Public Relations			
Computer Use			
Organizational Design			
Etc.			

TABLE 3.3 Drug Evaluation Scale

DRUG	NOT HARMFUL	SLIGHTLY HARMFUL	VERY HARMFUL	DISASTROUS
Cocaine				
Crack				
Hashish				
Amphetamines				
Steroids				
Morphine				
Marijuana				
Etc.				

Table 3.3 is another verbal scale that was used to determine the relative harmfulness of various controlled substances as perceived by undergraduate college students.

In both of these examples the subjects are presented a continuum of responses and will place an *X* in the preferred response column.

TABLE 3.4 Administrative Evaluation Scale	
CHARACTERISTICS	**RESPONSE**
Honest and sincere	1 2 3 4 5 6 7 8 9 10
Treats faculty with respect	1 2 3 4 5 6 7 8 9 10
Motivates faculty in job performance	1 2 3 4 5 6 7 8 9 10
A good communicator; knowledgeable in all HHP programs	1 2 3 4 5 6 7 8 9 10
Empathic toward faculty concerns	1 2 3 4 5 6 7 8 9 10
Maintains equity in faculty salaries	1 2 3 4 5 6 7 8 9 10
Knowledgeable about research, etc.	1 2 3 4 5 6 7 8 9 10

Tables 3.4 and 3.5 are examples of numerical scales. Table 3.4 lists characteristics of an administrator that are to be rated on a scale of 1 to 10, with 1 indicating a low rating and 10 a high rating. Table 3.5 contains a scale to be used by graduate students who have completed a program in HHP.

Tables 3.2–3.5 are modified versions of the original instruments, edited here to conserve space. Because human beings do the rating, the rating scale technique is susceptible to the **halo effect.** A person may like or be favorably disposed to the person being rated, and so they may give that individual high ratings on all of the scale items. On the other hand, a dislike for the person being rated could result in low ratings on all of the scale items. Thus, the validity of the rating scale is questioned.

Semantic Differential Scale. This is a technique that has been shown to be quite versatile and valid in measuring attitude and concepts. Research subjects are asked to make judgments on a concept based on the use of bipolar adjectives. They will respond by placing an X in one of the spaces between each pair of adjectives. Table 3.6 contains an example of the semantic differential where the concept to be rated is "athlete." The responses made by the subjects are converted to numerical values and are treated statistically. For a more detailed discussion of this technique, students are referred to Isaac and Michael (1976), Fox (1969), Best (1981), and Kerlinger (1973).

Rank Order Scales. In this technique the research subjects are asked to rank, usually in order of importance, a series of concepts or items. Table 3.7 presents an example of the rank order technique. The twelve qualities of conduct are to be ranked from 1 to 12, with 1 representing the most important quality and 12 representing the least important.

TABLE 3.5 HHP Graduate Program Evaluation Scale

PROGRAM FACTORS	INADEQUATE; UNSATISFACTORY	ADEQUATE; SATISFACTORY	OUTSTANDING; EXCELLENT
My overall degree program	1 2 3	4 5 6	7 8 9
The courses in my major	1 2 3	4 5 6	7 8 9
The courses in my inside minor	1 2 3	4 5 6	7 8 9
The courses in my outside minor	1 2 3	4 5 6	7 8 9
Academic advisement in the School of HHP	1 2 3	4 5 6	7 8 9
Career counseling in the School of HHP	1 2 3	4 5 6	7 8 9
HHP facilities (in terms of my program)	1 2 3	4 5 6	7 8 9
Library resources for my area of interest	1 2 3	4 5 6	7 8 9
Academic competence of HHP faculty in my area	1 2 3	4 5 6	7 8 9
Teaching effectiveness of HHP faculty	1 2 3	4 5 6	7 8 9
Methods of evaluating student achievement in HHP	1 2 3	4 5 6	7 8 9
My experience as grad assistant	1 2 3	4 5 6	7 8 9

Etc.

TABLE 3.6 Athlete

Kind	____ ____ ____ ____ ____ ____ ____	Cruel
Bad	____ ____ ____ ____ ____ ____ ____	Good
Beautiful	____ ____ ____ ____ ____ ____ ____	Ugly
Slow	____ ____ ____ ____ ____ ____ ____	Fast
Strong	____ ____ ____ ____ ____ ____ ____	Weak
Masculine	____ ____ ____ ____ ____ ____ ____	Feminine
Soft	____ ____ ____ ____ ____ ____ ____	Hard
Active	____ ____ ____ ____ ____ ____ ____	Passive
Wise	____ ____ ____ ____ ____ ____ ____	Foolish
Unsociable	____ ____ ____ ____ ____ ____ ____	Sociable
Graceful	____ ____ ____ ____ ____ ____ ____	Awkward
Small	____ ____ ____ ____ ____ ____ ____	Large

TABLE 3.7 Qualities of Conduct Scale	
Ambitious (hard working, aspiring)	_____
Broad-minded (open-minded)	_____
Capable (competent, effective)	_____
Courageous (standing up for your beliefs)	_____
Helpful (working for the welfare of others)	_____
Honest (creditable, commendable)	_____
Imaginative (daring, creative)	_____
Logical (rational, consistent)	_____
Obedient (dutiful, respectful)	_____
Responsible (dependable, reliable)	_____
Loving (affectionate, tender)	_____
Independent (self-reliant, self-sufficient)	_____

TABLE 3.8 Value Preferences Scale
VALUES
A prosperous life (wealth)   An exciting life (stimulating, active)
Salvation (saved, eternal life)   Human equality
Human freedoms   A world at peace
Family well-being   Social recognition
National unity   Inner harmony
Etc.

Paired-Comparison Scale. Several pairs of concepts are presented in this technique. The research subjects are asked to indicate which item of each pair is the most important by underlining or circling it. Table 3.8 is a paired-comparison example containing several pairs of value preferences. The subjects are to select which value of each pair is the most important or most preferred.

Likert Scale. This is a five-point scale designed to measure a particular attitude, belief, or judgment about something. The continuum of response runs

TABLE 3.9 Team Cohesiveness

I feel that being on this team gave me a chance to make friends.	SA A U D SD
Most of my teammates believe in things I do not.	SA A U D SD
The coach always tried to do the right thing for the team.	SA A U D SD
I didn't like the members of this team very much.	SA A U D SD
The coach of the team didn't really know basketball; she just got stuck with the job.	SA A U D SD
Most of my teammates were out for their own glory and cared little about the team.	SA A U D SD
I believe playing on this team was boring.	SA A U D SD
The other players on the team were willing to help me if I needed it.	SA A U D SD
I feel that I have some really good friends among my teammates.	SA A U D SD
I cared less what the coach or other players said; I believe in making my own decisions.	SA A U D SD

from strongly agree (SA), agree (A), undecided (U), disagree (D), to strongly disagree (SD). The subjects responding to a Likert-type attitude scale are asked to circle the letter of the point on the scale that represents their opinion, belief, or judgment. An example of the Likert technique appears in table 3.9. The ten items that appear in the table were excerpted from a longer instrument developed by Cotter in 1978 for use in her basketball team cohesiveness study.

If the Likert intervals (SA to SD) are presumed to be equal, a scoring system can be applied to allow the responses to be treated statistically. If the Likert intervals are not presumed to be equal, a sum of the scores is not legitimate and the scale may have to be analyzed item by item. Whether the items all measure the same or different concepts influences, to some degree, whether the sum of the item scores is correct. A discussion of this issue is beyond the scope of this book.

Questioning Techniques (Fox 1969; Best 1981)

Structured Questionnaire. Also called the *closed-ended questionnaire,* this instrument includes questions that can be answered with yes-no or true-false responses, or by selecting an answer from a list of suggested (multiple-choice) responses. The short, quick response format takes less time and effort from the subjects and tends to be fairly objective. The analysis of the data from this type of instrument is relatively simple.

The following examples from an instrument used in a breast cancer study, illustrate the structured type of item:

How would you classify your knowledge of breast cancer, in particular the various methods of detection?

_____ quite knowledgeable

_____ some knowledge

_____ very little knowledge

How have you learned about breast cancer? Check any appropriate answer.

_____ media (newspaper, T.V., radio, etc.)

_____ literature from cancer societies

_____ physician

_____ health course

_____ experience (yourself or family member)

Unstructured Questionnaire.   Also called the *open-ended* or *essay questionnaire,* this technique provides an either-or or multiple-response opportunity. Subjects answer freely in their own words. While this format tends to produce answers of greater depth, it takes considerable time on the part of the subject. It requires a highly motivated person to wade through several open-ended questions. This type of questionnaire is frequently used in exploratory situations, those in which the researcher is trying to gain information that may or may not exist in any particular manner, shape, or form. The unstructured item is not always easily tabulated, analyzed, and interpreted. The following examples from a study of applicants for an Assistant Athletic Director/Athlete Advisor position illustrate the open-ended item:

> How would you motivate a student-athlete who has demonstrated excellent athletic ability, but is very apathetic toward academic responsibilities?

> A coach has an athlete who appears marginally ineligible. He asks your assistance in getting this athlete eligible. What would be your response to the coach, the athlete, and any faculty involved?

Checklist.   A relatively simple instrument, the checklist is basically a very highly structured questionnaire. Usually, a long "laundry list" of items is presented and the subject is asked to check those that apply. Sometimes a yes or no response is necessary. A "things to do today" list or a "things to do to get ready for vacation" list are examples of the typical checklist. The example shown on page 87 appeared in a park and recreation interest survey.

Structured Interview.   In large measure, the structured interview technique is an oral questionnaire. The researcher poses the questions, along with the expected answers, much the same as the structured questionnaire. The questions are asked in order and no repetition is permitted. Questions other than those listed are not permitted. The questions and expected answers are written down in what is called an *interview guide.* Distinct advantages of this technique are that (1) less bias prevails because whatever is in the guide is asked without alteration, and (2) the interviewer may not need to know a lot about the research dynamics being studied. Public opinion

Your Leisure Interest

Do Now	Would Like to Do		Do Now	Would Like to Do
_____	_____	Little League baseball	_____	_____	Football
_____	_____	Slow-pitch softball	_____	_____	Square dancing
_____	_____	Community Center activities	_____	_____	Tennis
_____	_____	Attending sporting events (outdoors)	_____	_____	Swimming
_____	_____	Attending sporting events (indoors)	_____	_____	Boating
_____	_____	Fishing	_____	_____	Hiking
_____	_____	Family camping	_____	_____	Golf
_____	_____	Picnicking	_____	_____	Playground
_____	_____	Shuffleboard	_____	_____	Ice skating
_____	_____	Basketball	_____	_____	Horseshoes
		List below any others	_____	_____	Rifle range
_____	_____	_____			
_____	_____	_____			
_____	_____	_____			

pollsters frequently use this technique by employing high school or college students as interviewers. They are screened for good interpersonal skills (essential to this technique) and then are sent out to do the interviewing without a lot of information concerning the variables and dynamics involved.

Unstructured Interview.   This technique utilizes no set format of questions and expected answers. The open-ended question format applies in that the person being interviewed is supposed to answer in his or her own words and provide all relevant information in as long or brief a period of time as is necessary. The interviewer may have a guide with possible questions, but is not tied to it. Usually the interviewer will know the areas of the research dynamics being studied and will select questions from each one. There usually is no set order for the questions and they can be repeated to ensure complete understanding on the part of the interviewee. No question implies a particular response. One major advantage of this technique is that follow-up or clarifying questions can be asked to preclude misconceptions on the part of both the interviewer and interviewee. Good interpersonal skills on the part of the interviewers are important, but perhaps even more so is the amount of knowledge they have concerning the research dynamics to which the questions are tied. Limited knowledge about the research topic provides a dull, boring, and weak data collection interview. The more informed interviewers are, the better decisions or judgments they will make as the interview process unfolds.

Delphi Technique. This technique is unique in the questioning method employed and is used to get consensus from a defined group of individuals on a specific issue. Individuals respond to the questions to produce the collective input of the group. Then each one reviews his or her position based upon group trends and revises that position as warranted. Ultimately a group consensus is obtained. In brief, the Delphi technique is accomplished through the following procedures (Rubinson and Neutens 1987):

1. Identify group members whose consensus opinions are sought.
2. Use initial questionnaire to solicit concerns, goals, and problems for which consensus is sought (e.g., knowledge competencies needed for a particular field of study, such as adapted physical education teachers, health educators, outdoor educators, and exercise specialists).
3. Arrange initial results in a second questionnaire. Each member ranks these items in terms of importance.
4. Present a third questionnaire containing an initial trend toward consensus on each item along with each member's initial response. Again each item is rated.
5. Administer a fourth questionnaire. It contains the data obtained from the third questionnaire and each member's most recent ranking. A consensus trend appears as the items are ranked for the third and final time.
6. Present the data from the fourth questionnaire, representing the final group consensus.

The Delphi technique has not been extensively used in HHP, but has wide application potential for topics in those fields. Van Clief (1982) used the technique to identify the books that have significantly influenced or are likely in the future to influence the development of physical education in the public schools. The data for determining consensus were obtained from a group of active fellows and fellows emeriti of the American Academy of Physical Education. Only books written by American physical educators were considered.

Criteria for Selecting Methods and Techniques

The selection of the data gathering method(s) and technique(s) is always based on the type of data needed to solve the research problem, and many underlying factors must be considered. The researcher will examine the needs of the research in terms of (1) the demands on the subjects, (2) the cost in terms of energy, money, and time that will be required, and (3) personal ability to handle selected methods and techniques, including data analysis procedures. The process usually follows this sequence: Problem → Data → Approach → Method(s) → Technique(s). The problem of the research implies a certain kind of data obtained by the appropriate historical, descriptive, or experimental approach. The approach will incorporate one or more methods that will be carried out by one or more techniques. Once a technique has been determined, the instrument needed to collect the data must be determined.

The Data-Collecting Instruments

A **data-collecting instrument** is any paper-and-pencil test or measure, mechanical or electronic equipment measure, or physical performance test used to collect information (data) on the variable under study. The choice of the instrument to be used in the data-collection process involves deciding whether it will be one that has already been developed and will be used as it is, one that already exists but will be revised, or one that will be new and needs to be developed. This decision will be based on the needs of the research and what instruments are available.

Whenever data are to be collected, the researcher must keep in mind that, at a minimum, there are three characteristics or attributes data must have to be worth using in a research study: (1) objectivity, (2) reliability, and (3) validity. **Objectivity,** sometimes called *rater reliability,* exists if the same or similar scores would occur no matter who collected the scores. In other words, the data is not unique to the person who collects it. Objectivity of the data is estimated by having two or more people independently score the performance of each individual in a group as he/she performs. Then the scores of the two or more persons are compared as to agreement. An example for physical performance data is each of two people independently scoring each person in a group as to the number of sit-ups correctly executed as he/she takes a sit-up test. For paper-and-pencil test data each of two people would independently score the test. If there is good agreement, objectivity is demonstrated. An intraclass correlation coefficient is calculated to determine the degree of agreement. The maximum value of the coefficient is 1.0 and a value of at least .70 and maybe .80 would be required to indicate acceptable objectivity. (More on objectivity, including the calculation of an intraclass correlation coefficient, can be found in Baumgartner and Jackson [1995].) Once the objectivity of the data from a test or measuring procedure has been demonstrated, it is not necessary to estimate objectivity each time the test or measuring procedure is used. If the scores from a test or measuring procedure are found to be sufficiently objective, then reliability of the data is estimated.

Reliability is declared for the data to the extent that a test or measuring procedure yields the same or basically the same score for a person on two or more occasions. This could mean administering the test or measuring procedure two or more times within a day, called **internal consistency reliability.** This is commonly done with nonfatiguing physical performance tests and measures. An example is administering three trials, one after another, of a sit-and-reach test to measure flexibility. For knowledge tests or any paper-and-pencil test where a total score is obtained, internal consistency reliability is calculated as an indicator of consistency of performance across test items. If the test or measuring procedure is administered once on each of two or more days, **stability reliability** can be determined. An example is administering a one-minute sit-up test on one day and then administering the test again three days later.

Reliability for physical performance measures is estimated by calculating an intraclass correlation coefficient. Reliability for paper-and-pencil tests is commonly estimated by calculating the Cronbach alpha coefficient or a Kuder-Richardson coefficient. The maximum reliability no matter the technique used is 1.0 and usually a value of at least .70 is required to demonstrate acceptable reliability. Once the reliability of the data from a test or measuring procedure has been demonstrated it is not necessary to establish reliability each time the test or measuring procedure is used. However, reliability can be influenced by factors such as the gender, or age of the group tested, so be sure any previously reported reliability coefficients apply to the group used in your research. (More on reliability and the calculation of reliability coefficients can be found in measurement books like Baumgartner and Jackson [1995].) If the scores from a test or measuring procedure are found to be sufficiently reliable, then the data has the potential to be valid.

Validity is declared for the data from a test or measuring procedure if the data really are measures of what they purport to measure. For example, if you administered a paper-and-pencil test that was supposed to measure fitness knowledge and it really did measure fitness knowledge because the more fitness knowledge a person had the higher the person scored on the test, the test would be declared valid. Validity is not all or none, there are degrees of validity. Thus, to the extent that things other than fitness knowledge influenced scores on the test, the test would not be perfectly valid. Validity can be estimated using a variety of techniques too numerous to discuss here. Consult any measurement book for information on estimating validity. The important thing for a researcher to remember is that before data is collected make sure the test or data collection procedure will yield valid data. As a consumer of research, when reading a research report, check that the tests or measuring procedures are known and/or documented to yield valid data.

Selecting the Instrument

Selecting a research instrument for any project is usually the result of a thorough search of the literature. The researcher who wants to study the effect of improved physical fitness on the self-concept of adolescents will probably find that several tests measuring self-concept are available. Once it is determined that such an instrument exists, the next step is to assess its acceptability. We have just finished a discussion of certain characteristics of data. Some of these same criteria apply to the selection of the data instrument as well. Whether the instrument is *reliable* (measures consistently each time the test is used) and whether it is *valid* (measures what it is supposed to measure) are important characteristics in this part of the process also. In this case, an acceptable instrument would be shown to, in fact, measure self-concept the same way on repeated applications of the test. Quite frequently an instrument will be selected on the basis of its reliability and validity as reported by the researchers who have used it in earlier studies. If measures of reliability and validity are not provided, various statistical techniques can be applied to quantitatively determine the reliability and validity of the instrument. Measurement books such as Baumgartner and Jackson (1995) discuss these techniques. Sometimes, researchers must make their own determination of the reliability and validity of the instrument they plan to use. Part of determining validity is analyzing whether or not the instrument is *appropriate.* Can the subjects meet the demands of the instrument, or is it too hard or too easy for the ability of the subjects? The vocabulary of an instrument may be appropriate for one age group and not for another. The same can be true for certain physical performance tests. If the instrument is not appropriate, it will not produce valid data. Without reliability and validity the data are of no use in answering the research question.

In selecting an instrument, a researcher will also consider other criteria. The instrument should be *objective,* that is, provide a score for each subject that is "independent of the personal judgment of the scorer" (Best 1981, 200).

How easy the test is to administer, how much it costs in time and money, and how easy it is to score are other factors the researcher must consider. Ideally, the researcher selects the most reliable and valid instrument. In reality, however, if that test is difficult, time consuming, costly, and very demanding of the subjects, the researcher may instead select a test that is a little less reliable and valid, but is less difficult to handle, has a shorter administrative time span, is less costly, and is less demanding of the subjects.

Revising the Instrument

Quite often a researcher locates an instrument that is not quite acceptable for the intended research situation, in which case the instrument must be revised. Permission should be obtained before revising a paper-and-pencil instrument originally developed by someone else. Permission is sometimes needed to revise a physical performance instrument. When a standardized instrument is used or revised, permission from the instrument's publisher is required.

Changes in an original instrument may take many forms, but are usually done to better fit a particular group of subjects. Self-concept has been studied with different age groups, sexes, and races, and various kinds of disabled populations. Obviously, one instrument designed to measure self-concept cannot be used with all subject groups. The same can be said concerning the study of countless numbers of variables of a research interest. Collins, in her 1989 study of body figure perceptions and preferences among male and female preadolescent children, used a pictorial instrument modified from the original instrument developed in 1983 that used adult male and female subjects (Stunkard, Sorenson, and Schulsinger 1983). Basically, the major change was that Collins revised the Stunkard adult figure drawings to reflect the figures of children. She also used seven figures for each gender, while Stunkard used nine figures. Revising an instrument may change its reliability and validity, and new measures must be determined for the revised instrument if changes are major enough. Note: Reliability and validity of an instrument are often specific to the age and gender of the subjects.

Instrument Development

It is difficult and time-consuming to develop an instrument and this procedure is avoided by both veteran and beginning researchers whenever possible. The task is undertaken only when it becomes obvious that no paper-and-pencil, electronic or mechanical, or physical performance test or instrument exists to generate the needed research data.

The starting point for instrument development is, once again, the literature. All of the dynamics in the prospective research problem must be thoroughly understood, and what instruments are available to use as models must be known before the instrument development begins. Suppose a researcher is interested in determining the motivation of high school students for participating or not participating in athletics. The dynamics involved in this phenomenon are many and are comprised of intellectual, sociological, psychological, and physiological components. A complete review of the literature must include related research and conceptual articles reflecting each of those components and what instruments others have used. The knowledge accrued from such a review will provide the basis for determining the content of the instrument. That is, what type of questions and/or statements will contribute most in the attempt to measure the motivation students have, or do not have, for athletic involvement during high school?

The usual next step is to select the questions or statements and produce a tentative instrument. In writing these research items, the researcher is careful to see that each item will provide a reasonable estimate of each relevant component of the athletic motivation problem. If, for example, one of the components related to athletic participation is the student's perception of whether or not athletic participation will enhance the chances of being successful in life, then the researcher's task is to develop questions or statements that will provide an estimate of this component. If the students perceive that athletic participation will enhance their self-concept and status among their peers, the instrument should contain items that will provide a measurable estimate of these components.

Once the tentative instrument has been developed, it is then submitted to a jury of experts or committee of authorities. The researcher invites selected individuals, who are considered to have expertise in the problem area, to review the content of the instrument. These can be people who have taught, researched, or written in the problem area. The task of the jury members is to review the research questions or statements and revise them as needed. Which items should be rewritten? Should any of the items be deleted? Should items be added? Which items are most significant to the essence of the problem? Which are relatively insignificant? Needless to say, the work of the jury suggests careful attention to the elimination of instrument flaws. Submitting the proposed instrument to a jury of experts is an excellent way to increase the content validity of the measured tool.

Based on the reaction of the jury, the researcher revises the instrument. In most instances the instrument is submitted to the jury only once, but it may be necessary to repeat the procedure two or more times.

The next step in the instrument development process is the pilot study or preliminary investigation. The intended instrument is administered to subjects selected from the same population of subjects who will make up the actual research sample, but who are *not* sample subjects. The pilot study serves as a trial run of the instrument to see if it is in further need of revision. The objectives of a pilot study are (1) to determine whether or not the subjects understand the content items in the instrument, (2) to determine whether the instrument will provide the needed data, (3) to familiarize the researcher and any assistants with instrument administration procedures, (4) to obtain a set of data for trying out the proposed data treatment techniques, and (5) to first determine the reliability and then the validity of the instrument, since reliability is part of validity.

The researcher will further revise the instrument if the pilot shows change to be necessary. A pilot study may not always be needed, but is a valuable research tool. The knowledge that the instrument is sufficient and will yield reliable and valid data, that the planned instrument administration procedure is appropriate, and that the planned attack on the research problem is the proper approach are the typical payoffs for conducting a pilot study. The actual research study may not be completely without problems, but the prospects of severe trouble occurring are diminished by having performed a test run. With a successful pilot study, the researcher can claim a finalized instrument.

This discussion of instrument development happens to be for a paper-and-pencil instrument. However, the same basic steps occur in the process of developing any instrument. These steps are: (1) survey the literature, (2) develop a tentative instrument, (3) reflect upon and revise the instrument, (4) obtain opinions of experts concerning the instrument, (5) revise the instrument, (6) conduct a pilot study, (7) revise the instrument, and (8) use the instrument.

Summary

The research problem can be attacked using a variety of approaches. The researcher's intent, time frame of interest, and hypothetical deductions all play a role in the selection of the research approach. The term *variable* has a variety of connotations and is illustrated in detail. Data-collecting methods and techniques are determined by the selected research approach, and the research instrumentation relates to the techniques necessary to produce the needed data. Several examples have been provided to aid the student in applying these concepts.

Formative Evaluation of Objectives

Objective 1 Suggest one study that could be researched under each of the three research approaches.

1. Write out a statement of the problem for the following:
   a) a descriptive study.
   b) a historical study.
   c) an experimental study.

Objective 2 Group the significance of the terms used to describe (define) a variable.

1. Why can an independent variable be a dependent variable in another study? How does randomization help control for extraneous variables?

Objective 3 Know when it is appropriate to apply the different methods of collecting data.

1. Name a topic that could be an appropriate study for
   a) observation.
   b) measurement.
   c) questioning.

Objective 4 Know the various techniques available for each data-collection method.

1. What technique would be most useful in studying the health knowledge of junior high school students?

Objective 5 State the criteria for selecting the appropriate research instrument.

1. What are the three most important characteristics one should look for in selecting a research instrument?

Selection of Research Subjects: Sampling Procedures

Key Words

Cluster sampling
Deliberate sampling
Fishbowl technique
Multistage sampling
Nonprobability samples

Population
Representative sample
Sample
Sample size
Sampling unit

Simple random sample
Stratification
Systematic sampling
Table of random numbers

Objectives

While all steps in the research process are important, perhaps the most crucial to a successful investigation are the procedures used in the selection of research subjects. The researcher first identifies and defines the population from which information (data) is to be obtained. To study an entire population is difficult, if not impossible, hence the use of the sampling process. Considerations are given to such factors as sample size, how representative of the population is the sample, and the appropriateness of the subjects to the various research methods and tests. The process of sampling permits the researcher to generalize the results from a study of the sample to the larger population.

After reading chapter 4, you should be able to:

1. Identify and define a population from which a sample of subjects is to be selected.
2. Know how to determine the characteristics of the sample.
3. Know the various methods of selecting samples.
4. Know the various factors that are used to determine sample size.

The needs of the research problem usually dictate the type of subjects who will be selected for study. Quite frequently the research statement of the problem indicates what subjects will be used in an experimental or descriptive study. It is imperative that the researcher have a carefully thought out plan for selecting the subjects.

The subjects must be appropriate to the methods, techniques, and instrumentation that will be incorporated in the study so they can produce the needed research data. Subjects should be selected who may be expected to be available throughout the duration of the study. The number should be large enough to (1) assure reliability of the research results and (2) permit a reasonable number of subjects to be available to produce data in the event of subject mortality (e.g., injury, absence, dropout for any reason).

Obviously, the realities of the research setting and the practical needs of the researcher often affect the subject selection process. A physical fitness study involving children may need a large number of subjects, whereas a mountain climbing study on the relationship of nutrition and altitude may involve few subjects. A researcher studying selected mechanical aspects in pole vaulting cannot select just any pole vaulter. The objective would be to study the high-level, world-class vaulters; the availability of these athletes is very likely to present a problem for the researcher.

Population and Sample

A major reason for doing research is to obtain information that can be applied to a large group of people. This could be accomplished by studying an entire group, but this is often impractical, if not impossible, to do. For example, if we really wanted to know the physical fitness status of all preadolescent children in the United States, we could fitness test all members of that group. However, this would not be possible in terms of the number of researchers needed to collect the data, the tremendous amount of money needed to finance the project, and the exorbitant time and energy the project would require.

The term **population** refers to an entire group or aggregate of people or things having one or more common characteristics. Often, a population is the focus of a research effort. Populations can be made up of people, animals, objects, organisms, deeds, attributes, materials, or any other defined element. We can talk about a population of fitness test scores, attitude scores, and personality traits. All dance majors in the nation's colleges and universities, all coaches of all sports, all female high school coaches, all physical education teachers, all elementary school physical education teachers, all college Division I football coaches can be referred to as populations. The point is, researchers can define or describe a population any way they choose to suit the particular research purpose. The variable of diet, for example, could be studied among older Americans, athletes, the mentally disabled, various socioeconomic groups, teenagers, and many other populations.

Populations, then, can be defined in numerous ways. They can be infinitely large, as would be the case of the fitness test of all high school students; or they can be finite, such as the number of dance majors reporting to class at a particular college on a particular day. As a general practice, populations are considered finite.

Because it is often difficult, if not impossible, to study an entire population, the process of sampling is undertaken. A **sample** of the members of a population is selected as a representative subgroup of that larger population. The researcher observes and analyzes certain characteristics of the sample of subjects to get an idea of what those characteristics may be like in the entire population. From the information (data) obtained from the sample, the researcher then makes inferences about the population. The mean blood pressure score for a sample of cardiac rehabilitation subjects is used to approximate the mean blood pressure for the entire population of such subjects enrolled in a rehabilitation program. These statistics, then, are used to estimate the population information (parameters).

The crucial element in the selection of a sample from a population, is that the sample be **representative,** or similar to, the population on the characteristics being investigated. If a researcher uses just a few exercise science majors to find out what may be true about a very large number of exercise science majors, then it is imperative that the researcher be as certain as possible that the small group of majors is representative of the total population of exercise science majors. Said another way, whatever variable is being studied in a particular population (e.g., attitude, behavior, self-concept, fitness, motivation, etc.) should be present in the sample drawn from that population. A researcher may want to make generalizations about the performance of all the children who take the AAHPERD fitness tests each year. To be representative, and for the generalizations to be valid, the sample would have to include subjects from all geographic areas of the country, all races, and all socioeconomic levels. A more usual practice is for a researcher to study a sample from a smaller population. There is a population of children in Indiana who take the AAHPERD fitness tests each year. In studying the fitness characteristics of a sample of these children, the researcher could infer, or generalize, the results back to the Indiana population. It would be invalid to generalize to the entire United States population because children from the other forty-nine states were not included in the sample. It is important to remember that the results of data from any sample may not be generalized outside the population from which the sample is drawn.

Sample Selection Methods

Random Selection

Randomization in sample selection is important to the quality of the research for three reasons: first, to help ensure the representativeness of the sample to the population about which generalizations will be made; second, to show that the researcher was unbiased as to which members of the population were selected in the study; and third, to equalize characteristics among groups in research studies requiring multiple groups, such as experimental and control groups. If each group is representative of the population, the groups will start the research equal in ability, and the research will be safe from criticism about which subjects were selected and placed in each group. Random sampling is a basic requirement underlying inferential statistical tools.

The **simple random sample** is obtained when every individual or element in the population has an equal chance of being selected, and the selection of one person does not interfere with the selection chances of any other person. This process is considered to be bias-free because no factor is present that can affect selection. The random process leaves subject selection entirely to chance.

Two different procedures may be used to obtain a random sample—the fishbowl technique and the table of random numbers. In the **fishbowl technique,** the names of every individual in a population are written on a piece of paper. The pieces of paper are placed in a bowl, box, hat, or similar container, and the number of pieces of paper corresponding to the number of subjects needed in the sample is drawn from the container one at a time. If we wanted to study 50 exercise science majors from a population of 300 majors, the names of the 300 majors would be placed in a container. One name at a time would be drawn until the sample of 50 was filled. This technique can be accomplished in two ways. If, after each name is selected, it is put back into the container, the method is called *random selection with replacement.* If the names are not replaced after they are drawn, this is called *random selection without replacement.* There is not a lot of difference between the two procedures when the population size is large, but without-replacement selection does not strictly meet the definition of the random selection process. In the exercise science sample, each major has 1 chance in 300 of being selected. If the names are not replaced, the probability of each subsequent name being drawn increases (1 in 299, 1 in 298, etc.). So, if a name is selected, it should be replaced. If it comes up again, put it back into the container. Each person in the population then continues to have the same opportunity, or percentage of chance, to be selected. Despite the statistical correctness of random selection with replacement, most researchers sample without replacement since an individual cannot be used as a subject again after once being selected.

Perhaps a more convenient and sophisticated way to select a random sample, or to assign subjects to groups, is to use a **table of random numbers.** Many tables have been produced in which the numbers (0–9) are randomly ordered. Table 4.1 is an excerpt from a table of random numbers. Such tables are relatively simple to use. Just assign a number to the members of the population, then use the columns of numbers to pinpoint those members of the population who will be selected for the sample.

To illustrate, let's say we wanted to study 20 of the 40 national governing bodies (NGBs) that manage the Olympic sport competition under the aegis of the United States Olympic Committee (USOC). We are interested in NGB management, marketing, and fund raising practices. To select our sample of 20 NGBs, the members of the entire population would be numbered from 1 to 40. Since we have 40 NGBs, and 40 contains two digits, we need to refer to two adjacent columns. With eyes closed, we place a pencil on the table of numbers to select the column in which to begin the selection process. We will also use the column to the left of the pencil-determined column. Columns 9 and 10 turn out to be the starting place for our selection of the sample. Column 9 shows a 5, and column 10 shows a 3 for a double digit of 53. Since we have no NGBs numbered above 40, we skip 53. The next double digit is 26, so the NGB numbered 26 is selected. Following down in the two columns, we see the NGBs 21, 9, 33, 4, 18, and 10 are also selected. To complete the process, we will utilize every next pair of columns until 20 NGBs are selected. Any number higher than

TABLE 4.1 Excerpt from a Table of Random Numbers

COLUMNS

1	2	3	4	5	6	7	8	9	10	11	12	13	14	15
0	2	5	6	0	1	5	9	5	3	7	6	4	3	5
0	0	2	1	0	4	5	5	2	6	2	3	7	9	4
6	3	6	0	6	4	9	3	2	1	5	0	5	3	4
8	0	9	5	1	0	0	4	0	9	3	8	2	7	0
2	0	1	5	1	2	3	3	8	2	0	1	6	2	5
1	1	8	0	5	0	5	4	3	3	8	0	8	2	7
0	8	4	2	2	6	8	9	5	1	6	4	5	0	9
3	1	0	6	0	1	0	8	0	4	5	7	1	8	2
5	4	1	7	8	4	5	6	1	8	9	9	3	3	7
1	0	5	1	8	2	1	6	1	0	8	4	8	7	6

40 is skipped. If a number comes up that has already been selected, it too is by-passed. Hence, we end up with a randomly selected sample of 20 NGBs and can be more than reasonably confident that the selection process was free from bias.

Stratified Random Sampling

A big help in ensuring a representative sample is the process of **stratification.** This is accomplished by dividing the population into various strata or subgroups, based on some characteristic that is important to control in the study, and then selecting a set number of subjects from each strata. The following is an example from a study of how the high schools in a given state financed the girls' athletic programs.

SCHOOL SIZE		
Small	**Medium**	**Large**
0–499 pupils	500–999 pupils	>1000 pupils

Let's say that there are 400 schools in the state and the researcher decides to study financing practices in a sample of 100, or 25 percent of the schools, and randomly selects that number. There are many more small schools than medium or large ones, and just by luck the selected sample contains 80 small schools, 15 medium schools, and 5 large schools. The resultant data on how schools in the state finance the girls' athletic programs would probably be unbalanced in favor of the small schools and would not fairly represent the financing strategies of the medium and large schools. This problem could be overcome, or at least minimized, by first stratifying the schools by size, then taking a proportional random number of schools from each strata. In our example above, there are 250 small schools, 125 medium schools, and 25 large schools. Since the researcher wants a final sample of 100 schools (25%), proportional random sampling (taking .25 × the number of schools in each strata) would yield, roughly, 63 small schools, 31 medium schools, and 6 large schools. Thus, the final sample of 100 schools is quite representative of the total population of 400 schools. Any generalizations or inferences from the sample to the population stand a better chance of being more valid than if proportional stratified random sampling had not been used. While not completely foolproof, this procedure is considered to be the most efficient way to achieve representativeness.

Computer programs can also be used to select random samples. The program called Random Numbers, developed by Stephen Silverman of the University of Texas, has been quite successful. It is described in some detail in Thomas and Nelson (1985). Many packages of statistical computer programs include a random numbers program.

Systematic Sampling

When some "system" is applied to the selection of subjects we call the procedure **systematic sampling.** In a study of a population of public and private schools in a large city, the researcher would prepare an alphabetized list of the schools and then select every fifth school on the list. In another situation a researcher may decide to select every one hundredth person listed in a telephone directory. In another case a researcher may simply be situated at a particular location and stop every fifteenth person and ask each a brief set of research questions.

While systematic selection approximates a random sample, it does not strictly satisfy the definition of random sampling and, hence, is not entirely bias-free. In the schools example above, if every fifth school is selected, schools 4 and 6 have no "equal chance" of being selected. Many parochial schools, because their names begin with *S* and are listed near the bottom of the roster of schools, will not be selected. Subtle biases may also be present in systematic sampling. For example, in a study to determine homeowner attitude toward services provided by the city, this sampling technique might result in obtaining corner lot homeowners who may have different feelings and impressions than those who live in the middle of the block.

Systematic sampling is quick, efficient, and saves time and energy. This is particularly true when populations exist on a definitive list or roster. In this instance, it is simply convenient to select every *n*th element of the population, as opposed to using a table of random numbers, which usually is a little more time consuming. It can also be argued that systematic sampling provides for a broad sampling across a population and, therefore, results in a more accurate sample (Sax 1979).

Cluster Sampling

Also referred to as area sampling, **cluster sampling** is particularly appropriate in situations where the researcher cannot obtain a list of the members of a population and has little knowledge of their characteristics, and where the population is scattered over a wide geographic area. Let's say that a researcher wants to survey 1,000 teachers out of a population of 4,600 teachers in forty-six schools in a large city. Each school has 100 teachers. If the teachers are selected at random, the subjects in the sample would be scattered all over the city. The expense in time, money, and energy in designing a plan to get to the 1,000 teachers is enormous. The researcher decides to randomly select twelve schools from the population of schools, and then survey the 100 teachers in each school. Allowing for certain factors of subject mortality, the researcher reasonably expects approximately 1,000 teachers to respond. The teachers in each school represent a cluster.

In general, cluster sampling is more practical and less costly. However, it is not entirely bias-free. In this example, the schools are selected at random, not the teachers who are of interest in the investigation. The schools are the **sampling unit** because they are what was sampled. Conclusions and inferences are always stated in terms of the sampling unit. Since schools are the sampling unit, the mean score of the teachers in a school is the score for a school, with a sample size of 12, not 1,000. An alternative to using all 100 teachers in the twelve schools would be the process of **multistage sampling.**

Multistage Sampling

In the first stage a random sample of twenty-four schools is drawn and in the second stage a random sample of 50 teachers from each of the twenty-four schools is drawn. Now teachers are the sampling unit. Multistage sampling is superior to simple random sampling because all teachers belong to a school so at stage 1 all teachers had an opportunity to be selected.

Deliberate Sampling

With this method, the researcher knows that specific characteristics exist in a certain segment of a population. Since these traits are extremely critical to the results of the investigation, the researcher using **deliberate sampling** selects those subjects who contain the characteristics. Biomechanics researchers oftentimes purposely select excellent performers in a sport when they are trying to determine correct kinetic and kinematic parameters. Such factors are found in the top gymnasts, swimmers, basketball players, and other athletes, but they are probably absent in beginners or lower-level performers. Since this selection process is always biased, its use is encouraged only when the research advantages are superior to both the statistical and public relations aspects of bias-free selection (Fox 1969).

Nonprobability Samples

As indicated earlier, if a researcher is to justify generalizations about the population from which the sample is drawn, the sample must be selected at random. The random sample is a chance sample and follows the laws of probability. Some samples do not.

Samples not selected at random are called **nonprobability samples.** Examples are intact classes, volunteers, a typical group, or a typical person. The results of these kinds of samples frequently do not reflect accurately the traits of the population in which the researcher is interested. They may not, then, be representative of the population and can lead to faulty conclusions.

Suppose a researcher wants to study fifth-grade pupils on some physical fitness variable. These students belong to a class made up of four sections of 30 pupils each for a population of 120 prospective subjects. The researcher's plan is to select 30 subjects from the 120 at random. However, the school principal says, "No, the random selection would mean that some pupils from each section might be selected in the sample, and if you indiscriminately pull them out of their respective sections for testing purposes you will disrupt the school schedule. Instead, select just one section, intact, and make arrangements to do your testing before or after the school day." The question is, how representative of the characteristics of all of the fifth graders in the school is this one fifth-grade section? How representative is it of similar fifth-grade populations? The point is, intact or available groups impose a serious restriction on the researcher's ability to generalize the data obtained to the larger population from which the sample was drawn.

The use of volunteers can introduce an element of bias into an investigation. Say a researcher visits four college personal health classes and asks the students to volunteer to be in a study on the sexual behavior and characteristics of undergraduate college men and women. Twenty-five of the 150 students volunteer. How representative are four classes of a population of undergraduate men and women? Maybe the population should be the 150 students in the four classes. How representative of the 150 are the 25? The sample of 25 volunteers may be biased. What caused 25 students to accept the invitation to participate in the study and 125 to decline? The problem with volunteers is that they may be different from the nonvolunteers on the characteristics that are the focal point of the study. They usually possess special kinds of characteristics, which permit them to volunteer and which tend to bias the sample. Similarly, the selection of one individual elite swimmer or one group of elite swimmers, based upon the assumption that they are typical of all elite swimmers, provides for an element of bias also. Selecting subjects in this manner does not permit all elite swimmers an equal chance to be studied; the law of probability, or chance, has not been permitted to operate. To generalize from the "typical" subject to, perhaps, several hundred, would be stretching a point, to say nothing about the limits it would place on the researcher's ability to gain statistical significance when generalizing from the "sample" of one (or one "typical" group) to a larger population.

Sample Size

Sample size is difficult to determine with any degree of certainty. Beginning re-searchers, particularly students, often believe that a large sample will produce better data and more valid conclusions based upon these data. Regardless of size, the cru-cial factor is whether or not the sample is representative of the population. A well-selected and controlled small sample is better than a poorly selected and controlled large sample. Sample size is influenced by population size. Fifty subjects out of 100 may be representative, but 50 subjects from a population of 1,000,000 would not be representative.

In the 1936 presidential election, the *Literary Digest Magazine* predicted that the Republican candidate, Alfred Landon, would defeat the incumbent Democrat, Franklin Roosevelt. The prediction was based on responses to the magazine's survey of 10 million United States voters, 2 million of whom responded. President Roose-velt won the election in a landslide, carrying forty-six of the then forty-eight states. While one might say that 2 million respondents is a large sample, it is obvious that the majority opinion of these people did not represent the entire population of eli-gible voters. The sample was drawn from telephone and automobile registration lists. In 1936, in the depths of a depression, a lot of people did not have telephones or automobiles. Those who did possess them had money and probably aligned them-selves with the Republican party. The sample was biased and unrepresentative of the political leanings of Mr. and Mrs. Mainstream America.

In contrast, George Bush, in 1988, through the use of the computer, was pre-dicted to be the presidential victor with less than 5 percent of the votes cast. The sample on which the prediction was based was obtained through careful stratifica-tion of the voting population on several characteristics previously known to be related to voting practices, followed by proportional random sampling. This sample was unbiased and representative.

The size of the sample does become important in the statistical applications used to analyze the data produced by the sample, and in making inferences from the sample to the population. In general, the larger the sample, the more statistical power gener-ated by the statistic being used. A long-standing convention in experimental research is to consider thirty per group as the minimum acceptable sample size. Another guide-line is that the sample size never needs to exceed 50 percent of the population.

Sample size will also depend on the research approach utilized. Experimental studies will typically employ fewer subjects than will descriptive studies. Samples in experimental research are usually quite "captive" and, depending on the data-collecting demands, result in less subject mortality than in descriptive research. In the descriptive approach, especially when sending survey instruments through the mail, subject mortality, or attrition, can be quite large. The practice in descriptive research is to select a large enough sample so that if attrition does take place (i.e., people fail to return a completed survey instrument or questionnaire), an ample amount of data will still be produced.

Nonresponse in questionnaire studies must not be taken lightly. If 500 questionnaires are sent and only 100 are returned, what does this mean? How representative is the sample of 100 of the larger population from which the 500 prospective subjects was drawn? What selective or systematic factor is operating to cause 400 people to decline the opportunity to participate?

Some years ago at Indiana University, a researcher planned a study of male high school basketball officials. The study was an attempt to determine the physical fitness ability of these men to withstand the demand of officiating basketball games. Included were measures of several fitness variables, one of which was heart rate as determined by an electrocardiographic radiotelemetry heart rate system. The population of male basketball officials in the state at that time was 1,000. The researcher's desire was to select at random 10 percent of the officials, believing that 100 would be a representative sample from which to generalize back to the population of 1,000. So, 100 officials were sent invitations to participate in the study; 12 accepted, 88 declined. If 100 could be representative of 1,000, could 12? Obviously concerned, the researcher wrote to each of the men who declined the invitation in an attempt to ascertain the reason(s) for the declinations. Among the reasons given were: (1) they thought the radiotelemetry device would interfere with their ability to officiate without distraction, (2) they were just too busy, and (3) they could not afford the time to come to the university lab for a treadmill exercise designed to reproduce the demand of running up and down a basketball court to enable the researcher to collect gases. Hence, in this case, the data-collecting procedures operated in a manner that caused subject attrition. The researcher changed his mind about conducting an inferential study and opted for studying the 12 subjects as planned, and then presenting the results as they related to that group using descriptive statistics. It might be added that the study was conducted successfully and contributed to several states increasing the physical fitness standards for officials (Holland 1970).

Probably as important as sample size is the appropriateness with which the sample is selected. Random sampling, as indicated earlier, is the best approach to sample selection because the laws of probability operate in such a way that sampling error in both large and small samples can be estimated. Such estimates give researchers a gauge of how confident they should be that the results they obtain are accurate (Best 1981). The selection process, the types of variables being studied, how the data on those variables are collected, the proposed statistical procedures, and elements of public relations may all operate to dictate sample size.

Whenever a sample is used, it is logical to wonder what the results might have been if all of the people in the population had been included. An appropriate sample usually provides a good estimate of what the results would have been. All estimates involve some degree of error; the goal is to minimize that error. The researcher never knows exactly how much error is present, but it can be at least partially controlled by obtaining a sample that is in proportion to the total number of people in the population. Let's say, for example, that a researcher wants to survey parental opinion on whether or not sex education should be taught in the elementary school. The percent of yes responses will be determined. The researcher wants to be able to say with 90 percent certainty that the sample percent comes within 5 percentage points of what the findings would be if all of the parents had been surveyed. Although the researcher knows there will be some variation in the percent of "yes" opinions from the sample to the population, if there is high confidence (90%) that this variation is small ($\pm .05$), faith in the sample percentage increases.

In this example, if 3,000 parents made up the population, the sample would have to include 341 parents. While several attempts have been made to develop a foolproof computational formula for determining the exact size of a sample, none presently exists. However, many statistics books do present various procedures for determining the sample size needed based on the confidence limits set by the researcher. Tables 19 and 20 in *Tables for Statisticians* (Arkin and Colton 1963) address sample size for percent of population having a given attribute. Table 4.2 presents a

TABLE 4.2 Determining Sample Size from a Given Population*

N	S**	N	S	N	S
10	10	220	140	1,200	291
15	14	230	144	1,300	297
20	19	240	148	1,400	302
25	24	250	152	1,500	306
30	28	260	155	1,600	310
35	32	270	159	1,700	313
40	36	280	162	1,800	317
45	40	290	165	1,900	320
50	44	300	169	2,000	322
55	48	320	175	2,200	327
60	52	340	181	2,400	331
65	56	360	186	2,600	335
70	59	380	191	2,800	338
75	63	400	196	3,000	341
80	66	420	201	3,500	346
85	70	440	205	4,000	351
90	73	460	210	4,500	354
95	76	480	214	5,000	357
100	80	500	217	6,000	361
110	86	550	226	7,000	364
120	92	600	234	8,000	367
130	97	650	242	9,000	368
140	103	700	248	10,000	370
150	108	750	254	15,000	375
160	113	800	260	20,000	377
170	118	850	265	30,000	379
180	123	900	269	40,000	380
190	127	950	274	50,000	381
200	132	1,000	278	75,000	382
210	136	1,100	285	1,000,000	384

Note: *N* is population size.
  S is sample size.
* Krejcie, Robert V. and Margan, Daryle W. (1970). Determining sample size for research activities. *Educational and Psychological Measurement,* 30, 607–610. Reprinted by permission.
** Sample size for 90% confidence that the difference in the population and sample percentage is no more than .05.

table that was developed by Krejcie and Margan (1970) for determining sample size. It is based on 90 percent certainty (confidence) that the sample and population percentages do not differ more than .05. Tables for other situations can be found in books devoted to statistics or sampling procedures.

Summary

Sample size is important, but probably not as important as the representativeness of the sample to the population. Data from previous studies in the problem area and from pilot studies can provide the researcher with some indication of how large a sample needs to be in order to produce significant results. A sample of adequate size will be one that permits the study to be sensitive enough to determine a statistically significant difference if, in fact, it exists, and to be able to properly generalize the results.

Formative Evaluation of Objectives

Objective 1   Identify and define a population from which a sample of subjects is to be selected.

1. What difficulties would a researcher encounter if the research idea was to study selected health knowledge concepts in all American seventh-grade children as subjects?

Objective 2   Know how to determine the characteristics of the sample.

1. Why should a sample include characteristics that are also in the population from which the sample was drawn?

Objective 3   Know the various methods of selecting samples.

1. What are some of the problems involved in sampling? What methods of sampling are usually applied to obtain an unbiased sample?

Objective 4   Know the various factors that are used to determine sample size.

1. Is accuracy in a research study enhanced by selecting a large sample from a population? Why or why not? How do researchers attempt to procure a representative sample?

part

II

TYPES OF RESEARCH

Research can be classified or typed in a variety of different ways. Some authors use a three-classification system: experimental, descriptive, and historical. Other authors use a system with more than three classifications, which essentially splits the three classifications previously mentioned into more parts. Classifications can be developed based on a variety of criteria such as the methods used, the intended use of the research, and the type of setting in which the research takes place. Classifications of research serve more as a convenient way of presenting research than anything else. Many research studies do not fit neatly under one research classification but have characteristics of several research classifications. The point to remember is that all well-conducted research is good research. There is no hierarchy to these research classifications.

In this book, types of research are discussed under five chapter headings. Chapter 5, "Experimental Research," deals with a type of research that is very traditional and commonly conducted. It is research to find new ways of doing things in the future. Chapter 6, "Descriptive Research," encompasses many different research approaches. It also is a very traditional and commonly conducted type of research to describe the present situation. Chapter 7, "Historical Research," describes research conducted to show what happened in the past. It is not a common type of research in HHP but is slowly becoming more prevalent.

Chapter 8, "Creative Activities," covers research undertaken in order to create something new and unique, such as a new dance, technique or piece of equipment, computer program, or art form. It is a common type of research in a department of fine arts, but a relatively new type of research in HHP. Chapter 9, "Qualitative Research," is a common type of research in the social sciences, but a relatively new type of research in HHP. The methods in qualitative research differ considerably from the methods commonly found in experimental research.

5

Experimental Research

Key Words

Analysis of covariance (ANCOVA)
Block design
Central tendency error
Covariate
Counterbalanced design
Dependent variable
Designs
Double-blind study
External validity

Halo effect
Independent variable
Internal validity
Matched pairs design
Overrater error
Physical manipulation
Placebo
Pre-experimental design
Quasi-experimental design

Research hypothesis
Selective manipulation
Single-blind study
Statistical techniques
True experimental design
Underrater error
Variate

Objectives

This chapter contains information concerning experimental research. You should be familiar with how experimental research is conducted and the major issues in conducting this type of research.

After reading chapter 5, you should be able to:

1. Understand what experimental research is and how it is conducted.
2. Know the threats to validity and how to control them.
3. Recognize the types of designs commonly used in experimental research.

Experimental research is a traditional type of research and is conducted in most disciplines. It is virtually the only type of research performed in the sciences. In all cases, experimental research is conducted to increase the body of knowledge in the discipline and to suggest what procedures should be followed in the future. For example, a researcher who compares the effectiveness of two or more teaching or training methods, drugs, or techniques is trying to determine if there is one that is best and should be used in the future. The scientific method discussed in chapter 1 is always followed in experimental research. Finally, experimental research always involves manipulation of the experimental unit (e.g., human subject, animal subject). Consider the typical methodological study where each group of subjects receives a different treatment. The treatment received by a subject has the potential to change (manipulate) the subject. Isaac and Michael (1981) state that the purpose of experimental research is to investigate cause-and-effect relationships by subjecting experimental groups to treatment conditions and comparing the results to control groups not receiving the treatment.

Steps in Experimental Research

In order to conduct a research study in a systematic manner, the researcher should follow a definite, step-by-step procedure, starting with initiating a problem area and ending with dissemination of the research findings. Isaac and Michael (1981) have defined a procedure similar to the fourteen steps that follow.

Step 1   The first step is *stating the research problem,* clearly identifying both the problem to be researched and the purpose of the research. The research should not continue without a clear statement of the purpose because all subsequent steps and the entire conduct of the study are based on the statement of purpose.

Step 2   The second step is *determining if the experimental approach is appropriate.* Experimental research is conducted for the future and involves some manipulation of the subjects by applying an experimental treatment. Not all aspects of the research have to be experimental, but the major thrust and conduct of the research is experimental.

It is interesting to note that a study comparing existing groups (e.g., physical fitness differences between boys and girls) is often considered experimental research, but there is no manipulation of the subjects. However, if the difference between boys and girls in terms of leisure time pursuits is being studied, the research is more apt to be classified as not experimental. In these two situations, the research will be conducted the same way no matter how it is classified.

Step 3   Step 3 is *specifying the independent variable(s) and the levels of the independent variable(s).* An **independent variable** is used to form the experimental groups and is unaffected by the experimental treatment. The levels of the independent variable are the number of different values it will take in the research study. For example, if four treatment groups are used in a study, the independent variable is treatment, and there are four levels. If the independent variables are training days with three levels and training time with four levels, the design is two-dimensional and each of the twelve groups receives a different combination of the two treatments, as presented on page 112. Group 1 trains three days a week for thirty minutes each training day, while group 12 trains five days a week for sixty minutes each time.

		MINUTES OF TRAINING TIME PER DAY			
		30	40	50	60
NUMBER OF TRAINING DAYS PER WEEK	3	Group 1			
	4				
	5				Group 12

Essentially, it is during this step that decisions are made concerning the basic design of the study.

Step 4   Step 4 is *specifying all the potential dependent variables.* **Dependent variables** are the variables that could be measured during the research study to generate the data for analysis. Scores of subjects on these variables are dependent on the treatment they received. One or more dependent variables are identified at this step. The number and type of dependent variables are influenced by the statement of the research problems in step one.

Step 5   Step 5 is *stating the tentative hypotheses.* Experimental research requires a written **research hypothesis** that is either accepted or rejected based on the findings of the research study. The hypothesis is based on personal belief, presently accepted beliefs, and/or what the research literature supports. Since the researcher is supposed to be unbiased as to the outcome of the study and, in many cases, has no special insight as to outcome of the study or present beliefs, the research hypothesis is often one of equality. That is, the research hypothesis states that all groups are equal in ability at the end of the study, or, if a single group is measured before and after the experimental treatment, the hypothesis states there is no change in the ability of the group. However, a research hypothesis of inequality is also common. For example, if the research is comparing a traditional method with a new method and the researcher thinks the new method is better, the research hypothesis will be stated accordingly.

This statement is considered tentative because hypotheses very often have to be modified as the planning of the study progresses. Further, tentative hypotheses need to be established at this early stage because they influence some of the later steps in the research process.

Step 6   Step 6 is *determining the availability of measures for the potential dependent variables,* which were identified in step 4. These measures must have acceptable validity and reliability. Ideally, these measures already exist and are easily identified based on the researcher's knowledge and/or review of the literature. Often, the researcher will have to modify an existing measure to meet the needs of the study and to make the measure appropriate for the subjects in the study. Such modification is acceptable as long as the measure, as changed, remains valid and reliable. Sometimes the researcher will have to develop an entirely new test, instrument, or procedure to obtain the measure for a dependent variable. This is time-consuming since validity and reliability of the new measure must be determined before it is used. If the researcher decides a measure neither exists nor can be developed, the potential dependent variable is eliminated from further consideration.

Step 7   Step 7 is *pausing to consider the success potential of the research.* Based on all steps up to this point, does it seem that the research can be successfully conducted? If the research has little success potential, the project should be dropped before considerable time and energy is invested. Many things can be considered here. Certainly the time, expense, and difficulty of doing the research are concerns, and availability of subjects is often a major consideration. The possibilities for establishing the levels of the independent variable(s) (see step 3) realistically and ethically must be taken into account. Also, the availability of measures for the dependent variables influences the success potential of a study.

Step 8   The eighth step is *identifying the full potential of intervening variables.* Variables should be classified into the following groups: (1) should be controlled; (2) can be permitted to vary systematically; (3) can be ignored because of their relationship to variables classified as (1) or (2); and (4) can be left alone. Variables that can affect the outcome of the study must be controlled. Ways of controlling variables are discussed in this chapter. Systematic variables are not a danger to the outcome of the study because they vary in a known manner or in the same manner for all subjects and groups in the study. Maturation of the subjects is an example. If two variables are highly related, controlling one of them will control the other. Height and weight are an example. Variables that the researcher does not believe can affect the outcome of the study can be left alone. Care should be exercised to make sure that all important intervening variables are identified and that they are not misclassified as unimportant.

Step 9   Step 9 is *making a formal statement of the research hypotheses* and is a refinement of step 5 based on information gained and changes made in the study during steps 6 through 8. Issues related to stating hypotheses are addressed under step 5 and should be reviewed here. The research hypotheses stated at step 9 are important because the execution of the whole study is geared toward eventually providing the researcher with evidence for accepting or rejecting the hypotheses.

Step 10   Step 10 is *designing the experiment.* This is usually a time-consuming step in experimental research because it involves considerable planning and identification of procedures for conducting the study. Even the smallest details of the day-to-day conduct of the study must be carefully considered. Insufficient planning at this step is the downfall of many experimental research studies. Planning for data collection, sample selection, and data analysis all take place at this step. *Before* any data collection takes place, it is important that each research hypothesis be stated and that analysis techniques for all the data to be collected are known to exist. The value of conducting a pilot study at this step cannot be overemphasized.

Step 11   Step 11 is *making a final estimate of the success potential of the study.* It is good to pause before the experiment begins and check whether all stages of planning have been conducted adequately. Are there any aspects of the research study that could seriously limit the quality of the experiment in terms of potential conclusions? Particularly, are the procedures and controls in the potential study going to produce valid results addressing all of the research hypotheses?

Step 12   Step 12 is *conducting the study as planned in steps 1 through 11.* There are likely to be aspects of the study that could be improved, but if the planning of the study has been thorough, no major problems will compromise the quality of the study. During the implementation of the study, constantly verify that the integrity of the experiment is being maintained. This step terminates with the final data collection.

Step 13   Step thirteen is *analyzing the data* according to the data analysis plan. The need for some analysis not in the original plan may arise during the course of the data analysis. This additional analysis is acceptable as long as it does not seem to be an effort to obtain findings in support of what the researcher wants to prove.

Step 14   The fourteenth and last step is *preparing a research report.* This report should, at minimum, contain the procedures used in the study as well as the major findings of the study. The report may be little more than a record of the research that the researcher will later use for reference when the memory of the details of the research is less clear. On the other hand, the report could be as extensive as a master's thesis.

Internal and External Validity

Validity was defined and discussed in chapter 3 in terms of a measurement. Experimental research involves two other important classifications of validity. The first classification is **internal validity.** Internal validity deals with how valid the findings are within, or internal, to the study. Did the experimental treatments make a difference in

the study in that the treatments caused the subjects in the study to change in ability or are the changes in the ability of the subjects due to other factors (see "Threats to Internal Validity" later in this chapter)? If the treatments caused the change in the ability of the subjects, then internal validity can be claimed.

The second classification, **external validity,** is the degree to which findings in a research study can be inferred or generalized to other populations, settings, or experimental treatments. Particularly, external validity is concerned with whether the findings for the sample of subjects in the study can be inferred to the population they represent and to other populations. In other words, are the findings in the research study unique to the subjects in the study, or do the findings apply to other groups? If the findings in a research study can be inferred or generalized to other populations, settings, or experimental treatments, external validity can be claimed. A study using inmates in a prison might lack in external validity. Good internal validity is required to have good external validity, but good internal validity does not guarantee good external validity.

Control of all variables operating in an experimental research study is highly desirable but seldom, if ever, accomplished. The researcher would like all subjects to be treated the same in terms of all variables (e.g., sleep, food, exercise) except for the experimental or treatment variable, which is allowed to vary among subjects. Too much control can harm external validity, but not enough control destroys internal validity. Having so much control that the research setting is unique or totally removing the research from the setting where it will be applied destroys external validity. Excellent control is possible in prisons and military installations, but findings on subjects in these places may not apply to subjects in other situations.

Controlling Threats to Validity

Campbell and Stanley (1963) discuss twelve factors that can threaten the validity of an experimental research study. Isaac and Michael (1981) and Van Dalen (1979) also discuss these potential threats in detail. The first eight factors threaten internal validity and the last four factors threaten external validity. Obviously, a researcher tries to control as many of both types of these factors as possible in an experimental research study.

Threats to Internal Validity

History. History refers to specific things that happen while conducting the research study that affect the final scores of the subjects in addition to the effect of the experimental treatment. Suppose that subjects participate in an activity or program outside of the research study but that this activity is very similar to the experimental treatment. If this outside participation increases their final scores, it makes the experimental treatment seem more effective than it really is. A second example

is the atypical occurrence, such as an epidemic, local disaster, or one-time emphasis on the research topic in the community, that occurs in the lives of the subject during the research study and that affects their final scores.

Maturation.   Because they grow older during the experimental period, the performance level of the subjects changes and this change is reflected in their final scores. Seasonal changes might also be considered here. Example 1: As young subjects grow older during the fifteen-week experimental period, their physical performance level changes no matter what the effect of the experimental treatment. Thus, change in the performance of a treatment group from pretest to posttest may be inflated by maturation. Example 2: Between September when the research study begins and December when the study ends, subjects become less physically fit due to less daily activity because they are in school all day and the weather is bad. This loss of fitness counteracts the effect of the experimental treatment. A control group (group receiving no treatment) can be a check on the maturation threat.

Testing.   The act of taking a test can affect the scores of the subjects on a second or later testing. For example, subjects are pretested, then the experimental treatment is administered, and finally the subjects are posttested. One reason why subjects do better on the posttest is because they learn from the pretest. The pretest is like a treatment. This poses a real problem if the pretest and posttest are the same knowledge or physical performance test. Baumgartner (1969) tested subjects with several physical performance tests, retested them two days later, and found that scores had improved from the initial test to the retest.

Instrumentation.   Changes in the adjustment or calibration of the measuring equipment or use of different standards among scorers may cause differences among groups in final score or changes in the scores of the subjects over time. This suggests that researchers need to check the accuracy of their measuring equipment regularly and frequently and make sure a standard scoring procedure is used. Any difference in the test scores of several treatment groups or change in the test scores of the subjects in a group over time (pretest to posttest) must be due to differences among groups or a change in the subjects over time and not due to changes in the calibration of the equipment or scoring procedure. Testing equipment and scoring procedures must be held constant for each subject in research environments involving multiple pieces of the same equipment, multiple scorers, or multiple days of data collection.

Statistical Regression.   The tendency for groups with extremely high or low scores on one measure to score closer to the mean score of the population on a second measure is called statistical regression. This tendency may be mistaken for experimental treatment effect. For example, a high IQ and a low IQ group are formed. An experimental treatment is applied to both groups for twelve weeks. Then

a physical ability test is administered to both groups, and it is found that they are equal in physical ability. This equality may be due to the regression effect or to the treatment effect. Using random sampling procedures to form groups eliminates the threat.

Research studies in which the research question is whether groups that differ in one attribute differ in terms of another attribute may have similar problems. For example, do disabled and nondisabled populations differ in their beliefs concerning use of leisure time? No treatment is applied in this example, so random samples from the two populations are obtained and a score for beliefs about the use of leisure time is obtained for each subject. The finding that the two populations do not differ in their leisure time use beliefs is due to the regression effect.

Selection.   The way subjects are selected or assigned to groups can be biased. This may result in groups that are not representative of a population, groups that are not equal in ability at the beginning of the experiment, and/or groups that differ at the end of the experiment for reasons other than differences in the integrity of the experimental treatments. Random selection of subjects and random assignment of subjects to groups usually controls this threat. Thus, following the random sampling techniques outlined in chapter 4 and using sample sizes that are sufficiently large for the research situation will control this threat. When subject selection is a threat it is often due to small sample size per group and/or failure to use one of the necessary alternatives to simple random sampling when required for the research setting.

Experimental Mortality.   This particular threat to internal validity is created with the excessive loss of subjects so that experimental groups are no longer representative of a population or similar to each other. Some subject loss is to be expected in a research study, but if many subjects of the same type drop out of a group it can considerably change the characteristics of the group and the outcome of the study.

Interaction of Selection and Maturation or History.   The maturation effect or history effect is not the same for all groups selected for the research study, and this influences final scores. This problem may arise when each group is an intact pre-existing group rather than a randomly formed group. For example, if the groups differ considerably in age or background, this may affect how they respond to the experimental treatments. Also, if groups start out unequal in ability due to maturation or history, they may not have the same potential for improvement as a result of the experimental treatments.

Threats to External Validity

Interaction Effect of Testing.   This effect occurs when the pretest changes the group's response to the experimental treatment, thus making the group unrepresentative of any particular population and certainly unrepresentative of a population that has not been pretested. There is always the danger that administering a test before the experimental treatment (pretest) changes the subjects. For example, the pretest may make the subjects more aware of the need to increase their knowledge or performance level, causing them to respond to the experimental treatment more positively than they otherwise would.

Interaction Effects of Selection Bias and Experimental Treatment.   The subjects or groups selected in a biased manner react to the experimental treatment in a unique way so they are not representative of any particular population. High IQ or high skill level or metropolitan subjects may not react to a particular treatment in the same way as low IQ or low skill level or rural subjects and, thus, are not representative of them. If the population is well defined before the sample is drawn, this threat should be minimal. The problem (threat) can easily occur when a convenient group is used in the research and an attempt is made to define a population that fits the group.

Reactive Effects of Experimental Setting.   The experimental setting is such that the experimental treatment has a unique effect on the subjects or groups that would not be observed in some other setting. Thus, the results of the study are not representative of any particular population. If any element of the experimental procedure alters the normal behavior of the subjects, then the effect of the experimental treatment may be altered and it will not have the same effect on a different group of subjects. For example, subjects may think the experimental treatment or drug is supposed to cause a change in their behavior or performance, so they react or perform differently for reasons that are not due to the treatment. Subjects who react to the researcher in a unique manner provide another example. Conducting the research in a lab rather than in the natural setting is a third example.

Multiple-Treatment Interference.   Multiple-treatment interference is the effect of prior treatments on the response of the subjects or groups to a present treatment. This makes their response to the present treatment unique and not representative of the way any other population would respond to the present treatment. This effect can occur when the same subjects are used in several related studies. For example, the same high performance level runners are used in three different studies dealing with the physiological responses to running. Are their responses in the third experiment influenced by participating in the two previous studies? Researchers should check on the background and experiences of potential subjects to control this threat to external validity.

Types of Designs

Designs are the variety of ways a research study may be structured or conducted. Campbell and Stanley (1963) present the advantages and disadvantages of many types of design in terms of how each controls the threats to validity. They classify designs as being either pre-experimental, true experimental, or quasi-experimental. Only a few representative designs are presented here since it is impossible to present all the designs that the reader may encounter.

The **pre-experimental designs** are weaker than true experimental designs in terms of control. Pre-experimental designs have no random sampling of subjects, are usually one group or two unequated groups, control few threats to validity, and have many definite weaknesses. The one-group pretest/posttest design is an example. It requires that a group be tested before the experimental treatment is administered and again after the experimental treatment has been administered. For example, fifty subjects are administered an initial (pretest) fitness test. Then the subjects are administered the experimental treatment which, in this case, is doing prescribed exercises one hour per day, three days per week for eighteen weeks. Finally, the final (posttest) fitness test is administered. This is the same fitness test used for the pretest. If the group improved in fitness from the pretest to the posttest, the experimental treatment is judged to be effective. But all of the change from the pretest to the posttest may not be due to the experimental treatment. The change could be partially or totally due to the threats to validity of history, maturation, testing, instrumentation, selection and maturation or selection and history interaction, interaction effect of selection bias and experimental treatment, or interaction effect of testing. Only the threats to validity of selection and experimental mortality are definitely controlled in this design. Another example is the use of intact classes. All pupils in one class receive treatment A and all pupils in another class receive treatment B. There is no random sampling of subjects or random assignment of subjects to treatments, so it is not known if the two treatment groups started the study equal in ability. If the treatment groups are unequal at the end of the study it may be because (1) the treatments were not equally effective, (2) the groups were unequal at the start of the study, or (3) some combination of the two previous reasons.

The **true experimental designs** are recommended over other classifications of designs because they offer good control. True experimental designs always have random sampling of subjects, random assignment of subjects to groups, and all threats to internal validity controlled. The pretest/posttest control group design is an example. It is an extension of the pre-experimental design just presented. Here, the experimental group is tested before and after the experimental treatment is administered. The control group is tested at the same times as the experimental group, but receives no treatment that changes its ability. Each group is a random sample from a population. Provided the experimental and control groups are equal in ability on the pretest, if the experimental group performs better than the control group on the posttest, the result should be due to the experimental treatment. This design controls the eight threats to internal validity but does not control the interactive effect of testing. Another example is the use of two experimental groups and a control group. From a population some members are randomly assigned to each of the three groups, but all members of the population are not selected as subjects. Further, the two experimental and one control treatments are randomly assigned to groups. Assuming the three groups are equal in ability at the beginning of the study, differences among the three groups at the end of the study should be due to differences in the effectiveness of the three treatments.

Many times, the researcher will conduct the research in the setting where the research will actually be applied, but the situation will lack the control required for the true experimental design. The researcher quite often controls the data collection times and who is tested, but does not totally control when and to whom the experimental treatment is administered. Further, random assignment of subjects to groups is not always possible. These situations lead to quasi-experimental designs.

The **quasi-experimental designs** are fine as long as the researcher understands what the designs do not control. These designs lack either random sampling of subjects or random assignment of subjects to groups. Quasi-experimental designs are much better than pre-experimental designs. The nonequivalent control group design is an example. It is just like the pretest/posttest control group design except subjects are not assigned to groups by using random sampling procedures. Instead, the experimental and control groups are existing groups, like classes or facilities, that are similar in characteristics and may be equal in ability. The pretest will indicate how similar they are before the experimental treatment is administered to the experimental group. This design controls the threats to validity of history, maturation, testing, instrumentation, selection, and experimental mortality; but it does not control threats to validity of the interaction effects of maturation and history, or the interaction effect of testing. Thus, this design does not have as much control as the true experimental design—the pretest/posttest control group design.

Designs have been discussed in terms of how they control the threats to validity. Also, designs can be discussed in terms of their complexity and ability to answer research questions. Simple designs answer one research question and more complex designs answer several research questions. To present various designs in an abbreviated form, X is used to represent a treatment is administered and O is used to represent data is collected. For example, $O_1 X O_2$ indicates that the subjects are tested initially (O_1), a treatment is administered (X), and subjects are tested once again (O_2). Presented in Table 5.1 are examples of designs ranging from simple to complex. In designs 1 and 2, the research question is simply whether some treatment will cause a change in the scores of a group; design 2 is the better design because it uses a control group. Designs 2 and 3 are both two-group designs but have different research questions. The fourth design is a combination of designs 2 and 3. Design 5 is essentially design 3 extended to three or more groups. Design 6 is presented primarily as a lead-up to design 7. Design 7 is superior to design 6 because more information is obtained in the form of combinations of A and B treatments. The A treatment and B treatment in designs 6 and 7 are two different treatments. For example, A treatment is three methods of instruction, and B treatment is two different number of weeks of instruction. In this example, design 7 is used because combinations of treatments A and B are possible. However, if A treatment is three ways of teaching first aid and B treatment is two ways of teaching sex education, the two treatments cannot be combined, so design 6 is used.

TABLE 5.1   Example Research Designs in Ascending Order of Complexity

DESIGN	RESEARCH QUESTION	DESIGN*	REMARKS
1	Is treatment effective?	O_1 X O_2	A group is tested before and after a treatment; compare means for O_1 and O_2 to see if O_2 is better
2	Is treatment effective?	O_1 X O_2 O_3 O_4	Treatment group gets X and control group gets no treatment; sometimes O_1 and O_3 not collected; if means for O_1 and O_3 are equal, groups started equal; compare means for O_2 and O_4 to see if O_2 mean is better
3	Which treatment is better?	X_1 O_1 X_2 O_2	One group receives X_1 and another group receives X_2; compare means for O_1 and O_2 to see if equal
4	Is each treatment effective? Which treatment is better?	O_1 X_1 O_2 O_3 X_2 O_4	One group receives X_1 and another group receives X_2; if means for O_1 and O_3 are equal, groups started equal; compare O_1 and O_2 means and compare O_3 and O_4 means to see if treatments are effective; compare means for O_2 and O_4 to see if one treatment is better
5	Which treatment is better?	X_1 O_1 X_2 O_2 X_3 O_3	Same as design 3 but more than two groups; compare means of O_1, O_2 and O_3
6	The two questions are:		
	(1) Which A treatment (A_1, A_2, A_3) is best?	A treatment X_1 O_1 X_2 O_2 X_3 O_3	See design 5; compare means of O_1, O_2, and O_3
	(2) Which B treatment (B_1, B_2) is better?	B treatment X_1 O_1 X_2 O_2	See design 3; compare means of O_1, and O_2
7	The three questions are:		
	(1) Which A treatment (A_1, A_2, A_3) is best?	X_{11} O_{11}** X_{12} O_{12} X_{21} O_{21}	A treatment: Compare means of $(O_{11} + O_{12})$, $(O_{21} + O_{22})$, $(O_{31} + O_{32})$
	(2) Which B treatment (B_1, B_2) is better?	X_{22} O_{22} X_{31} O_{31} X_{32} O_{32}	B treatment: Compare means of $(O_{11} + O_{21} + O_{31})$, $(O_{12} + O_{22} + O_{32})$
	(3) Which combination of the A and B treatments $(A_1B_1, A_1B_2, A_2B_1, A_2B_2, A_3B_1, A_3B_2)$ is best?		Combinations: Compare means for O_{11}, O_{12}, O_{21}, O_{22}, O_{31}, O_{32} See designs 3, 5, and 6

There are six groups, each receiving one of the six combinations of A and B.

	B_1	B_2
A_1	A_1B_1	A_1B_2
A_2	A_2B_1	A_2B_2
A_3	A_3B_1	A_3B_2

*X = treatment is administered O = data is collected
**X = is the treatment for the A B treatment group

Validity in Summary

Two classifications of validity and the threats to each classification have been discussed. In many research studies maximum internal and external validity cannot be obtained due to constraints on finances, time, subjects, the research setting, or other resources. The researcher must decide what is most important, internal or external validity, and which threats to validity are more important to control than others.

As indicated earlier in the chapter, good internal validity is required to have good external validity. Campbell and Stanley (1963, 5) indicate that internal validity is the basic minimum for an experimental design. Thus, a research study must be designed in a manner that establishes good internal validity.

A researcher must consider the threats to validity while designing the study. After selecting a tentative design of the study, the researcher should determine which of the threats to validity exist, the seriousness of these threats, and how easy it is to control each threat. It is impossible to generalize to all research situations, but the strategy to follow is to modify the tentative design of the study to control the major threats to validity and those that are easy to eliminate. Minor threats and threats that are hard to eliminate may have to be uncontrolled. This strategy is much harder to accomplish when a major threat is hard to eliminate.

Cook and Campbell (1979) subdivide internal validity into statistical conclusions validity and internal validity, and subdivide external validity into construct validity of cause or effect and external validity. Discussion of statistical conclusion validity and construct validity of cause or effect requires background beyond the scope of this book. Advanced students may appreciate a discussion of the four types of validity.

Methods of Control

Control is vital in experimental research. The researcher wants to control the effect of all variables except the experimental variable. Although ideal, this degree of control is seldom if ever achieved in HHP research. Nevertheless, the researcher must control the effect of the variables that could have a major impact on the study. Control of variables can be obtained in several ways.

The best way to control the effect of variables is by **physical manipulation.** The researcher physically controls all aspects of the subjects' environment and experience throughout the experimental period. Thus, the amount of sleep, food intake, drug use, stimulation, stress, exercise, practice, or training is the same for all subjects unless one of these variables is the experimental treatment. For example, if each of four groups is being taught by a different method, teaching method is the experimental treatment. The method varies from group to group, but the researcher tries to keep all other variables constant for all groups. Controlling all variables except the experimental treatment is difficult unless the subjects happen to be prisoners, military recruits, or animals. The researcher tries to be sure each group receives the designated teaching method without any additional benefit from the method outside the experiment and without opportunity to benefit from the teaching method of another group. Since some variables cannot be physically controlled, the researcher might resort to other control methods.

Selective manipulation is commonly used to gain control and can take many forms. The intent of selective manipulation is to increase the likelihood that treatment groups are similar in characteristics and/or ability at the beginning of an experiment. By selecting only certain subjects, the researcher manipulates the treatment groups to gain control. **Matched pairs** and **block designs** are forms of selective manipulation. The population to which the results of the research study are inferred or applied is defined. Accessible members of this population are tested on one or more variables that the researcher wishes to control in the study. Based on this variable(s) subjects with similar scores are matched into pairs if two groups are needed or into blocks if more than two groups are needed in the research study. The same number of subjects are randomly assigned to each treatment group from each pair or block. This procedure produces groups that start the experiment basically equal in terms of the variable(s) used for matching.

The variable(s) used for matching should be ones the researcher feels must be controlled because the variable(s) can have a major effect on the outcome of the study. Some common matching variables are initial ability, age, height, weight, gender, and IQ.

> *Example 1:* The researcher wants to compare two teaching methods. She believes that gender may influence the effectiveness of a teaching method. So, the researcher assigns twenty boys and twenty girls to each teaching method using random sampling procedures.

This is different from subject pairing as presented earlier because it equates or balances the two treatment groups in terms of gender. If the researcher is willing to match subjects based on both gender and IQ, twenty pairs of boys and twenty pairs of girls could be formed with the two subjects in a pair basically equal in IQ score. From each pair, a subject is randomly assigned to each teaching method group. The groups are taught by the teaching method assigned to them, and then a test is administered to all subjects. Differences between groups are checked based on test scores.

> *Example 2:* The researcher is going to compare three different methods of developing strength in college males. Ninety-eight students are administered a strength test. Based on these initial test scores thirteen blocks with six students of similar strength in a block are formed. Two students from each block are randomly assigned to each group. Subjects train for ten weeks with the method assigned their group. Then the strength test is administered again to each subject. Based on this final test score, differences among groups are determined.

Another common form of selective manipulation to gain control is the **counterbalanced design.** These designs require that all subjects receive all treatments, but in different orders. However, these designs are limited to situations where it makes sense for subjects to receive all treatments. Counterbalanced designs are an alternative to designs where each group receives one of the treatments and differences among groups are examined to see if all treatments are equally effective. Campbell and Stanley (1963) and statistics books like Winer, Brown, and Michels (1991) and Keppel (1991) discuss counterbalanced designs.

A simple example of a counterbalanced design is the comparison of the effectiveness of two drugs, A and B. To conduct the study a sample of subjects is randomly drawn from a population. One-half the subjects receive drug A first and drug B later, while the other half of the subjects receive drug B, then A. The process sequence is the same in both cases: A drug is administered, the subjects are tested to determine the effect of the drug, a period of time passes to allow the drug to wear off and the subjects to return to normal, the other drug is administered, and the subjects are tested to determine the effect of the drug. Each subject receives a score under both drug A and drug B, so a comparison between the two drugs is possible. If there is an order effect so that the first drug taken influences the response of a subject to a second drug, the order effect is neutralized by counterbalancing.

Sometimes researchers conduct a study using only subjects of one rather than both genders, or subjects very similar in age or experience rather than more heterogeneous in terms of these attributes. For example, rather than use college undergraduate students as subjects, the researcher uses 18- or 19-year-old freshmen. These techniques might be considered selective manipulation.

Often, **statistical techniques** are used to gain control in an experimental research study. Statistical techniques are applied when physical manipulation or selective manipulation of variables is not possible. The researcher knows, at the beginning of the study before the treatments are administered, that the experimental groups differ in terms of one or more variables that must be controlled in the study. If these variables are not controlled, the integrity of the research study is seriously compromised. Sometimes the variables that must be controlled are the same ones that would be used to form blocks in the block design discussed under selective manipulation techniques. In this situation, the research setting is such that the subjects are already in groups so a block design cannot be used. The following is an example of this situation.

Treatment groups in the research study very often differ in initial ability. If the groups differ in ability at the end of the experiment, it is not known whether this is due to the initial inequality or difference in effectiveness of the treatments. A statistical technique commonly used in this situation is **analysis of covariance (ANCOVA).** Basically, the ANCOVA technique adjusts the differences among the groups in scores at the end of the study based on differences in initial ability among the groups. If differences among the groups are found after final scores are adjusted, the researcher concludes that all experimental treatments are not equally effective.

In the ANCOVA technique, one or more scores called the **covariates** are obtained at the beginning of the study. Covariates are used to adjust differences among groups in terms of a score called the **variate,** collected at the end of the study.

A statistical test of the differences among the groups in terms of the adjusted data is provided as part of the ANCOVA technique. The ANCOVA technique can be used with a variety of research designs and with as many covariates and types of covariates as the researcher desires. Extensive discussion of ANCOVA is found in Huck, Cormier, and Bounds (1974), Winer, Brown, and Michels (1991), Keppel (1991), and Dayton (1970).

Common Sources of Error

Many possible sources of error can cause the results of a research study to be incorrectly interpreted. When error is present, the outcome of the study is not totally due to the experimental treatment. These sources of error are more specific than the threats to validity discussed earlier in the chapter. All sources of error are not a concern in every research study. Those sources of error discussed in this section of the chapter do not cover all potential sources.

Hawthorne Effect

This source of error is named for a research study that was conducted at the Hawthorne Electric Plant in the 1920s. It was observed that having a group of workers participate in a research study caused them to feel special so they acted differently than the typical worker. The research study was conducted to determine how changes in the working environment would affect productivity. Results of the study showed that productivity increased no matter whether the change in the working environment was supposed to increase or decrease productivity. This points out that subjects in an experiment may perform in an atypical manner due to the newness or novelty of the treatment and because they realize that they are participating in an experiment. This suggests that, as much as possible, the subjects should be unaware that they are participating in an experiment and also unaware of the hypothesized outcome of the study. Particularly in studies comparing new and traditional methods (e.g., teaching, training), the researcher does not want the new method to seem superior to the traditional method due to the Hawthorne effect.

Placebo Effect

The subjects in an experimental treatment may believe the treatment is supposed to change them so they respond to the treatment with a change in performance. In a typical study to determine the effect of a drug, subjects are pretested, administered the drug, and posttested. The researcher wants any change in the performance of the group from pretest to posttest to be due to the drug and not due to the fact that the subjects think the drug is effective. In this example, the researcher has a second group (control group) that goes through the same procedure (pretest, drug, posttest) as the experimental treatment group, except the drug the control group receives is a

placebo, a drug that can have no effect on the subjects. Assuming the experimental and control groups were equal in pretest scores and that the psychological response to a drug is the same for both groups, superiority of the experimental group in posttest scores is due to the positive effect of the drug.

In some studies the experimental group receives a treatment and the control group receives nothing. This seems like a poor research technique since the control groups should be receiving some placebo if psychological response to a treatment is to be the same for both groups. The treatment for the control group should be one that cannot affect the test score used to compare groups at the end of the study.

"John Henry" Effect

In studies with an experimental group and a control group, the control group knows it is not supposed to be better than the experimental, so it tries harder and outperforms the experimental group. This might be called the "Avis effect" after Avis Cars—we are number two, but we try harder. Of course, there could be a reverse "John Henry" effect where the control group gives up. It is also possible for the experimental group to improve due to the treatment and for the control group to improve due to the "John Henry" effect, thereby making the groups equal in performance at the end of the study. Again, it seems better to keep the design and expectations of the study unknown to the subjects if possible.

Rating Effect

Several kinds of rating errors can occur. The **halo effect** is the tendency to let initial impressions or ratings of a subject or group influence future ratings. Where **overrater error** and **underrater error** occur the researcher tends to overrate or underrate subjects. Finally, there is **central tendency error** where the researcher tends to rate most subjects in the middle of the rating scale. Also, these rating errors can occur when subjects are asked to rate statements about beliefs, practices, or problems (see chapter 6). For example, each subject rates each of twenty-five statements about health practices on a 1-to-5 scale, with 5 being important and 1 being not important.

Rating errors can be minimized by not looking at previous ratings. Also, a rating scale with 4 (e.g., excellent, above average, below average, terrible) to 7 (e.g., very strongly agree, strongly agree, agree, neutral, disagree, strongly disagree, very strongly disagree) well-defined different values can minimize rating errors. Rating errors can be minimized if the researcher develops the rating process properly.

Experimenter Bias Effect

The bias of a researcher can affect the outcome of the study. Experimenter bias may influence methodology, treatment, and data collection. This bias is often in favor of the experimental treatment the researcher believes is best.

Some believe the researcher should not be involved in administering any of the treatments or collecting any of the data in methodological studies where each group receives a different method, such as teaching or training, over many weeks. This brings up an interesting dilemma when there are two or more groups in a methodological study. Should the same person administer the methods to all groups, or should different people administer the methods? If the same person administers all methods, the study could be criticized because the person may have biases and may not be equally effective with all methods. If different people administer each method, the study could be criticized because all people may not be equally effective with their methods. So, the situation is a no-win situation (similar to a "heads I win, tails you lose" coin flip). None of this discussion addresses whether the researcher is administering any methods. In many studies the researcher does not have a choice who administers the methods, but if choices exist the researcher selects the best procedure for the research setting.

When possible, the researcher keeps the subjects unaware of the purpose of the study and of their role in the study in order to eliminate any possible subject-caused error. Specifically, the subjects are unaware of whether they are receiving the experimental or control treatment. This study is referred to as a **single-blind study.** The research setting and procedures used in many studies often preclude the single-blind study. When both the subjects and those conducting the study (administering treatments and collecting data) are unaware of the purpose of the study and the way in which subjects are grouped, the study is referred to as a **double-blind study.**

Subject-Researcher Interaction Effect

Do subjects respond better to researchers of the same gender, do they respond better to researchers of the opposite gender, or does it make any difference? It is reasonable to assume that, in some research settings, gender of the subjects and researcher is influential and therefore contributes to error. What is important in any study is that the difference among groups in the research study and the effectiveness of the treatments in the study are not due to a subject-researcher interaction. The subject-researcher interaction effect should be minimal if the researcher functions with all groups in the same professional manner.

Post Hoc Error

This type of error is introduced by assuming a cause-and-effect relationship between two variables when such a relationship does not exist. For example: More people die in bed than any other place; therefore, beds are dangerous.

Measurement in Experimental Research

Experimental research almost always requires measuring the subjects involved with some test or procedure. Thus, questions like, What tests or procedures are available?, How are the reliability and validity of these measures determined?, How are these tests or procedures administered?, commonly arise. Guidance in answering these questions is often found in measurement books. Researchers collecting physical performance data should consult measurement books in physical education and exercise science like Baumgartner and Jackson (1995). If using some paper-and-pencil test or instrument to collect data, researchers might read measurement books in education and psychology such as Thorndike et al. (1991). Two excellent measurement books in health, which also contain considerable information on measurement in research, are Green and Lewis (1986) and Sarvela and McDermott (1993).

The newest tests, procedures, and techniques may not yet be in the measurement books, so they must be found in the research journals. Measurement specialists tend to conduct research dealing with improving or developing measurement tests, procedures, and techniques. Some researchers in all areas do measurement research on occasion.

Summary

Experimental research is characterized by subject manipulation with a treatment and tight control of the variables that operate in the research study. The potential variety of types of experimental studies is endless. For this reason, techniques for conducting experimental research are specific to the experimental study, and only topics common to all experimental research were addressed in this chapter.

Formative Evaluation of Objectives

Objective 1 Understand what experimental research is and how it is conducted.

1. What is the purpose of experimental research?
2. What is the importance of "control" in experimental research?
3. In experimental research there always is a hypothesis. What are some other things that always occur in experimental research?

Objective 2 Know the threats to validity and how to control them.

1. What are five common threats to the validity of research in your area?
2. What are the three most common techniques used in your area to control threats to the validity of the research?

Objective 3   Recognize the types of designs commonly used in experimental research.

1. What are two experimental research designs commonly used in your area?

2. What are the advantages of an experimental research design with a control group in it?

3. What are the advantages of a repeated measures design (pretest-posttest)?

6

Descriptive Research

Key Words

"After the fact" research
Closed-ended item
Completion item
Criterion referenced
Cross-sectional approach

Longitudinal approach
Multiple choice item
Norm referenced
Open-ended item
Percentile rank

Semistructured interview
Structured interview
Unstructured interview

Objectives

This chapter contains information about descriptive research. You should become familiar with the various types of descriptive research and the techniques commonly used in conducting descriptive research.

After reading chapter 6, you should be able to:

1. Identify the common types of descriptive research.
2. Identify techniques commonly used in descriptive research.

Whereas in the last chapter we found that experimental research focuses on the future, descriptive research is oriented toward the present. Descriptive research is conducted to describe a present situation, what people currently believe, what people are doing at the moment, and so forth.

Descriptive research is a broad classification of research under which many types of research are conducted. Some people mistakenly believe that experimental research is the only approach. Others mistakenly think that descriptive research is easier to conduct than experimental research. Any type of research is good if it is conducted properly, and all research is demanding. For the study to be conducted well, the researcher needs to have some formal training and practical experience in the research area. It is foolish to try to conduct a research study in physics without sufficient formal training. Likewise, it is an error to try to use the same techniques on elementary school-aged children that are used on adults.

Descriptive research is conducted by collecting information and, based on this information, describing the situation. Descriptive research can, but does not have to, include a research hypothesis. Consider a study in which 10,000 high school seniors are selected from a population and surveyed as to whether they smoke tobacco, and 38 percent indicate they do. The researcher reports that 38 percent of high school seniors in the population smoke tobacco. Using the same research procedures, the researcher could have hypothesized prior to conducting the study that 30 percent of high school seniors in the population smoke tobacco. In this case, the researcher reports the 38 percent and whether the research hypothesis is accepted or rejected.

Descriptive research is commonly conducted in physical education and may be the predominant research approach in health, recreation, and sports management. It is an approach commonly used in dance, as well. Descriptive research is conducted in kinesiology and exercise science, but not as commonly as in the other disciplines mentioned.

Types of Descriptive Research

The types of descriptive research are briefly described in this section to provide a general awareness of and broad appreciation for them. The types of descriptive research discussed are survey, developmental, case study, correlational, normative, observational, action, and ex post facto.

Survey

Survey research is the most common type of descriptive research. It involves determining the views or practices of a group through interviews or by administering a questionnaire. The questionnaire may be administered to a group by the researcher or mailed to the members of the group for them to complete and mail back to the researcher. Survey research will be discussed in detail later in this chapter.

Developmental

Developmental research usually deals with the growth and development of humans over time. For example, what are the growth and developmental changes each year from age 6 to age 18? More accurately, what are the growth and developmental attributes of each age group? Other developmental research might examine how organizations or professional groups develop over time.

There are two approaches to developmental research. One is the **longitudinal approach** in which a group is measured and observed on a regular basis for multiple years. For example, twice a year from age 6 to age 18 a large group of children is fitness tested. Based on this information, fitness standards are developed for each age level. The problem with this research approach is that it takes many years to complete, and it is difficult to keep track of the subjects over the many years that the study lasts. However, such studies are tremendously valuable. Presently, many epidemiologists wish there were more fitness data available on middle-aged adults as children to be able to answer questions concerning how fit children need to be in order to be fit as adults. As valuable as longitudinal studies may be, they are not a good choice for master's theses or doctoral dissertations due to the vast length of time involved.

The other approach to developmental research is the **cross-sectional approach.** Taking the earlier example of developing fitness standards for age groups with the cross-sectional approach, large samples of each age group are tested at the same time, and standards for each age group are developed. The assumption underlying this research approach is that each age group is representative of all other age groups when they will be or were that age. If this assumption is true, cross-sectional research will yield the same results as longitudinal research, but in a shorter time period. Cross-sectional research cannot always answer questions that longitudinal research answers. The earlier question by epidemiologists about fitness in children as an indicator of fitness in adults can only be answered with a longitudinal study.

Case Study

Case study research typically involves studying a person or event in great detail and describing what is found. A study of the training techniques or performance techniques of a highly skilled athlete is an example of a case study. It is assumed that less-skilled performers should use techniques of the highly skilled. A study of the way the Boston Marathon is organized and conducted for use as a model for how to organize and conduct a marathon is another example of a case study.

Being highly organized and very systematic in collecting the information needed to write the report is vital in this research approach. Essential to case study research is preparation by looking at literature on how to conduct case study research and at actual case studies for the techniques used.

Correlational

The purpose of correlational studies is to determine if a relationship exists between variables. The statistical techniques used are correlation and regression (discussed in chapters 10 and 11). To determine if a relationship exists between two variables, each subject must be measured on both variables. For example, to determine if a relationship exists between time spent practicing a task and ability in performing the task, a practice time and task ability score must be obtained for each subject. If the data analysis shows that the longer a subject's practice time, the better the subject's task ability score tended to be, the researcher concludes that a relationship exists and that practicing a task is beneficial.

Usually the variables in a correlational study are not ones that the researcher tries to manipulate as in an experimental study. In the previous example, the researcher just determined how much each subject practiced and how well each subject performed the task. Many correlational studies deal with the relationship between a subject classification variable (e.g., height, weight, gender, age, income,

TABLE 6.1 Example of Percentile Rank Norms for a Ten-Point Test											
TEST SCORE	0	1	2	3	4	5	6	7	8	9	10
PERCENTILE RANK	3	8	15	30	42	55	65	74	80	91	100

education) and a variable of interest to the researcher. For example, what is the relationship between age and beliefs concerning use of leisure time?

Sometimes correlational studies involve three or more variables, and the purpose of the research is to determine how well one of the variables can be predicted by some combination of the other variables. For example, how well can college grade point average be predicted by high school grade point average and SAT scores?

Correlational studies can be conducted to try to explain why subjects differ on a variable. This is a regression approach to a correlational study. Why don't all dancers execute a dance move with equal skill? Part of this difference in ability among dancers is explained by differences in amount of training, percent body fat, flexibility, and leg length to body height ratio. Wouldn't it be interesting to find that the leg length to body height ratio explained much of the difference among dancers in executing a move and that ability had little to do with things like amount of training, percent body fat, or flexibility?

Normative

Norms are standards of performance. The purpose of normative research is to develop performance standards. Performance standards are developed on a large representative sample from a population; these standards then are applied to other samples from the population.

Standards can be **norm referenced** or **criterion referenced.** The majority of standards have been norm referenced, but this discussion will consider normative research contributing to the development of either type of standard. Norm-referenced standards are designed to rank order individuals from best to worst and are usually expressed in **percentile ranks.** Test scores commonly achieved are presented in charts; for each test score there is a percentile rank indicating the percent of the subjects in the norming group who scored below that test score. Standards published with most physical fitness tests prior to 1980 and many other nationally distributed tests are norm referenced. An example of norm-referenced standards is presented in table 6.1. Measurement books such as Baumgartner and Jackson (1995) detail how to develop norm-referenced standards.

Criterion-referenced standards are a minimum proficiency or pass-fail standard. Drivers license test standards, Red Cross lifesaving and first aid certification standards are criterion referenced. Many physical fitness tests now have criterion-referenced standards. For example, if the criterion-referenced standard for passing the written drivers license test is 70 percent the examinee must answer at least 70 percent of the test questions correctly to pass. Any percentage from 0 percent to 69 percent is failing, and any value from 70 percent to 100 percent is passing.

Observational

This is research where the data are observations of people or programs. For example, five days a week for eighteen weeks a researcher observed a community recreation program and wrote down everything he observed. At the end of the eighteen weeks the researcher wrote a report based on those recorded observations.

With this type of research, data collection and analysis is quite time consuming and involves considerable technique. Formal training and practical experience are necessary before this type of research can be attempted.

Observational research has gained in popularity within HHP since 1980. It is discussed in detail in chapter 9 (Qualitative Research).

Action

Action research is conducted in the natural setting where it will be applied. Thus, it lacks some of the control possible with other types of research, but the results of the research are certainly correct for the setting. Action research is always conducted to try to find an answer to a problem that exists in the natural setting. Practitioners who constantly strive to do a better job are actually performing an informal type of action research. An example of action research could be the testing of a new approach to interest students or adults in starting a fitness program. Isaac and Michael (1981, 56–58) contrast formal research, action research, and the casual approach to solving problems; they characterize action research as less precise and demanding than formal research, but superior to the casual approach.

Ex Post Facto

Ex post facto research is research conducted using data that were generated before the research study was ever conceived. It is **"after the fact" research,** looking for relationships or explanations for certain things that presently exist by looking at data from the past. For example, looking at differences between heavy drinking and non-drinking 18-year-olds based on information kept on file about these individuals over the last eight years is ex post facto research.

Isaac and Michael (1981) present a thorough discussion of this research method, also referring to it as causal-comparative research. Best and Kahn (1989) warn that just because two variables are related does not mean that a cause-and-effect relationship exists, with one variable causing an effect on the other variable. Several research books in education (Wiersma 1991; Van Dalen 1979; Best and Kahn 1989) discuss this research approach in detail.

Survey Research

Survey research is the most common type of descriptive research performed in the Health and Human Performance area. For this reason, survey research is discussed further in this section of the chapter. The information presented in chapter 3 under "Measurement Techniques in HHP" and "Questioning Techniques" should be reviewed at this time. Particularly the information concerning scaling techniques (rating scales, semantic differential scales, and Lickert scale) and structured questionnaires applies to the discussion at this time concerning questionnaire construction and use.

In survey research, information concerning opinions or practices is obtained from a sample of people, representing a population, through the use of interview or questionnaire techniques. This information provides a basis for making comparisons and determining trends, reveals current weaknesses and/or strengths in a given situation, and provides information for decision making.

As with most types of research, information obtained by a survey has limitations. Survey information reveals, at best, what the situation *is,* not what the situation *should be.* Surveys that deal with behaviors or attitudes do not reveal the factors that cause or influence the behaviors or attitudes. Further, a survey cannot be used to secure all the information sometimes needed for decision making. Surveys are quite often limited by the sample used and the information obtained. Finally, the information obtained may be inaccurate or misinterpreted.

The many survey methods and techniques used with them make it impossible to discuss all methods and techniques in detail. The author's intent in this section of the book is to provide an overview of the methods and to discuss some of the more common techniques. Books are available on the survey method and the techniques involved with it. Sudman and Bradburn (1988) have written a practical guide to questionnaire design. Sage Publications (1996) list many excellent publications in their catalog dealing with survey research, survey construction, phone interviews, personal interviews, attitude measurement, and much more.

Preliminary Considerations in Planning a Survey

As in all types of research, the objective in planning the survey is to try to ensure that the data collected will be pertinent to the research question or problem. Survey research is performed no more easily or quickly than any other type of research. Sufficient training and experience in doing survey research, plus considerable planning, is necessary.

One consideration is whether the survey method is the most appropriate way to investigate the research problem. Survey research can be very time-consuming and financially expensive, so estimates of the time and cost should be made early in the planning stage. Finally, survey research can be conducted by phone interview, personal interview, administered questionnaire, or mailed questionnaire; planning should involve consideration of which survey method is best.

Survey Methods

Phone interviews are not often used by researchers in HHP as the primary data collection method. Personal interviews are becoming more prevalent. Administering a questionnaire to a group of subjects is a technique commonly used in the field. However, the mailed questionnaire to a sample of subjects is the method more often used than any other.

Phone Interview.   Marketing research, a form of survey research, and product sales commonly take place over the phone. Why do people in marketing research always call you at dinner time? Because you are likely to be home and probably have not been home all day. This is a phone interview technique: Call when people are home and are probably willing to talk to you. Don't call at 3:37 A.M., although people are usually home. When the phone is answered, the caller has about ten seconds to say something to get the person's attention, or the individual is likely to hang up. This is also a technique: What questions do you ask the person, and in what order do you ask the questions? How long can you hold a person's attention on the phone? Ask questions that require a short answer, and plan how to record the person's answers. So, there is considerable planning and technique in doing a phone interview. Much of the planning and technique for doing a phone interview is the same as that for doing a personal interview.

What are the advantages of a phone interview over other survey techniques? Phone interviews are quick and inexpensive when the sample is spread over a wide geographical area. But the method does not allow for very many questions to be asked, and recording the answers may be difficult. Talk to the survey researchers in business and sociology on campus who do phone interviews. Read the literature on phone interviews. Many of the educational research books address the topic. Babbie (1992) discussed phone surveys and noted that not all people have phones and listed numbers. This may bias phone survey results. However, Babbie indicated that random-digit dialing overcomes this problem and that this technique has gained popularity.

Personal Interview.   In the personal interview the researcher meets with each member of the sample, and based on their conversation, the needed information is obtained. If the sample is small and accessible, this is a feasible technique. When the information the researcher desires cannot be collected by asking a series of questions on paper (questionnaire), the personal interview must be used. For example, an interview is probably necessary to obtain information from a senior citizen about how things were fifty years ago.

What are some things to consider if the personal interview is selected as the data-gathering technique? One issue is how to contact potential subjects for an interview time. Another is the decision whether to use a **structured interview** (asking each subject the same specific questions), a **semistructured interview** (asking each subject the same general questions), or an **unstructured interview** (just letting the conversation develop). The decision is dependent on what information the researcher needs, whether questions can be formulated in advance, and what the subject is comfortable with or will tolerate. Still another decision is how to record the information provided by the subject. Tape recording the interview may be best because every word is permanently saved. An alternative is to take notes during the interview. Both approaches may be unacceptable to the subject or be so intimidating that the subject will not be open or totally truthful with the researcher. A sufficiently experienced or skilled interviewer may be able to just talk to people, and then write everything down after the interview is over and the subject is no longer present. The point is, personal interviews require much more planning and technique than many people realize.

Some of the advantages of the personal interview are completeness of response, ability to clear up misconceptions, opportunity to follow up responses, and increased likelihood that the respondent will be more conscientious with the interviewer present. Isaac and Michael (1981) favor the structured interview because it requires less training of the researcher and is more objective than the unstructured or semistructured interview. They also present some guidelines for interviews. Other useful references for those who desire additional information are Wiersma (1991), Rubin (1983), Henderson (1991), Babbie (1992), and Borg (1987).

Administered Questionnaire.   For a variety of reasons, the majority of survey research conducted in HHP uses a questionnaire as the data-gathering technique. A questionnaire is a series of questions or statements on paper. Each subject is given a copy of the questionnaire. The subject responds to the questionnaire and then returns it to the researcher. If the researcher can meet with the subjects, the questionnaire will probably be administered to all the subjects at one time or to several groups of subjects at several times. However, the most prevalent procedure is to mail or distribute the questionnaire to the subjects, who complete the questionnaire on their own, and then return it to the researcher. Since the majority of procedures are the same no matter whether the researcher administers the questionnaire or distributes it for completion, the majority of information about questionnaires is discussed in the section on distributed questionnaires. Information specific to administered questionnaires is presented here.

If the researcher is unable to get the subjects together at one time or in several groups to administer the questionnaire, the researcher may as well distribute the questionnaire. Often, a researcher seeks permission to administer a questionnaire to an intact group such as a class, school, agency, or exercise program. The other possibility is to organize the subjects so they come together in one or more groups to complete the questionnaire. In either case, a room or facility must be secured for administering the questionnaire. The facility must be large enough to easily accommodate the largest possible group and conducive to completing a questionnaire (i.e., is quiet, contains desks or tables providing a writing surface, has adequate seating, etc.). Some thought should be given about whether pencils and other materials need to be provided. Certainly, what to say to the subjects about the purpose of the questionnaire and how to complete it needs to be planned. How to pass out and receive back the questionnaires has to be thought through. The larger the group, the more important these plans become, particularly if the researcher has access to the room or facility for only a limited amount of time. A common pitfall is to think that a questionnaire that typically takes forty-five minutes to complete can be administered in sixty minutes. All subjects will not arrive on time, giving the verbal directions and distributing and receiving the questionnaire will take time, and some subjects will take more than forty-five minutes to complete the questionnaire.

Distributed Questionnaire.   When the sample is geographically spread or cannot be brought together as a group, the distributed questionnaire is used. Distribution may be by mailing it to the subjects or putting it in their mailbox at work, by handing it to the subjects in class or at work or in some location where they gather, or by having another person distribute the questionnaires for you in classes or on job sites. This will include some planned procedure for having subjects return the completed questionnaire to the researcher. Researchers distribute more questionnaires by mail than by any other method.

Good questionnaire research requires considerable planning and technique and is not something that just anyone can throw together quickly. Professional pollsters and marketing research experts conduct outstanding questionnaire research. Graduate students often do a poor job with questionnaires due to lack of knowledge and sufficient planning.

Everyone receives many questionnaires in the mail each year. The good ones are often completed and returned; the poor ones usually go in the trash. By way of example of the latter, the author once received a poorly xeroxed copy of a questionnaire. One question asked, "Do you belong to TAHPERD?" First, was the question referring to the Tennessee or Texas Association of Health, Physical Education, Recreation and Dance? Second, why would a person living in Georgia belong to either one? The questionnaire was a xeroxed copy of one that another researcher had developed for use in Tennessee. The questionnaire went in the trash.

The following discussion of questionnaire research assumes that the questionnaire is distributed and returned by mail. Questionnaire development, format, distribution, return, and examples are treated separately.

Questionnaire Development.   Questionnaires are used for a variety of purposes, and very often the purpose dictates the type of items (i.e., question or statement) used in the questionnaire. So, item type is one decision to be made in questionnaire development. An item is classified as **open-ended** if subjects have the freedom to respond however they choose. For example, the question "Why did you enroll in this adult fitness program?" is open-ended. A second type of item is **completion;** the subject fills in the blank. For example, "What is your age in years to the last year?" is a completion item. The third type of item is **multiple choice** or **closed-ended;** the possible responses to the item are provided and the subject selects the most appropriate response(s).

Following are two examples of a closed-ended item:

1. Select the response below that best reflects your feelings about the research course you are presently taking.

1. Great   4. Below average

2. Above average   5. Terrible

3. Average

2. Check all of the vehicles listed below that you own.

_____ 1. Car   _____ 4. Motorcycle

_____ 2. Truck   _____ 5. RV

_____ 3. Jeep   _____ 6. Van

Commonly, questionnaires are used to determine opinions or attitudes. Here is an example:

Indicate your degree of agreement or disagreement for each of the following items.

1. Being the best in a group is very important to me.

1. Strongly agree   3. Disagree

2. Agree   4. Strongly disagree

Each item must be carefully written so it is easy to understand and not ambiguous. This takes considerable time if done correctly since the questionnaire must be read and edited several times. Rules and hints on writing knowledge tests generally apply here. The reading level as well as the attention span of the subjects must be considered. Directions for responding to the questionnaire must be presented at the top of the first page of the questionnaire. An example question and response are often provided right after the directions. If the questionnaire is supposed to cover a content area or be all-inclusive, then care must be taken to develop items that cover the necessary area.

Reliability and validity of the questionnaire must be determined *before* it is used in the research study. Validity is the degree to which the questionnaire measures what it is supposed to measure. Just because you developed the questionnaire does not make it perfect. Validity is usually estimated by a jury of experts. The jury should have representation from content experts, questionnaire construction experts, and questionnaire use experts. Hopefully, the jury will find the questionnaire to be well constructed, covering the necessary content, and ready for use. Based on the input from the jury, the questionnaire may be revised and evaluated by the jury again, depending on the extent of the revisions.

Reliability is consistency of response. The researcher wants to be assured that the responses of the subjects to the questionnaire would not be different if the questionnaire was administered to them at some other time. As ideal as it might be to administer the questionnaire to some subjects on two different days to check for consistency of response, this is rarely done. Instead, researchers put several pairs of items in the questionnaire with items in a pair either similar or opposite. Items 6 and 33, below, provide an example of paired opposite items.

6. I like candy.   **33.** I don't like candy.

   1. Agree   1. Agree

   2. Disagree   2. Disagree

The questionnaire is administered and the responses to paired items are examined to see whether they are as expected. No matter whether the questionnaire is administered on two different days or on one day with paired items, an intraclass R as an estimate of reliability either for each item administered twice or for each pair can be obtained (see Baumgartner and Jackson 1995).

The goodness of the questionnaire should be determined before it is used to collect the research data. This is always the case with the validity of a questionnaire just discussed. Some researchers determine reliability using data from the research study. The problem with this is that if the reliability is poor, it is too late to make changes in the questionnaire to improve reliability. Unreliable data are no good, so all of it should be discarded.

As discussed in chapter 3 a pilot study is the best solution to this possible problem. The questionnaire is administered to a small number of individuals similar to the subjects who will take part in the research study, and the reliability for their data is determined. As part of the pilot study, it is a good idea to keep track of such things as how long it takes individuals to complete the questionnaire, whether the questionnaire appears to contain any ambiguous items, and any other factor that could affect the successful administration of the questionnaire. Based on the pilot study, the questionnaire is revised as needed.

Questionnaire Format.   The appearance and layout of the questionnaire is as important as the content. The questionnaire must be professional in the way it is typed, and in the quality of the paper and reproduction or people will not complete it. Items need to be arranged in rows or columns for a neat appearance, ease of completing the questionnaire, and ease of data entry into the computer, if necessary, for analysis. Demographic information such as age, gender, education, and income are often requested on the questionnaire. Since questions about age and income sometimes irritate subjects, demographic questions should be placed at the end of the questionnaire. Irritating questions at the end of a questionnaire are often left blank, but if they appear at the beginning of a questionnaire it may cause the entire questionnaire to go into the trash. In fact, any controversial item should be placed at the end of the questionnaire for the same reason (e.g., "Have you gained a lot of weight in the last five years?").

Answers to closed-ended items that will be computer analyzed need to be numerically coded. Subjects should be asked to check the appropriate item or circle the appropriate number.

Example:

Poor format

What is your gender? _____

Good format

Circle the number for your gender.

1. Female   2. Male

or

Check the number for your gender.

_____   1. Female

_____   2. Male

Closed-ended items are preferable to completion items. Also, it is better to provide choices in the form of nonoverlapping intervals rather than specific values, particularly on items that may have a large number of different values, for which the subject may not know the exact value, where the researcher does not need the exact value, or which may irritate the subject.

Example:

Poor format

What is your income? _____

Good format

What is your income?

_____   1. less than $12,000

_____   2. $12,001 to $18,000

_____   3. $18,001 to $27,000

_____   4. $27,001 to $40,000

_____   5. more than $40,000

Inform the subject whether one or multiple answers to an item are desired (see the earlier example on vehicles owned, p. 139). This is particularly important when the data are going to be computer analyzed because sufficient space must be allowed to accommodate all answers. When multiple answers are possible, each answer choice is treated as if it were an item: A one (1) is entered into the computer if that answer is checked, and zero (0) if it is not checked.

Questionnaire Distribution.   The biggest concerns with distribution are controlling the cost of getting the questionnaire to the subjects and trying to obtain a high rate of questionnaire return. The researcher can influence both. For example, the fewer the pages in the questionnaire, the less expensive it is to mail and the shorter it looks to the subject, the more likely that it will be returned. Generally, there is a tendency to ask too many questions on a questionnaire. No matter what the number of questions, reproduce the questionnaire on both sides of the page and use the smallest readable print size. Even the weight of the paper used can sometimes influence mailing rate.

The researcher is expected to provide a self-addressed stamped envelope for returning the questionnaire. Failure to do so will almost certainly decrease the rate of return. To minimize the postage on the return envelope, ask subjects to respond to all closed-ended items on a standardized answer sheet rather than on the questionnaire and to just return the answer sheet. Standardized answer sheets are often an efficient tool for organizing the data to be entered into a computer. However, if groups are not familiar with standardized answer sheets, their use will decrease questionnaire return rate or result in such poorly erased or completed answer sheets that data will be lost.

A good mailing list is an essential component of distributing a questionnaire. Lists are not always highly accessible. Lists with the name of a person rather than a title (e.g., "department head") are generally desirable. However, if the questionnaire is going to the person presently in the position and there is considerable turnover in the position, a title may be better than a personal name. Check into the advantages and disadvantages of bulk mail in comparison to first and second class mail in terms of cost, speed of delivery, and forwarding because considerable cost reduction is possible with bulk mail.

Researchers can do a number of things to try to improve the percentage of questionnaires returned. To give some idea of the extent of this problem, the expected rate of return is 50 percent; perhaps 80 percent return may be expected from professional subjects who have an interest in the questionnaire results; but only a 10 percent return is likely when surveying the general public. For this reason researchers tend to send out enough questionnaires to ensure a desired number of returns. However, a small percentage of returns makes the goodness of the results questionable. Are the people who returned the questionnaire really a representative sample of the target population? Would the results have been different if more people had returned the questionnaire? It is important to motivate people in every way possible to return the questionnaire. A cover letter with the questionnaire explaining why the study is being conducted and its importance to humanity will improve the return rate. A cover letter signed by an influential person also increases the return rate. Offering to share the results, giving money, a catchy saying ("a penny for your thoughts," and enclose a penny), all help to motivate people to return the questionnaire.

Sending the questionnaire out at a time when people are likely to have time to complete and return it is good strategy. Sending questionnaires to coaches in the middle of their season or to anyone just before Christmas is not wise. Also, one to three follow-up letters sent at two- to three-week intervals after the first mailing, reminding people to return their questionnaire, increases the percentage of returns. Having people put their name on the questionnaire before they return it makes follow-up easier and is to the advantage of the researcher. However, some subjects will not return the questionnaire or will not be totally truthful in completing it if they have to put their name on it. If there are any highly personal items on the questionnaire or any items dealing with illegal activities, do not request the subject's name on the questionnaire.

Example:

How often do you smoke pot?

1. Weekly
2. Monthly
3. Several times a year
4. Never

Law enforcement agencies have been known to confiscate questionnaires dealing with illegal activities. Generally, it is better not to ask for names on questionnaire returns unless you really need them.

Questionnaire Return.   Most survey studies require the use of a computer to analyze the volume of scores. A fifty-item closed-ended questionnaire returned by 350 subjects generates 17,500 scores. So, when questionnaires are returned, scan them to be sure they are ready for data entry. Even if names are on the questionnaires, give each questionnaire an identification number, enter that number and questionnaire data into the computer, check the information for data entry error, and then destroy the questionnaire. Of course, open-ended questions must be analyzed by hand.

Anticipate that some items on all questionnaires will not be answered because subjects will accidentally skip or decline to answer certain items. This is acceptable as long as only a few items on each questionnaire are left blank and it otherwise seems that the subject completed the questionnaire accurately. Some researchers put items on a questionnaire to check for accuracy of subject response and reject those questionnaires that fail the accuracy check. For example, a drug use questionnaire includes a long list of drugs and requests subjects to check the ones they use. Kerosene is on the list of drugs and a subject checks it; the questionnaire is rejected. Unexpected responses to open-ended items are sometimes found. The same drug use questionnaire contained this item: "Is there a big drug problem on campus?" One subject responded, "No!! You can get it anywhere." The questionnaire was not rejected.

Attitude scale questionnaires usually check for accuracy by stating some items positively (e.g., Smoking is okay.) and some items negatively (e.g., Drinking alcohol is evil.) to produce a varied response to items within subjects. In this case, a researcher rejects the returned questionnaire if visual inspection shows that the majority of the items are answered with the same response; it appears that the subject just checked answers without reading the items.

Questionnaire Examples

I. *Poor format*

Listed are activities taught in the physical education department. Please check the activities you have taken at the university. If you check an activity, then please check the skill level you presently have in the activity. "B" is beginner, "I" is intermediate, and "A" is advanced.

ACTIVITY	TAKEN	SKILL LEVEL		
		B	I	A
Archery				
Bowling				
Golf				
Dance				
Swimming				
Tennis				

NOTE: This is a poor questionnaire because much space is wasted, and there is no numerical coding of responses.

Improved format

Listed are activities taught in the physical education department at the university. Please use the following code to indicate your status for each activity.

CODE: 0—Did not take activity
    1—Took activity; presently have beginner level skill
    2—Took activity; presently have intermediate level skill
    3—Took activity; presently have advanced level skill

_____ Archery   _____ Dance
_____ Bowling   _____ Swimming
_____ Golf   _____ Tennis

II. *May I have about five minutes of your time?*

I need your assistance.

This is my dissertation research. The purpose of the study is to determine what faculty members think are important attributes in a department head. Using the scale shown below, please rate the importance of each attribute of a department head. Then return your ratings in the enclosed addressed, stamped envelope.

Importance Rating Scale

Not Important At All							Extremely Important
1	2	3	4	5	6	7	

Attributes

_____ Friendly
_____ Professional
_____ Organized
_____ Good looking

III. *Using the key below, rate each task by putting an "X" in the face that best represents your feeling.*

KEY   ☺ I know that I have the ability to perform the task.

☺ I am not sure that I have the ability to perform the task.

☹ I know that I don't have the ability to perform the task.

1. How do you feel about your ability to dribble a ball without your opponent getting it away from you? ☺ ☹ ☺

2. How do you feel about your ability to do a front roll? ☹ ☺ ☺

Note: This questionnaire can be scored 3–2–1 from smile to frown; the faces follow no pattern from item to item; faces can be used with young children.

IV. *What are the four biggest problems in our discipline today?*

Note: This is an open-ended question because the researcher does not know all the problems and probably does not have enough space on the questionnaire to list all the problems.

V. *What was your undergraduate degree major?*

VI. *An example of a questionnaire is presented in example 6.1.*

EXAMPLE 6.1
Example Questionnaire

The AAHPERD Fitness Tests Opinionnaire

The American Alliance for Health, Physical Education, Recreation, and Dance (AAHPERD) presently distributes the Youth Fitness Test (used by the President's Council on Physical Fitness and Sport) which was introduced in 1957 and the Health Related Physical Fitness Test which was introduced in 1980. AAHPERD must decide whether to continue to distribute the two tests, combine the two tests into one test, or discontinue one test. Numerous groups and committees have given AAHPERD their recommendations. However, public school physical education teachers have had very limited input on this important issue. This is your opportunity to make your views known. What AAHPERD does will influence what fitness tests are available to you in the future.

Funded by: Georgia Association for Health, Physical Education, Recreation, and Dance

Endorsed by: American Alliance for Health, Physical Education, Recreation, and Dance; State Consultant for Physical Education, Georgia Department of Education

This opinionnaire should take less than 15 minutes to complete. Please complete each question and return it today in the stamped, self-addressed envelope.

Thank you,

Dr. Ted Baumgartner
The University of Georgia

EXAMPLE 6.1
Continued

For your information, the Youth Fitness Test is considered a motor fitness test (fitness to participate in physical activities). The Health Related Physical Fitness Test is considered a fitness test for healthy living (throughout life). The items in these two tests and what each item is supposed to measure are presented below:

Attribute Measured	Youth Fitness	Health Related
Cardiorespiratory endurance	Distance run	Distance run
Abdominal strength	Sit-ups	Sit-ups
Arm and shoulder-girdle strength	Pull-ups or flexed-arm hang	
Leg power	Standing long jump	
Body composition		Skinfolds
Flexibility (of lower back and hamstrings)		Sit-and-reach
Speed	50-yard dash	
Agility	Shuttle run	

1. Are you aware of the Youth Fitness Test (due to college classes, reading, workshops, etc.)? (circle number)   1. Yes   2. No

2. Have you administered the Youth Fitness Test within the last three years? (circle number)   1. Yes   2. No

3. Does your school or school system require that you administer the Youth Fitness Test on a regular basis? (circle number)
    1. Yes   2. No

4-a. If you were given the choice, would you administer the Youth Fitness Test on a regular basis? (circle number)   1. Yes   2. No
    3. I do not have enough information about the test to decide.

4-b. If you answered *no* above, circle *one* or *more* reasons why you do not plan to use the test. (circle number(s))

    1. Too time-consuming   2. Too unfamiliar
    3. Lack of equipment   4. Not in line with program objectives
    5. Not sufficiently motivating 6. Not valid
    7. Not enough space   8. Other (specify) _____
    _____

5. Are you aware of the Health Related Physical Fitness Test (due to college classes, reading, workshops, etc.)? (circle number)
    1. Yes   2. No

EXAMPLE 6.1
Continued

6.   Have you administered the Health Related Physical Fitness Test within the last three years? (circle number)   1. Yes   2. No

7.   Does your school or school system require that you administer the Health Related Physical Fitness Test on a regular basis?
(circle number)   1. Yes   2. No

8-a.   If you were given the choice, would you administer the Health Related Physical Fitness Test on a regular basis? (circle number)
1. Yes   2. No
3. I do not have enough information about the test to decide.

8-b.   If you answered *no* above, circle *one* or *more* reasons why you do not plan to use the test. (circle number(s))

1. Too time-consuming	2. Too unfamiliar
3. Lack of equipment	4. Not in line with program objectives
5. Not sufficiently motivating	6. Not valid
7. Not enough space	8. Other (specify) _____

9.   Do you administer some kind of fitness test in your physical education program at least once a year? (circle number)

| 1. Always | 2. Usually |
| 3. Seldom | 4. Never |

For each fitness test item listed below, please indicate if you feel the item should be part of a fitness test battery. (circle a number under *Yes, No,* or *No Opinion*)

	YES	NO	NO OPINION
10. Distance run	1	2	3
11. Sit-ups	1	2	3
12. Pull-ups (boys)	1	2	3
13. Flexed-arm hang (girls)	1	2	3
14 Skinfolds	1	2	3
15. Standing long jump	1	2	3
16. Sit-and-reach	1	2	3
17. 50-yard dash	1	2	3
18. Shuttle run	1	2	3

Finally, we would like to ask a few questions to help us interpret the results and to give you a chance to make comments and suggestions.

1.   Is your school located in a rural or urban area? (circle number)
1. Rural   2. Urban

EXAMPLE 6.1
Concluded

2.   What is the student population of your school? (circle number)
     1. 0–100   2. 101–500   3. 501–1,000
     4. 1,001–1,500   5. Over 1,500

3.   What is your school called? (circle number)

     1. Elementary school   2. Middle school/Junior high school
     3. Senior high school   4. Other (specify grade levels) _____

4.   What percent of your teaching time is spent teaching physical
     education, *not* health education or other subjects? (circle number)
     1. 0–20   2. 21–40   3. 41–60   4. 61–80   5. 81–100

5.   What is your age? (circle number)
     1. 20–29 years   2. 30–39 years
     3. 40–49 years   4. 50–59 years   5. 60 years or older

6.   What is your gender? (circle number)   1. Female   2. Male

7.   What is the highest degree you hold? (circle number)
     1. Bachelors
     2. Bachelors plus 25 quarter (17 semester) hours of graduate credit
     3. Masters
     4. Masters plus 15 quarter (10 semester) hours of graduate credit
     5. Specialist
     6. Doctorate

8.   Are you usually (presently or the majority of the time) a member of the
     Georgia Association for HPERD (GAHPERD) and/or the American
     Alliance for HPERD (AAHPERD)? (circle number)

     1. No, neither organization   2. Yes, GAHPERD
     3. Yes, AAHPERD   4. Yes, both organizations

9.   Is there anything else you would like to tell us with regard to fitness
     testing? If so, please use the space below.

Questionnaire Summary.   Research using a questionnaire as the data-gathering
instrument is quite common in HHP. Considerable information has been presented
concerning construction and use of a questionnaire. For people who will seldom use
a questionnaire, it may be too much information. But for people who will use a questionnaire in their research, it is probably not enough information. A number of excellent sources are available for those who desire more information. All of the following
are enlightening: Isaac and Michael (1981, chap. 4); Wiersma (1991, chap. 7); Best

and Kahn (1989, chap. 6); McMillan and Schumacher (1984, chap. 6); Rubin (1983, chap. 10); Tuckman (1988, chap. 10); and Rubinson and Neutens (1987, chap. 5). Books specific to survey methods and mail surveys such as Babbie (1990), Dillman (1978), and Weisberg and Bowen (1977) are excellent sources.

Summary

This chapter has discussed the purpose of descriptive research and the many types of descriptive research. At a minimum, the student should now have an understanding of why descriptive research is conducted and some of the common types of descriptive research. Students who may conduct or consume descriptive research should have a basic understanding of each type of descriptive research. This chapter was an introductory overview of descriptive research. Considerably more expertise is required to actually conduct a descriptive research study or knowledgeably critique the descriptive research of others than can be gained by reading this chapter.

Formative Evaluation of Objectives

Objective 1   Identify the common types of descriptive research.

1. What are three types of descriptive research commonly conducted in your area?

2. What are several types of descriptive research commonly conducted in HHP?

Objective 2   Identify techniques commonly used in descriptive research.

1. What are four techniques commonly used in descriptive research in your area?

2. When using a questionnaire in a research study, what are five things to do that will increase the likelihood of a successful study?

Historical Research

7

Key Words

external criticism
internal criticism

primary sources

secondary source

Objectives

The historian always hopes to produce a record of the events that have occurred in the past or to generalize from past events those things that may control behavior in the present or future. Historical materials often explain the way the professions in HHP have evolved, the way they are organized, highlight the leaders of the professions, and show what activities and problems have surfaced over the years in the professions.

After reading chapter 7, you should be able to:

1. Define historical research.
2. Compose a statement of the problem for a prospective historical study.
3. Distinguish between the external and internal criticism of a historical study.

The Nature of Historical Research

Using the historical approach, the researcher endeavors to record and understand events of the past. In turn, interpretations of recorded history help to provide better understanding of the present and suggest possible future directions.

Historical researchers, like those conducting experimental and descriptive research, are interested in discovering facts, trying to get at truth. While historians do make observations, they do so through the eyes of other people, those who witnessed a historical event or who wrote about it. Historical studies, like all research studies, involve the collection of data. These data are verified and interpreted following specific standards and then are presented as a report deemed acceptable after critical examination by others.

Historical research is important in HHP. These fields have a common past. A thorough study of the past can lead to an understanding of what each field in HHP has inherited and now serves as its roots. Each field has a history and a heritage from which its depth, tradition, and even its present is derived. History repeats itself. Why we do certain things today is based on what has happened to us in the past. What data may exist concerning the origin, growth, and development of the HHP disciplines? What problems were present and how were they solved? What societal and cultural pressures have affected HHP? What movements have come and gone? Which movements have remained and what form do they now take? Who were the pioneer leaders in each field of HHP? What were their contributions? If all of HHP was once under the umbrella of Physical Education, what was the genesis of the separation into what are now many well-defined fields of study? Who were some of the individuals responsible for the separatist movement? What are the historical justifications for changing the name *Physical Education* to *Kinesiology?* What trends, events, and relationships have dictated this name change?

In seeking data to answer these and other critical questions concerning past HHP history, we will discover that events occurred, ideas surfaced, and people came and went. More importantly, however, a study of the past can let our professions know how they have been shaped by it. What HHP is and what it might become in the future depends largely upon the impressions professionals hold about what HHP used to be and how it developed to the point where it is today. The historical approach is oriented to the past and the researcher seeks to cast light on a question of current interest by conducting an intensive study of material that already exists. Historical research can pull all the information in many scattered sources together in one source. Historical research can put on paper what lies in the memories of older people who were present at historical events. If it is not recorded, the information is lost when these people die. Information from individuals who have for many years attended the Masters Golf Tournament in Augusta, Georgia, can shed much light on that historic event and, in fact, the history of golf in the United States.

It frequently is the case in historical research that the collected data cause us to construct new interpretations of an event or person based on the information gained as a result of study. The assassination of President John F. Kennedy, the matter of whether or not President Zachary Taylor was poisoned, and the origin of the game of baseball are examples of past events whose interpretation has been altered based upon new data. Other historical research is more dramatic and gets higher visibility in seeking to find material not presumed to exist. A good example is the discovery of the Dead Sea Scrolls in 1947 by a group of Bedouins (Best 1981). This was an exciting happening, but such occurrences seldom take place.

Data Control and Interpretation

Historical research differs from other scholarly work because its subject matter, the past, is difficult to capture. This, in turn, makes interpretation of the past unique and difficult. Historical researchers, like those in experimental and descriptive research, utilize data. However, the researcher of history encounters problems with data that are different than those of the other approaches as Fox (1969, 407) pointed out:

1. These data already exist and new data cannot be generated, only found.

2. These data cannot be controlled in the same way they are controlled in the other research approaches.

3. Whatever data are found must be analyzed without clarifying the questions being asked.

In experimental research, for example, we often are concerned about the possible effects of extraneous and intervening variables and we try to control them. This is not possible in historical research. Many factors may have affected the historical data, but the historian can exercise no control over these factors. Typical of the factors that might have affected a document or event are memory, politics, censors, greed, jealousy, ulterior motives, ideology, ego, bias, and discrimination. Thus, historical researchers are faced with two problems in the development of their data. The researchers lack the basic elements of control necessary to produce data of the kind and form they wish, and then they must apply some frame of reference to the data if those data are to be meaningful (Fox 1969, 407).

The historical researcher cannot interpret words and events by using present day terminology. All interpretations must be done according to the meanings of that time. The researcher's task is to take information from a given time period and examine and interpret it from within the societal and cultural perspectives of that period. The meaning of words and use of terms change with time. Using the term *sports medicine* in interpreting the meaning of some athletic training event of fifty years ago would be improper because that term, while in vogue now, did not exist in 1942. Even the term *athletic training* would have to be used in the context of that time and not the way we interpret it today. It is important that the researcher becomes saturated with the educational, political, economic, environmental, and cultural habits of the period being studied. The better the researcher's background knowledge of the time period being studied, the better will be the interpretation of the facts and the more reliable the final report.

Sources of Historical Data

To provide data about the past the historian must obtain considerable reliable information. To obtain this information, the researcher will consult two categories of material: **primary sources** and **secondary sources.**

Primary Sources

Primary source material consists of original documents or remains of documents and physical artifacts, or people who can provide eyewitness evidence where there is no intervening account of an event between its occurrence and its use by the historical researcher. A primary source is connected directly to the event; it is firsthand information. In table 7.1 are presented some examples of various kinds of primary sources.

TABLE 7.1 Primary Sources

OFFICIAL RECORDS	CORRESPONDENCE AND WRITINGS	RELICS AND REMAINS	OTHERS
Laws and acts	Memoirs	Buildings	Photographs
Charters	Autobiographies	Monuments	Folklore
Licenses	Contracts	Sculptures	Ballads
Minutes of meetings	Diaries	Implements	Myths
Committee reports	Original speeches	Costumes	Dances
Budgets	Original manuscripts	Skeletons	Ceremonies
Medical records	Lecture notes	Inscriptions	Anecdotes
Court proceedings	Written eyewitness	Coins	Superstitions
Tax rolls	accounts	Paintings	Video recordings
Wills		Museum pieces	
Attendance records		Facilities	
Certificates		Apparatus	
Diplomas			
Honors and awards			
Report cards			

Primary sources are of the utmost importance. "They are the basic materials of historical research" (Van Dalen 1959, 471). The historian always tries to obtain original material. The use of secondary kinds of informational sources when the primary ones are available constitutes a major mistake in this research approach.

Secondary Sources

Secondhand accounts of historical happenings, hearsay evidence, for example, constitute secondary source material. An interpreter is placed between the researcher and the historical event. This person is not tied directly to the event and, consequently, is not an eyewitness. Typical secondary sources are textbooks, newspapers, abstracts, almanacs, encyclopedias, and bibliographies. It should be noted that a source can be primary in one situation and secondary in another. This is particularly true in the case of textbooks and newspapers. Textbooks in recreation and park administration are normally considered a secondary source. However, if they are used to determine the depth and breadth of the content of such books, they are considered to be primary sources. Stories and written materials change and get taken out of context when repeated or rewritten over time. The good historical researcher has little faith in secondary sources, though they should be studied and checked out for correctness. Sometimes the lack of primary sources will lead the researcher to secondary sources, but this is the exception rather than the rule. In general, a secondary source cannot be depended upon to yield historical truth.

Evaluating Historical Data

Historical data, once gathered, must be critically evaluated to determine whether or not it can be considered as fact and, consequently, as historical evidence. This is a difficult and complicated procedure as the researcher attempts to determine such factors as authenticity, genuineness, worth, and accuracy.

External Criticism

The researcher uses **external criticism** to determine the authenticity, genuineness, and validity of the source of the data. Many questions are asked about the author, the time and place in which the document was written, the prevailing conditions of the era in which it appeared, and whether or not the document was a hoax or a forgery. Is the document on the concept of the right-to-life genuine? Did Dr. Jones really write the right-to-life paper? If he did write it, was he competent? Was he a truthful person? What motives did Dr. Jones have when he came out strongly against abortion and birth control devices and substances? Did his religious beliefs influence his stance on the concept? On what scientific studies did he base his stand? Is this Dr. Jones's original piece of work or a duplicated version?

In applying external criticism, researchers use several methods as pointed out by Rubinson and Neutens (1987, 200):

1. Physical and chemical tests of parchment, paper, cloth, wood, ink, paint, or metal are used to determine the age and authorship of a data source.
2. Tests of signature, script, handwriting, spelling, and type are used to check authenticity.
3. Consistency in language use, in knowledge and technology of the time period, and documentation are observed closely.

Historians today also enlist the aid of the computer in the authentication of historical data. Such was the case in November 1985 when the manuscript of a poem was discovered. The poem languished unnoticed in the Bodlein Library at Oxford University for 230 years. The poem, a love lyric of nine stanzas, was attributed to William Shakespeare. In an attempt to authenticate the poem as Shakespeare's creation, computer concordance was used. This technique reviewed all of Shakespeare's work and told exactly how often and in what context he used every word he ever wrote. Shakespearean scholars were immediately active with their criticism. Many agreed that the poem was too awful to be genuine and that the quality of lines like "Star-like eyes win love's prize when they twinkle," cast serious doubts about Shakespeare's authorship. They thought the poem was unconventional, that the rhythm was clumsy and the rhymes forced, and the style was utterly unlike Shakespeare's early style. One expert, quoted in an article that appeared in the *Bloomington Herald-Telephone,* 8 December 1985, doubted the poem's authenticity and added this comment, "It is something that a hack of some ability would write."

Internal Criticism

Internal criticism assesses the meaning of the content of the document. Interpretations are made to determine the value of the historical data, and the document or event is closely examined to establish its accuracy and worth. Did the event actually occur? If so, did it take place as it was described? How consistent is the writer's account with other reports about the same event? In the right-to-life example, one would seek to determine if Dr. Jones's statements were representative of health, medical, and historical facts. He may have been the true author of the document, but he may have twisted the truth, either accidentally or on purpose. Many of the statements may reflect bias and prejudice, thus negating the accuracy and value of the account. The author's motives for writing a document or describing an event should be carefully examined. It should not be surprising that the writings of medical science researchers and tobacco company researchers differ with regard to the effects of smoking on health. Have the environmentalists taken liberty with the truth when they produce scathing literature concerning the "facts" of human destruction of the environment? Whether the historical event took place is usually quite easily established, but affirming that it happened *as described* is often difficult. In most instances two or more independent sources, preferably primary ones, are needed to verify a historical fact.

Historical researchers, then, use both types of criticism, but especially that of internal criticism. It must be applied to documents, events, and published and unpublished studies in an attempt to avoid conclusions that may end up being quoted and requoted widely, disseminating a great deal of false information over a long period of time.

Oral History

Oral history research is conducted through taped interviews with individuals who are in a position to be able to recall their involvement and perceptions of various events and movements. Much excellent historical data has been obtained by interviewing people who have made contributions to the fields of HHP. Since 1985, the Oral History Research Center at Indiana University has conducted interviews with current and retired faculty members. Data were gathered from the current faculty members on their perceptions of issues as broad as the quality of life of today's professor, as well as more personal concerns regarding rewards and recognition, research and teaching, and strategies and opportunities for career development. Interviewing retired faculty will add a historical dimension enabling the origins of today's academic priorities and problems to be traced and preserving the memories of those who came before.

There are many ways to handle interviews and the information they provide. For oral history purposes, these seem to be the major considerations:

1. All taped oral history needs to be written down and preferably edited by the person who provided the account.

2. When using the interview technique the content should be written from the researcher's notes, verbatim as much as is possible.

3. The questions asked and how they are asked are most important. Leading questions should not be asked. The researcher should aim to draw out the individual's personal views and feelings, avoiding any tendency respondents may have to say what they think the interviewer wants to hear.

4. Interviewing can be tiring for the person interviewed. Several sessions with the same person may be necessary, but should last no longer than about one hour.

5. Let the person to be interviewed know in advance what topics will be covered so that some preparation can be made.

6. The person conducting the interview should have read the literature concerning the topic(s) about which questions will be asked.

7. The interviewer should always be at ease to help make the person being interviewed as comfortable as possible.

8. The interviewer should avoid "small talk." Discussions should adhere to questions concerning historical problems only.

9. Avoid confrontation and second-guessing the person interviewed. Argumentation is not acceptable in oral history interviews.

In analyzing data from oral sources, a strict application of external and internal criticism should be observed. Information provided by the oral source can be very subjective and opinionated. Some people have a tendency to embellish past events to make a better story. With older people, memory can be a problem. The researcher should make every effort to maintain historical standards, at the center of which is objectivity, when evaluating the data and writing the oral history report.

Biographical Research

Biographical historical research presents yet another avenue for the professional in a field of HHP to gain further insight into the background of that field. Studying the life, career, and contributions of former leading scholars, teachers, coaches, administrators, dancers, health educators, and recreators can provide a better understanding of the philosophies and movements that are the foundation of current thought and activity in the Health and Human Performance arena. Nevins (1938, 349) stressed biographical study because it "humanizes the past and enriches personal experiences of the present in a way that history can seldom do." Appropriately, the subjects of biographies have been leaders with outstanding professional credentials, their legacies preserved through careful and objective evaluation of their contributions to their respective fields. At the same time, the heritage of each HHP field will be kept and maintained.

Biographical research emphasizes the use of primary source materials and applies external and internal criticism to evaluate the data. Grosshans (1975) completed an excellent biography on Delbert Oberteuffer and his contributions to the fields of health and physical education. Besides extensive personal interviews with Oberteuffer, she talked to his family members, childhood friends, fellow students, professional colleagues, and former employees. In determining the worth of the data obtained from these individuals, Grosshans applied these questions, originally formulated by Van Dalen (1964):

1. Was the position, location, or association of the contributor favorable for observing the conditions he reported?
2. Did emotional stress, age, or health conditions cause the contributor to make faulty observations or an inaccurate report?
3. Did the contributor report on direct observation, hearsay, or borrowed source material?
4. Did the contributor write the document at the time of the observation, or weeks or years later?
5. Did the contributor write from carefully prepared notes of observation or from memory?
6. Did the contributor have biases concerning any person, professional body, period of history, old or new teaching methods, educational philosophy, or activity that influenced his writing?
7. Was the objective of the contributor to win the approval of succeeding generations or to please or antagonize some group?
8. Did the contributor contradict himself?
9. Are there accounts by other independent, competent observers that agree with the report of the contributor?

The biographer encounters many of the problems typical of most historical research. The following list represents some of the items that can become problematic in a biographical study:

1. Faulty memory of the primary source people.
2. Inability to interview a primary source person of great potential value.
3. Failing to discover a potentially strong primary source person or document.
4. Responses of a living subject of the biography could be biased and could color those of other primary source people.
5. Including too much detail or controversial aspects of the subject's private life might be offensive to family members and colleagues.

6. Difficulty in striking a balance between being too sketchy and including too much detail.

7. Challenge of organizing the data and presenting it in a smooth-flowing narrative.

Hypotheses in Historical Research

Historical studies do not always begin with a hypothesis. If the researcher has no reason or basis for predicting what may or may not be found, then the study will be hypothesis-free. More frequently, however, the researcher develops hypotheses about what the historical data are expected to show. In a 1978 study of the influence that L. B. Sharp, an early leader in the American outdoor education movement, had on the lives and careers of selected educators and youth leaders, Piercy (1978, 3) hypothesized that (1) there is evidence of Sharp's influence on these educators and leaders, and (2) the educators and leaders consider Sharp's personality to be a major asset in his ability to lead. If the gathered evidence supports the predictions, they thus are confirmed. However, they are rejected if the evidence refutes them.

Hypotheses may be formulated in many HHP historical studies. Here are a few examples:

1. The media has had no significant effect on the growth in girls' and women's athletics since Title IX.

2. Increased leisure time in the United States in the past forty years has had no significant impact on the physical fitness of citizens.

3. Socialist thought had a profound influence on the municipal recreation and athletic programs during the period from 1900 to 1960.

4. Religion has had no significant effect on school health education curricula and practices.

Hence, hypotheses are formulated in an attempt to explain historical phenomena. The goal in testing these hypotheses is to extend our knowledge base concerning historical events, people, and occurrences. Historical research must teach.

Historical Research in HHP

Interest in historical research in HHP has flourished in recent years. In each associated field a group of scholars is devoted to the cultural history of that field of study. Physical education developed a sport history discipline that led to the formation of the North American Society for Sport History (NASSH) in 1973. The publication outlet for sport scholars is the *Journal of Sport History.* An increasing number of sport historians are producing a large body of accurate and insightful work. Many of these researchers reside in major universities offering graduate HHP programs through which students can pursue advanced degrees in history. The curricula for these degrees include courses in history, anthropology, sociology, psychology, and philosophy to collectively provide a broad background for quality historical research.

Great strides have been made in recent years by health education and recreation educators to increase interest in historical research. Each field maintains archives and holds symposia dealing with historical research. Societies similar to NASSH are quite likely to be organized in these fields. The majority of historical studies conducted by HHP graduate students have been sport history reports, biographical sketches of leaders, and treatments of the historical development of agencies, organizations, and athletic conferences. A major and continuing limitation for graduate students interested in engaging in historical research has been a lack of sufficient time to complete a historical project. It is difficult to predict in advance just how long the project will take. The search for new data could take years, and the development of concepts and insights in relationship to the data takes additional time. Graduate students, in most instances, do not have the financial resources to permit them to spend an indefinite period completing a degree. Hence, many graduate students in HHP, while they may be interested in history, opt to do experimental or descriptive research projects which usually consume less time than historical work. The fields of Health and Human Performance offer a wide range of topics for historical research. Following is a brief list of varied topics that have been studied by professionals, including students, in those fields:

1. *A Century of Women's Basketball* (Hult and Trekell 1991).
2. "Hanya: Portrait of a Pioneer: The Story of Dancer/Choreographer Hanya Holm" (Andrews and Drake 1991).
3. "George Warren Donaldson: His Professional Philosophy, Influences and Contributions to Outdoor Recreation" (Stoner 1990).
4. "Prized Performers, but Frequently Overlooked Students: The Involvement of Black Athletes in Intercollegiate Sports in Predominantly White University Campuses, 1890–1972" (Wiggins 1991).
5. "The Growth of National Women's Tennis, 1904–1940" (Lumpkin 1977).
6. "William Buckingham Curtis: The Founding Father of American Amateur Athletics, 1837–1900" (Wettan and Willis 1977).
7. "One hundred sixty Years of Rugby Football (1823–1983)" (Caruthers, Fleming, and Willis 1982).
8. "Elmer Dayton Mitchell: Father of Intramurals" (Reznik and Stevenson 1980).
9. "A History of Intercollegiate Soccer in the United States of America" (Baptista 1962).
10. "The Origin and Development of Adapted Physical Education in the United States" (Bishop 1963).

11. "The History of the Indiana State Board of Health from 1922–1954" (Absher 1978).

12. "A History of the Evolution of Health Education as a Specialized Area of Professional Education in Indiana Colleges and Universities, 1816–1973" (Scheibner 1974).

Format for Historical Research

Most theses, whether they take the experimental, descriptive, or historical approach, contain the same basic elements. The historical research format, however, differs somewhat from the other types.

Chapter 1 usually contains the statement of the problem; purpose of the study; need, significance, or justification for the study; delimitations of the study; limitations of the study; and hypotheses (if applicable).

Chapter 2 usually contains sections more often seen in chapters 2, 3, and 4 of descriptive and experimental studies. These include nature of information needed; sources of data; procedures for collecting data; and organization and analysis of data.

Following chapter 2, the researcher may have any number of chapters, each one containing a different aspect of the historical event or person. The final chapter is usually similar to a typical chapter 5 in descriptive and experimental research, including such elements as the summary, implementations, conclusions, and recommendations. Typically, historical theses have more than five chapters.

A good reference for the historical research format is the study by Grosshans (1975) titled "Delbert Oberteuffer: His Professional Activities and Contributions to the Fields of Health and Physical Education." Following is the table of contents from that study, presented as an illustration of the practical application of the historical research format. The study is available through the Indiana University Library.

Sample Format for Historical Research

Chapter

1 INTRODUCTION

Statement of the Problem

Purpose of the Study

Need and Significance of the Study

Delimitations of the Study

Limitations of the Study

2 REVIEW OF RELATED LITERATURE AND PROCEDURES

Nature of Information Needed

Sources of Data

Procedures for Collecting Data

Organization and Analysis of Data

3 OREGON CHILDHOOD

Childhood and Early Education

Reed College and W.W. II

4 THE MAKING OF AN EDUCATOR

The Undergraduate Years

The Master's Degree Year

Teaching at the University of Oregon

Earning the Ph.D.

A Job in Ohio

The "First" Book

5 AN OPPORTUNITY IN OHIO

State Supervisor of Health and Physical Education

The Ohio Course of Study

The Move Across Town

6 DELBERT OBERTEUFFER AT THE OHIO STATE UNIVERSITY

Introduction

Katharine Hersey Oberteuffer

The Graduate Program

Committee Participation

The Fullington Committee

The Council on Instruction

Basic Tenets in the Classroom

Student Reactions

The Influence of Delbert Oberteuffer Upon His Students

Chairmanship Responsibilities

Faculty Appointments

Basic Service Program

Summarization of Chairmanship

The Resignation

The Retirement

7 PHYSICAL ACTIVITIES CULMINATING IN THE GULICK AWARD

Fundamental Viewpoints in Physical Education

Physical Education

Author and Orator

8 EARNING THE HOWE AWARD IN HEALTH EDUCATION

Fundamental Viewpoints in Health Education

ASHA Editorship

The Separation of the ASHA–APHA National Conventions

The Leader

9 FORMULATION OF LIFE-LONG POINTS OF VIEW

John Freeman Bovard

Harry Alexander Scott

Jesse Feiring Williams

10 DELBERT OBERTEUFFER: AN APPRAISAL

Post Retirement Honors

The Public Speaker

Gratifying Moments as a Public Speaker

"The Judge"

Other Job Opportunities

Professional Strengths and Weaknesses

Major Contributions to Health Education

Major Contributions to Physical Education

11 SUMMARY, IMPLEMENTATIONS, CONCLUSIONS, AND RECOMMENDATIONS

Summary

Implementations

Conclusions

Recommendations

BIBLIOGRAPHY

APPENDIX

Appendix A: Copy of Interview Questions Used by the Investigator in Personal Interviews

Appendix B: List of Personal Interviews Conducted by the Investigator

Appendix C: List of Persons Contributing Data Through Personal Correspondence

Appendix D: Copies of Letters Used in Collecting Data

Appendix E: Unpublished Materials Utilized in the Study

VITA

Summary

Historical research is characterized by searching for facts about past events. This information is most often used to (1) understand the past and (2) help to understand the present and provide future directions. Data in historical research cannot be controlled in the same way as in descriptive and experimental research. The reliability and validity of historical data are tested through the processes of external and internal criticism. An attempt has been made in this chapter to show how the typical historical research format differs from that used in the other research approaches.

Formative Evaluation of Objectives

Objective 1   Define historical research.

1. To what does the term history refer?
2. How does it relate to your special area of HHP?

Objective 2   Compose a statement of the problem for a prospective historical study.

1. Write a statement of the problem for a historical study in some aspect of your special area of HHP.

Objective 3   Distinguish between the external and internal criticism of a historical study.

1. How is external criticism implemented? Internal criticism?
2. Select a historical research topic and illustrate how you would employ each type of criticism.

Creative Activities

Key Words

Creative activity

Creative research

Objectives

This chapter contains a discussion of creative activities as an alternative to conducting research. You should be aware that in some areas creative activities are performed rather than conducting research.

After reading chapter 8, you should be able to:

1. Identify when creative activities are used as an alternative to conducting research.
2. List activities that are commonly considered creative.

Introduction

If a person develops or produces something new, unique, or beautiful, some people call it **creative research;** others call it **creative activity.** Creative research, or creative activity, is given a chapter of its own in this text because it is important to be aware of the possible alternatives in situations where research is a job requirement.

In the first edition of their introduction to research text, Thomas and Nelson (1985) included a chapter titled "Creative Research." This may have been the first time creative research was included as a research classification in such a text. The chapter was eliminated in their second edition.

At many colleges and universities, promotion is based partially on research productivity in the form of research publications. However, at many of these institutions the promotion guidelines list the requirement as "research or creative activity." That reference has allowed faculty members in fine arts departments to substitute creative activities for research productivity. Generally, faculty members outside fine arts departments have not been allowed to make this substitution.

So, what is creative research or creative activity in a fine arts department? For an artist, it is producing a beautiful picture; for the sculptor or potter, it is producing a beautiful object. Creative activity for the musician is playing beautiful music or writing beautiful music. The individual in dance or drama who performs at a very high level or produces outstanding dances or plays is engaging in that particular form of creative activity.

Creative research or creative activities are not restricted to a fine arts department. The writer who produces a best-seller or the poet who produces an outstanding poem or book of poetry would seem to qualify as having been creative. There are numerous examples of creativity, some of which will be discussed later in the chapter.

At the University of Georgia the graduate faculty in the School of Health and Human Performance met to discuss what constitutes research. They decided that creative involvement should be considered a creative activity and not referred to as creative research. Further, the group recognized that creative activities, as an alternative to research productivity, may be appropriate in the department of dance. So, for the rest of the chapter the term used will be "creative activity."

People in health and human performance who publish in research journals about their creative activities are credited with doing research, although it may not be called creative research. Thus, it seems that writing for publication about a creative activity conducted in a manner that resembles research seems to be an important criteria for determining whether a creative venture is considered creative activity or research. Within the historical-descriptive-experimental system of classifying research, most creative activities leading to publication are descriptive. Isaac and Michael (1981) present nine basic methods of research: (1) historical, (2) descriptive, (3) developmental, (4) case or field, (5) correlational, (6) causal-comparative, (7) true experimental, (8) quasi-experimental, and (9) action. Again, creative activities best fit under their descriptive method heading. They describe the purpose of the descriptive method as being to portray, in a systematic, factual, and accurate manner, a situation or area of interest. Thus, creative activities described factually and accurately might be considered research. Most of the creative activities typical of fine arts departments (creating a beautiful object or performance) probably could not or would not be described in a journal article, and thus would not qualify as research. Thus, creative activities are accepted as an alternative to traditional research productivity in certain situations.

Examples in HHP

Earlier in the chapter it was suggested that creative activities take place in the health and human performance discipline. Many faculty members in dance, as members of dance departments or physical education departments housed within schools or colleges of HHP, engage in the same type of creative activities as dance faculty members in fine arts departments. They may be very skillful performers or be skilled at choreographing dance movements. The development of large and complex computer programs for computer-assisted instruction or for some application could be considered a creative activity. Developing, perfecting, or performing a new gymnastic move or routine could be classified as a creative activity. In fact, if a mechanical analysis of a new gymnastic routine was conducted, it would be considered research. Finally, developing a new piece of equipment or a new procedure is certainly creative. Usually, a description of the procedures followed and the results obtained in developing the new equipment or procedure is published, so it qualifies as research.

Procedures and Evaluation

Procedures for executing a creative activity and evaluating that activity vary considerably depending on the type of activity and the context within which it takes place. First, we will discuss how procedures and evaluation take place in fine arts departments because they have been doing it for a long time and may serve as a model. Then, procedures and evaluation in other departments will be discussed.

Fine Arts Departments

In fine arts departments the artist, sculptor, and potter produce their art object. Their art objects are displayed at shows or exhibits where one or more well-qualified judges or critics evaluate the art object. The quality of the art object is established based on these evaluations. The more art objects a person produces and the higher the evaluations of these art objects, the more highly a person is judged in terms of their creativity or capability. One problem in this procedure occurs when the art object is very heavy or large in size; a two-ton statue or mural is difficult to transport to a show or exhibit.

The music, dance, and drama person in fine arts may face a slightly different situation. These people may either perform themselves or produce the music, dance, or play that others perform. If they themselves perform, their situation is the same as that of the artist, sculptor, and potter. If on the other hand, they produce an artistic work that others perform, how the artistic work is evaluated is dependent on the skill of the performers. Highly skilled performers can make an average artistic work look great, and average skilled performers can make an excellent artistic work look average. In addition, problems and great expense arise with transporting instruments, costumes, props, and backdrops (not to mention large groups of people) great distances to regional and national competitions for judges to evaluate the artistic work. More will be said about some of these problems when discussing procedures for developing a dance and having it evaluated.

Dancers choreograph a dance. This involves selecting the music for the dance and developing the dance by recording each step and movement every dancer will execute. This takes a vast amount of time and energy. Once this stage has been accomplished, the dancers are taught the dance and are rehearsed until they are ready to perform. Some time prior to performance, the costumes for the dancers must be selected and obtained, the lighting of the dance must be established, and props and scenery or backdrops for the dance must be built or bought. Ultimately, the dance must be performed and evaluated if the choreographer is to receive credit for creative activities.

As indicated earlier, the skill of the dancers affects how well the dance is executed. Also, the budget for the dance costumes, scenery, music, and lighting influence how the dance looks. Ideally, a well-qualified and recognized dance critic would be readily available to evaluate the dance on its merits alone, allowing for the ability of the dancers and any budget restraints affecting the appearance of the dance and dancers. However, such resources are uncommon on many university campuses, so less-qualified and less-recognized dance critics are used. Or, dance critics are used who have outstanding credentials but apply the same standards they use to evaluate professional dance company performances. Budget restraints usually make it difficult to take the dance to regional or national competition. Asking another member of the dance faculty to evaluate the dance choreographed usually causes problems because the person is not a recognized authority, others suspect the evaluation is overly high, the choreographer thinks the evaluation was too critical and faculty personal relations may suffer. Some choreographers choose to have the dance professionally taped and then mail it to a recognized authority for evaluation. Not only is this a tremendous expense for the choreographer, but much of the quality of the dance is lost on a tape.

Other Departments

Development and evaluation of computer programs may vary considerably depending on the type of program developed. However, generally a large amount of time is spent in developing, correcting, and refining the program. Finally, a user's manual and possibly a sample printout for the program are developed. If the program is intended for computer-assisted instruction, formal construction procedures and evaluation techniques are typically required. Programs designed to perform a particular function, such as calculate a particular statistic or needed value (e.g., percent body fat or center of gravity) or store a particular set of information (e.g., all information about participants in an exercise program) are usually evaluated in terms of need for the program, correctness of the program, ease of use when inputting information, ability to catch user mistakes in following the directions, completeness of the printed output, and quality of the program directions and description manual. Two examples of computer programs developed in the area of health and physical performance are Kramer (1970), who developed a computerized system for analyzing and evaluating performance data, and Prusoczuk and Baumgartner (1986), who developed a program to calculate and sum T scores for multiple measures on each person. A T score program by Ross and Dill (1986) and a modification of that program by Gaunt (1987) have also been developed. Generally, a journal article or paper presentation on the computer program are required to get credit for it as research or a creative activity.

Research and creative activities dealing with developing new equipment or procedures can occur in numerous ways depending on the situation and what is being developed. Generally, the equipment or procedure is developed and refined. Then the goodness of it in terms of validity, reliability, objectivity, practicality, and usefulness is determined. To receive much credit for the research or creative activity an article about it must be published or a presentation about it must be made at a professional meeting. A few examples are presented below.

Baumgartner (1978) developed a modified pull-up as an alternative to the traditional pull-up because so many people cannot execute even one pull-up. Green, East, and Hensley (1987) developed a golf skill test battery because a good test battery was needed. McClenaghan and Williams (1986) developed a system to quantify dynamic stability. Brennan (1983) developed some measures of dance creativity and determined their reliability. Numerous other examples of test development can be found in the published literature as well as numerous references to unpublished tests.

Standards and Documentation

What follows are excerpts from The University of Georgia Guidelines for Appointment, Promotion, and Tenure (1995) in regard to creative activities. Notice that "the standard" is for creative activities in the fine arts, architecture and landscape design, and the performing arts. Notice that research or creative activities are expected of all faculty, and high quality is more important than quantity.

The Standard

Creative activities include innovative work in the fine arts, for example, the production of original paintings, sculptures, ceramics, musical compositions, novels, plays, poetry, and films; the development of plans for projects in architecture and landscape design; and fresh interpretations in the performing arts of music, drama, and dance.

Inquiry and originality are central functions of the University. Faculty are to discover new ideas, to fashion new interpretations of enduring ideas, and to participate in the application of these ideas. Consequently, faculty should conduct research or engage in other creative activities appropriate to their disciplines and to the missions of their promotion/tenure units, and they should disseminate the results of their work through media appropriate to their disciplines.

Faculty whose work assignments include research or other creative activities should clearly demonstrate high quality in these endeavors. The University distinguishes between the routine and the outstanding as judged by the candidates' peers at The University of Georgia and elsewhere. The principal standard should always be quality, rather than quantity.

Documentation

Evidence of creative activities includes, but is not limited to, the sources listed on page 170. In joint endeavors, the evidence should specify the extent of each person's contribution.

1. Honors and awards for creative activities.
2. Generation of creative products and values.
   a. Exhibitions of art works at important galleries when juries of recognized artists or critics select work on the basis of rigorous review.
   b. Performances in prestigious recitals or productions when appropriate judges select performances on the basis of stringent auditions.
   c. Membership on editorial boards reviewing publications, juries judging art works, or juries auditioning performing artists.
3. Acknowledgment of creative activities.
   a. Membership on teams making artistic recordings of important events or engaging in the delivery of technology through involvement in development projects.
   b. Special fellowships for artistic activities.
   c. Invitations to testify before governmental groups concerned with creative activities.
   d. Appointments as consultants to state, national, and international groups engaged in artistic endeavors.
   e. Selection for membership on the Graduate Faculty.
   f. Assessment of quality by recognized leaders in the discipline.
4. Obtaining grants related to creative activities.
   a. Competitive grants and contracts to finance the development of ideas, when these grants and contracts are subject to rigorous peer review and approval.
   b. Membership on panels reviewing proposals for grants and contracts.
5. Election to offices, committee activities, and important service to professional associations and learned societies, including editorial work and peer reviewing as related to creative activities.
6. Departmental and institutional governance and academic policy and procedure development as related to creative activities.

Evidence of the creative activities listed is not all-inclusive but is excellent in that it clearly indicates there are many ways to document productivity.

Creative Activities for Graduate Students

Since research or creative activities are accepted for college professors it would seem that, in some situations, creative activities should be acceptable for graduate students. Creative activities for graduate students can be developed using the same guidelines set for faculty and using the Master of Fine Arts (MFA) requirements. Most MFA programs require a creative project and a paper explaining the project. The creative project must be evaluated. The paper must explain how the final outcome of the creative activity (e.g., dance, art piece) was developed and provide background on why the final outcome was developed in the manner it was. Every aspect of the development of the final outcome of the creative project is defended based on literature review, experience, trying several alternatives, and so forth. Depending on the situation, it would seem that an evaluation of the creative activity of a college professor could require an assessment of the outcome and a document explaining the creative activity, just as is required of a graduate student.

Summary

One objective of this chapter was to make the reader aware that, in some situations, there is an alternative to research called creative activity. In fact, some publications and presentations about creative activities suggest that certain research could be classified as creative. However, creative research might really be a form of descriptive research.

A second objective of this chapter was to explain what constitutes creative activities in fine arts departments and what might be considered creative activities in other departments. Some of the issues and problems associated with creative activity, as an alternative to research, were presented.

Formative Evaluation of Objectives

Objective 1   Identify when creative activities are used as an alternative to conducting research.

1. In what areas and in what situations are creative activities used as an alternative to conducting research?
2. How often are creative activities used as an alternative to conducting research outside of the arts areas?

Objective 2   List activities that are commonly considered creative.

1. What are five activities that are usually considered creative?
2. Are there any activities in your area that might be considered creative?
3. If a person conducted an activity that might be considered creative but the person published an article in a journal about the activity, would this activity be classified as creative or conducting research?

Qualitative Research

Key Words

Confirmability
Core variable
Credibility
Critical theory
Dependability
Ethnographic research
Feminist theory
Field notes
Field research
Focus group interviews

Grounded theory
Inductive
Interpretation
Interview schedule
Key informants
Member checks
Naturalistic inquiry
Non-participant observers
Participant-observers
Phenomenology

Probes
Reflective field notes
Structured interviews
Symbolic interaction
Thick description
Transferability
Triangulation
Typology
Unstructured interviews

Objectives

After reading chapter 9, you should be able to:

1. Define qualitative research and its most frequently used synonyms, such as ethnography, naturalistic inquiry, and field research.

2. Outline differences between qualitative and quantitative studies.

3. Identify major theoretical frameworks in qualitative research.

4. Outline the general process for conceptualizing a qualitative study, framing the research question, collecting and analyzing data, and writing up a research report.

5. Describe the features of trustworthiness of qualitative data, including credibility, transferability, dependability, and confirmability.

6. Identify questions that can be used to evaluate the quality of a qualitative research article.

The inclusion of a separate chapter on qualitative methods in research methods texts in health and human performance (HHP) areas is a rather recent phenomenon. It reflects an increased appreciation for the fact that some research problems are best answered using qualitative methods. A tutorial appearing in *Research Quarterly for Exercise and Sport* (Locke 1989) served to introduce qualitative methods to its readership, and entire issues of such journals as *Health Education Quarterly* (Steckler,

McLeroy, Goodman, McCormick, and Bird 1992) have been devoted to the subject. Workshops on qualitative methods are common occurrences at national HHP conventions, and textbooks on qualitative research, especially in leisure studies, have been published (Henderson 1991).

When there is a need to understand the context of a phenomenon, or a desire to learn the subject's (or respondent's) perspective, qualitative methods can help the researcher generate detailed descriptive data using **naturalistic inquiry.** The term "naturalistic" in qualitative research denotes being in the natural environment or gathering data on natural behavior. There have been significant numbers of qualitative research studies conducted in HHP since 1980. A variety of problems and questions are addressed in these studies, including questions about teaching and educational organizations, program evaluations, organizational policies such as those to prohibit smoking, and the meaning of such concepts as health, leisure, and movement, to name only a few. The settings in which these studies occur are both domestic and international and include communities, schools, gymnasiums, clinics, and worksites.

The purpose of this chapter is not to provide a primer on the methods and techniques of qualitative research. The terminology itself has no agreed-upon usage, and there is some confusion and disagreement among researchers about appropriate vocabulary and terms. Neither is the chapter designed to be a definitive overview of the philosophy of the paradigm (or research approach), because there is considerable variety in the theoretical perspectives used by qualitative researchers in a number of fields including anthropology, sociology, psychology, and education. Rather, the purpose of this chapter is to describe qualitative perspectives and methods commonly used in HHP and to provide illustrative examples to which the student can refer for further information.

Introduction

Qualitative research is a relative newcomer to education. Until very recently, traditional research methodology in HHP was mostly positivistic-quantitative, objective, deductive, inferential, confirmatory, and outcome-oriented (Cook and Reichardt 1979). This is because these fields have been dominated by the predictive power of the natural science model of scientific inquiry, with less emphasis on historical, philosophical, interpretive, and other social science methodologies. Consequently, randomized field experiments using quantified observations were considered ideal, and most researchers devoted most of their attention to experimental designs and the quantitative methods associated with them.

By the early 1980s, there was growing dissatisfaction with the traditional methods among some researchers, particularly for program and curriculum evaluation. For example, conventional experimental designs were difficult to operationalize into program designs in the field, and they were often unable to detect unexpected positive and negative program outcomes. Curriculum evaluators were sometimes unable to explain why a particular curricular innovation worked, just that it did. Thus researchers in HHP turned to methods used by social scientists that could detect unexpected processes and outcomes, and could be modified according to field conditions.

In addition, some of these researchers began studying phenomena in the natural environment, from the perspective of participants themselves. For example, Griffin (1983, 1984, 1985) conducted a series of studies focusing on student participation in physical education. She developed **typologies,** or categories, of boys' and girls' participation patterns, providing an understanding of behavior styles in the physical education class. Bain (1985) studied students' experiences in a fitness and weight control class. Lawson (1983, 1986, 1989) focused on teacher socialization and working conditions in physical education. Harrington (1986) studied the concept of status conflict and who controls the gymnasium.

These researchers and others used a number of social science concepts, theories, and methods that have generally been grouped under the broad term of *qualitative research.* This type of research refers to the techniques of observing, documenting, analyzing, and interpreting attributes, patterns, characteristics, and meanings of specific, contextual features of phenomena under study (Leininger 1985). Qualitative research methodology has been referred to as holistic, inductive, dynamic, subjective, humanistic, exploratory, and process oriented (Cook and Reichardt 1979).

The Nature of Qualitative Research

The term *qualitative research* is an umbrella term referring to several research traditions and strategies that share certain commonalties. There is an emphasis on process, or how things happen, and a focus on attitudes, beliefs, and thoughts—how people make sense of their experiences as they interpret their world. The researcher is the primary research instrument, and the researcher's insight is the key instrument for analysis. Qualitative strategies enable the researcher to record and understand people in their own terms. Research questions are not framed by delineating variables or testing hypotheses, but most often come from real-world observations, dilemmas, and questions (e.g., Why is this program working well in one school, but not in another?). The data collected consist of detailed descriptions of people, events, situations, and conversations. Depth and detail are revealed through direct quotations and careful descriptions of behavior. This material is usually supplemented by other data such as analysis of official documents, memos, records, photographs, and interviews with additional persons in order to cross-check and fill information gaps. Qualitative researchers collect data through sustained contact with people in their natural settings. They do not consciously intervene in any way or take action to change the situation under investigation. Data are analyzed **inductively;** the researcher builds concepts, explains processes, and develops hypotheses, rather than beginning with hypotheses and analyzing them deductively as in quantitative research. As situations and dilemmas arise during the research process, the investigator records self-reflective field notes about these situations because they may influence data analysis.

Qualitative research is the term most commonly used in HHP to refer to this type of study, but several other terms are often used to describe the study of people, systems, and phenomena in their specific contexts. **Ethnographic research** is sometimes used synonymously with *qualitative approach,* although others use the term to denote a specific type of qualitative research, directed at observing and describing human society and culture. Some researchers, particularly anthropologists, deplore the use of the term ethnography for anything other than long-term participation in and description of a culture, but its use as a synonym for qualitative research in other fields, particularly education, is widespread (see Wolcott [1980] and Rist [1980] for a discussion of this issue). Qualitative research is frequently called naturalistic inquiry (Guba and Lincoln 1981) and **field research** because data tend to be collected in the field by people engaging in and observing natural, ordinary, everyday behavior (Burgess 1982). The exact use of these terms and others such as *interpretive, ecological,* and *descriptive* vary among individuals, disciplines, and settings with no consensus at present. Throughout this chapter we use *qualitative research* and *qualitative methods* as if these terms were agreed-upon and universally understood, but no such implication is intended.

Differences between Qualitative and Quantitative Studies

Both quantitative and qualitative research operate under assumptions that serve as the foundation of their methodologies. While researchers tend to subscribe to one method or the other in formulating their studies, it is important to note that many of the assumptions of both exist along a continuum (Goetz and LeCompte 1984). However, for practical reasons, it is helpful to dichotomize the two paradigms in order to compare and contrast them. Major differences between the two paradigms are listed below (Cook and Reichardt 1979; Merriam 1988; Steckler, McLeroy, Goodman, Bird, and McCormick 1992):

1. The quantitative paradigm uses experimental and quasi-experimental designs and statistical techniques to collect numerical data on a representative population sample. The qualitative paradigm applies anthropological and sociological research methods to understand relevant social phenomena. Data are in the form of words and phrases, and samples tend to be small and nonrandom.

2. The focus of quantitative research is on quantity (how much, how many). The goal of a quantitative investigation is hypothesis testing, prediction, or confirmation. Research is focused on outcomes, and the reliability of measures (e.g., scales, tests, surveys, or questionnaires) is stressed. The focus of qualitative research is on quality (the nature of something; its essence). The goal of qualitative research is

hypothesis generation, understanding, or discovery. Research is focused on elicit-ing an "insider's" view of the group under study, and the researcher is the primary instrument for data collection and analysis. The primary role of the researcher is to be responsive to the context, or situation, to observe, and to ask open-ended ques-tions to determine how people make sense of their lives.

3. Design characteristics of quantitative studies are predetermined and structured. In contrast, qualitative study design characteristics are flexible, evolving, and emer-gent. Procedures and methods often change with the situation.

4. Researchers using quantitative methods distance themselves from the people they are studying in order to maintain objectivity. Qualitative researchers are actively involved with their subjects, immersing themselves in a culture by observing people and their interactions, participating in activities, and asking questions.

5. Quantitative researchers use methods that provide factual, reliable data at the end of the research study that are usually generalizable to a larger group (population). Qualitative methods generate richly detailed data about the group being studied and provide contextual understanding. Results are not generalized to a reference population, although findings can often be applied as an explanation for the behavior of other groups.

Both the qualitative and quantitative paradigms have weaknesses, which to a certain extent are compensated for by the strengths of the other. Qualitative and quantitative researchers have attempted to justify the use of their methods by finding fault with the other. In reality, whether one uses the methods of the qualitative or quantitative paradigm depends on the nature of the research question; in general, questions that ask "who," "what is," "when," and "where" are likely to be answered by using quantitative techniques. Questions that ask "how," "what," and "why" may be more suited to qualitative methods. The research tools of each method are supe-rior to the other under different circumstances. Some studies have several research questions and employ both quantitative and qualitative methods (see Ennis, Ross, and Chen [1992], for example).

Theoretical Frameworks in Qualitative Research

Theory can be confirmed or generated through qualitative studies by providing a strategy for collecting, describing, or explaining data (Henderson 1991). According to Denzin (1978), the function of theory is to give order and insight so that theory and research guide each other. The organizing framework used will take the researcher in a particular direction. Several theoretical frameworks from different disciplines provide guidance for qualitative studies, and five of the most commonly used perspectives are described here. For a comprehensive review of other theoreti-cal perspectives, consult Henderson (1991) and Goetz and LeCompte (1984).

Symbolic Interaction

The **symbolic interaction** perspective has influenced the research of sociologists and anthropologists since the turn of the century, and is used by qualitative researchers as a basis for interpretive research. It assumes that all human experience is mediated by **interpretation** (Blumer 1969), and it suggests that people do not act according to predetermined responses, but rather they interpret meaning and define things through interaction with others. It is based on three premises: (a) that individuals act toward phenomena according to the meaning those things hold; (b) that the meanings are derived from social interactions with others; and (c) the meanings are adjusted according to the individual's interpretation of those interactions (Denzin 1978). Through participant-observation, the researcher focuses on how these interpretations lead to behavior in situations they are studying. How individuals interpret some phenomenon, how important or unimportant it is, the words used to describe it—all are indications of how people impart meaning to objects, people, and events, and this in turn determines how people act. For example, West (1989) used a symbolic interaction perspective to study what physical activity meant to fourth graders from diverse cultural backgrounds. Through participant observation and interview, she determined that competence, commitment, excitement, compliance, and social status were significant in the children's perceptions of self. These perceptions determined the degree of involvement in physical activity, and were defined and redefined by social interaction with the teacher and with other children. Thus, for the children in this study, the opportunity to enhance quality of life through physical activity was facilitated, restricted, or denied through this social interaction. The study generated hypotheses about the success or failure of physical activity that can be further tested using quantitative methods.

Phenomenology

The goal of **phenomenology** is to describe and clarify subjects' experiences without any previous assumptions as to their meanings. The researcher attempts to gain entry into the conceptual world of their respondents (Geertz 1973), working very hard to bring no preconceived ideas about that world to the study. The concept of phenomenology has influenced the work of sociologists for a century and today offers an important framework for interpretive research. Phenomenologists often use no interview schedule, preferring to maintain maximum flexibility to pursue information in whatever direction appears to be appropriate. Most questions derive from the immediate situation, allowing the interviewer to "go with the flow" (Patton 1980). As Wilson (1977, 249) states, "those who work within this tradition assert that the social scientist cannot understand human behavior without understanding the framework within which the *subjects* interpret their thoughts, feelings, and actions." The strength of this perspective is that it allows the researcher to be highly responsive to individuals and situations. By not assuming they know what things mean to the people they are studying, they often gain extraordinary insight into events and interactions. A weakness is that interviews can be lengthy and may occur over a long period of time.

Williamson's (1990) study of how physical education teacher educators (professors) perceive their relationship with public school professionals (physical education teachers) used a phenomenological perspective. No list of specific questions was used when interviewing participants; instead, over three separate interviews, participants shared their thoughts about the experience of being a teacher educator in physical education. The study revealed professors' awareness of an implicit hierarchy between themselves and school teachers that created a social barrier to collaborative relationships. Based on the perspectives, Williamson was able to make recommendations to overcome the perceived dissonance.

Grounded Theory

Grounded theory is more of a framework for *developing* theory than a theoretical perspective itself. Developed and refined by Glaser and Strauss (1967) and Glaser (1978), grounded theory is a sophisticated form of data collection and analysis that uses comparison as an analytic tool to generate concepts and hypotheses. These concepts and hypotheses are interrelated and grouped to form a whole, much as one constructs a picture shaped from parts individually collected and examined. Parts grouped together form a **core variable,** most often a social process; the analysis then traces the emerging process to identify its stages, dimensions, and characteristics. The final goal is middle-range theory in a specific content area such as pain management. The theory is identified as "grounded" because it emerges from the categories of data. It is particularly useful in areas that lack theoretical development and where there is little previous research.

An example of grounded theory research is Mullen's (1978) groundbreaking work on recovery after a heart attack, using the process of "cutting back" to explain much of what goes on in a patient's adjustment to life after a myocardial infarction. The process of "cutting back" is described in phases given such names as immobilization, estimating and explaining damage, resumption, figuring the calculus of cutting back, and new normal—adjusting to a new identity.

Morgan and Laing (1991) used a grounded theory perspective to clarify the relationship of the concepts of grief and role strain in spouses (caregivers) of persons with Alzheimer's disease. One group's process of grief was described using core variables of "coming to terms," where the spouse exercised such strategies as accepting, letting go, minimizing, protecting, normalizing, adjusting, and preparing. Another group's process of role strain was described as "hanging on," where strategies used by spouses were resenting, organizing, venting, delegating, and ignoring. These two groups emerged during the data analysis process; the nature of the couple's previous relationship was the strongest predictor of the group to which the spouse would later belong. McLachlan (1992), in a study of how family leisure is constrained in families who

Conceptualizing the Research. Ideas for study come to qualitative researchers as they ponder interesting, curious, or puzzling phenomena, which they observe, discover, or stumble across (Marshall and Rossman 1989). This leads to further observation, discussion, and reading, and is the first step in formulating the research question or questions. Studies of physical education classes, school health curricula, leisure program administration, organizational climate, and high school coaches begin with an observation of some phenomenon in its natural context and a desire to observe and record what happens. A plan begins to form from hunches. Some plans are more structured than others, and the particular research tradition from which the researcher is working, as well as the researcher's previous experience, affects how the study is conceptualized. Intuition about the importance of the problem, a feeling of "how interesting it will be to learn about this!" often play an early role. Typical questions at this stage are "What specific approach should I take?" and "What kind of data will I collect?". Ideas about how to gain access to the desired research setting also start to form.

Framing the Research Question(s). The researcher does not begin with a hypothesis to test. Qualitative research starts with observations in the real world that merge to form ideas and give rise to such questions as (1) What does the term "leisure" mean to people? (2) How do leisure patterns change over the course of life? (3) Why is a curriculum not working in this school, even though it is considered highly effective and is nationally respected? (4) What happens to elite athletes or dancers when they suffer a career-ending injury? (5) What is life like for a well-known high school or college coach? (6) What is different about the participants in a health promotion or adult fitness program who finish the course as opposed to those who drop out? Qualitative research questions usually begin with "what," "why," and "how." Most likely, initial research questions will be wide-ranging inquiries that will be refined and reworked as the research unfolds. In a cross-cultural study of the self-care behavior of Danes and Americans with multiple sclerosis (McLaughlin and Zeeberg 1993), for example, the original questions were phrased around whether Danes use alternative therapies to manage their symptoms and promote their health away from the physician. The underlying rationale for the question was based on the fact that Denmark is a social welfare state and all health care is provided for by the government, theoretically negating the use of other kinds of health care. As the study progressed it became clear that Danes used a variety of self-help and self-care strategies including self-medication. Additional questions were framed to learn *why* this occurs, since cost was not a factor. Thus, the approach of qualitative research is one of discovery, rather than the testing of *a priori* explanations and hypotheses.

Collecting Data. Qualitative researchers utilize the data collection strategies of direct observation, focused interviewing, document analysis, photographs, and supportive quantitative data. A strategy is chosen that will most clearly reveal the perspectives of the persons under study; the goal of the researcher is to produce **"thick"**

have a child with Down syndrome, used both phenomenological theory and grounded theory to generate a conceptual framework illustrating the leisure constraints.

Critical Theory and Feminist Theory

These two theories are concerned with the relationship between the researcher and those with whom studies are being conducted. The roots of **critical theory** are in neo-Marxism; as a research perspective it is concerned with the political beliefs of both the investigator and subjects, the purpose of which is to discover what should be done to improve the world of those being studied (Reason and Rowan 1981; Graham 1991; Henderson 1991). Empowerment and emancipation are possible results of the research, often precipitating social action on the part of both researcher and participants. Bain's research project (Bain, Wilson, and Chaikind 1989) of empowerment of a group of overweight women involved in an exercise program is an example.

Feminist theory has influenced qualitative research in the last decade. Because the qualitative paradigm is concerned with feeling and emotion as well as experience, qualitative methods are attractive to feminists who study women's experience from a woman's point of view. Feminism is used as a framework for a qualitative approach in Dixey's (1987) study of women's leisure, which examined why the game of bingo was such an important activity to a group of working class women. As the reasons emerged from the analysis, it became clear that the context in which the activity took place reflected their roles as women. Similarly, Dempsey's (1990) study of women's leisure activity in a rural community demonstrated the relationship of the men's power and how women and their activities were excluded and defined as inferior.

Methods in Qualitative Research

The Process of Qualitative Research

Although the particular theoretical perspective used in the research study will influence the way data are collected, analyzed, and interpreted, the following is a general guide to the process of qualitative research studies. Keep in mind, however, that even the most carefully planned study can end up being designed in the course of its execution. Becker (1970) notes that the finished report is the result of hundreds of decisions made during the research, as unanticipated contingencies interrupt data collection and analysis, as data having nothing to do with the original research questions are collected, and as unexpected findings stimulate new ideas to explore. Thus, a research outline often turns out to be a tentative plan. The following hardly constitutes a recipe for doing field research, but rather is a suggestion for ingredients. The stages are not necessarily sequential but often blend together as the phenomenon to be studied is conceptualized and as data are collected and analyzed.

description, a term coined by Geertz denoting the richest, most comprehensive description possible (Geertz 1973).

Direct observation.   The researcher usually spends extensive periods of time in the natural setting of the participants, observing the events, processes, and activities in which they are involved. The degree to which the researcher takes part can range anywhere from complete observation to complete participation, but most often falls somewhere between the two extremes. Those who become involved in the social system of the setting have the advantage of familiarity with the environment and developing participants' trust; in this role, researchers are called **participant-observers.** Anthropologists who go to a new country, begin to learn the language, and participate in the culture are an example. Researchers who study aspects of the organizations in which they work also fall into this category, but they must exercise caution in negotiating the thin line between involvement in the daily setting and remaining detached enough to observe the process without bias. **Nonparticipant observers** enter the setting as outsiders to observe events and behavior. They are removed from the social process and must find **key informants**—individuals who are especially knowledgeable about what goes on and who are willing to talk with the researcher and provide explanations. Nonparticipant observers must find ways to negotiate and gain access to the setting, as well as earn the trust of participants. Both observers collect **field notes,** the rough, sometimes unorganized, record of the world they are studying. Field notes are the written accounts of what the researcher sees, hears, experiences, and thinks about in the course of collecting data in a qualitative study (Bogdan and Biklen 1992). Field notes are the detailed log of the developments of the study, providing the rich description upon which analysis is based. These notes can be portraits of participants, reconstructions of conversations, descriptions of the setting, and accounts of particular events and activities. Experienced qualitative researchers write notes down as quickly as possible, at least in outline form; then, they transcribe the notes *the same day* while ideas and details are still fresh.

Researcher's written observations of their own behavior, along with their hunches, insights, and revelations are called **reflective field notes.** Since the researcher is the measuring instrument, reflective field notes are used to document efforts to reduce bias, observed effects of the researcher on the setting, and anything else that might affect the data being gathered (for an in-depth analysis on the method of writing field notes, see Bogdan and Biklen [1992]). These notes may appear as a paragraph in the final manuscript, serving as an audit trail to help the reader judge the quality of the research.

Focused interviewing.   Methods of interviewing, too, range on a continuum from formal **structured interviews** to informal, casual **unstructured interviews.** Formal interview structures so rigidly controlled that respondents cannot tell their stories in their own words fall outside the range of qualitative interviewing. Qualitative structured interviews usually employ an **interview schedule,** a guide consisting of a list of open-ended questions flexible enough for the researcher to note unexpected responses and proceed with further exploration. Interview guides are particularly useful in multisubject and multisite research for gathering comparable data.

Casual interviews are often used in observational studies when the researcher needs clarification about what is happening or wishes to document feelings. Some studies, however, use interviewing, including open-ended interviewing, as their main data collection device. For example, the phenomenological researcher encourages respondents to talk generally about the area of interest, probes to expand on topics the respondent brings up, and focuses on issues of interest to the respondent; the subject thus defines the content of the interview. Qualitative researchers select structured or unstructured interviewing based on their research goal. Frequently, both types of interviewing are used at different stages of the same study.

Interviewing requires an ability to put respondents at ease, a skill that requires patience and practice (see Spradley [1979] for a comprehensive guide). Most interviews begin with small talk, then progress to an explanation of the study, a discussion and signing of the informed consent form, and an overview of the way the interview will proceed. Gorden (1975) noted the importance of the opening question in a focused interview:

> There are several important and unique functions of the opening question. It may be broad enough to delineate the entire topic of the interview, or it may select a single point of departure. In either case, it should be clearly connected with the explanation of the interview so that the respondent is immediately aware that the interviewer is pursuing the stated purposes. If possible it should ask for information which is relatively easy for the respondent to give so that there is no chance of ego threat at the outset. The opener may also begin with a point on which the respondent feels particularly qualified to speak, thus appealing to his need for recognition. A well-phrased question might also demonstrate sympathetic understanding of the respondent's problems. (p. 279)

The use of **probes** conveys the researcher's interest in the respondent's statements. They also establish a basis for follow-up with further specific and focused questions in pursuit of the respondent's insights on the social process. Probes include such phrases as "That's interesting, tell me more about it," or "What do you mean by that?"

For short interviews, some researchers rely on memory and wait until later to write down answers. This allows for a very informal conversation with little distraction, but data can be easily lost or distorted. A comprehensive record of the interview can be created by taking notes or using a tape recorder. Taking notes can provide an adequate record, but it can slow the interview down and be distracting to both interviewer and respondent. Tape recording provides a complete account, but makes some respondents uncomfortable enough to inhibit their answers; some individuals refuse to give permission to tape record, and transcription of tapes can be time-consuming and expensive. Researchers who rely completely on tape recording are sometimes horrified to find that the interview is lost because the machine did not work properly. On occasion, the most useful information is obtained after the recorder is turned off.

In some cases it is desirable to interview groups of people to obtain insights into group perceptions, language, and beliefs. Known as **focus group interviews,** they are conducted by a skilled facilitator who guides discussion about topics that are important to the group being studied. Keller conducted focus groups to learn about senior citizens' perceptions of health in old age in order to develop a quantitative instrument (Keller et al. 1987). McLaughlin and Owen (1986) conducted focus groups of teachers who used a high blood pressure curriculum for sixth graders in order to understand what was important to the teachers, what went well, and what did not. Focus groups stimulate participants to freely express their beliefs, feelings, and needs, and are increasingly used in program and curriculum evaluations.

Document analysis.   The researcher is the main producer of field notes and transcripts, but information produced elsewhere can also provide useful data. Bureaucratic agencies such as schools and health agencies produce written reports of internal and external communication that can help the researcher understand how the agency or school is defined by its workers and provide potential insight into internal rules and regulations. Documents such as newsletters, news releases, students' records, minutes from meetings, codes of ethics, and philosophy statements offer insight and understanding into the "official" perspective of the agency or school.

On occasion, personal documents written by respondents can also yield useful information. Intimate diaries and personal letters sometimes turn up in the course of interviewing or observation. Often a respondent will volunteer that the documents exist. These materials can be especially valuable in clarifying what respondents have experienced.

While historians depend heavily on documents, qualitative researchers are more likely to use them to augment information gained from observation or interviews. In profiling a teacher, for example, a journal of the teacher's early experiences can prove invaluable in gaining insight into the teacher's perspectives.

Photographs and Videos.   Researchers use photographs to learn how people interpret their world. They are often available at schools and agencies in the form of newspaper releases and yearbooks, and can provide a useful sense of people no longer present, offering a historical rendering of the setting and participants. They may be helpful in adding to the evidence when used with other data. Researchers also take photographs and video recordings in the research setting. They can simplify the collection of factual information and serve as a record of events; they can give an idea of how people use a space such as a playground. Photographs and videos taken in the field can be a way to help the researcher remember detail, such as room layouts or classroom members. Showing a photograph to respondents can stimulate their insights and serve as a source of data.

Supportive Quantitative Data.   Quantitative data such as attendance counts, numbers of athletic injuries, achievement scores, and epidemiological data can be useful to the qualitative researcher. Such data can suggest trends of increase or decrease, provide descriptive information about the population, and be extremely useful in exploring the perceptions of respondents by asking whether respondents agree or disagree with the information presented. Most qualitative researchers use quantitative data in their studies to explore the context of the setting and the people.

Triangulation (Denzin 1978) is the process of cross-validation among researchers, research methods, and data sources. Cross-checking across different methods such as observations, interviews, and physical evidence contributes greatly to the study's validity. Flaws of one method can often be overcome by using another method; through cross-checking, events and processes for which data is insufficient can be clarified. For example, statements about program participation can be checked against records, or observations in a gymnasium can be clarified by interviewing instructors.

Triangulation among data sources assesses the accuracy of statements from such sources as administrators, students, and faculty. In constructing explanations, agreement among data sources helps ensure the adequacy of the analysis. If data are inconsistent, cross-checking is necessary to determine whom to believe. Triangulation among researchers involves checking the findings of other researchers who are taking similar measures at the same time, or following up a finding with another researcher to confirm it (Miles and Huberman 1984).

However one chooses to collect primary data, it is important to clearly state the researcher's role, because it is one aspect of gaining entry into the field. For example, if the role selected is one of a nonparticipant observer, officials at the research site will want to know exactly what this will involve (e.g., attending formal and informal meetings with respondents, being in the room with classroom activities, conducting casual interviews with students, and examining records and files). Since gaining entry to the field in most cases requires formal permission to conduct the study, most qualitative researchers write proposals that spell out exactly what data will be collected, how confidentiality of data will be handled, and how the setting stands to benefit from the results of the study. Maintaining good field relationships is crucial, and the researcher should attend to building trust and confidence.

Analyzing Data.   Qualitative researchers begin analysis of data almost immediately, and it proceeds along with data collection. Transcripts of conversations or written observations are examined to generate a tentative coding system from which categories of phenomena are derived. When a category is formed, all the incidents and conversations that appear to fit are compared. New categories are formed from old ones when some incidents initially coded for the old one do not fit. Once major categories are in place, the researcher then searches for trends and differences and inductively begins to synthesize explanations and phenomena. Explanations are checked and cross-checked for accuracy and understanding, and are modified to support new information. The researcher usually continues to observe or interview until no new information for codes and categories is obtained, that is, until the data are "saturated" (Goetz and LeCompte 1984). For a basic, helpful guide to data analysis, see Bogdan and Biklen (1992).

Writing Up the Research. Spradley (1979) asserts that what qualitative researchers do when they write their study is a translation. This is shaped by the evidence the researcher has collected and is supported by the words of the respondents. Papers are often written in first person and in active voice. No formal conventions are used to establish truth in a qualitative research paper (Bogdan and Biklen 1992). The task of the writer is to convince the reader of the plausibility of the presentation by quoting respondents, presenting short sections from field notes, and explaining triangulation methods. Alternative explanations, points of view of a minority of respondents, and problems in the study are frequently included to help the reader determine the accuracy and truthfulness of the research. Although the discerning reader will often have questions about the study, a well-written manuscript allows a reader who may not know anything about the phenomena to "see" it through the researcher's explanations and supporting data.

Trustworthiness of Qualitative Data

Qualitative studies are often criticized for their lack of "rigor," for making suggestions rather than reaching conclusions, and for lacking reliability and generalizability. Qualitative researchers tend to think about rigor differently than quantitative researchers, but qualitative studies can be rigorous. Lincoln and Guba (1985) suggest that qualitative data can be evaluated in terms of its "trustworthiness," and that the features of trustworthiness parallel the terminology of quantitative data, including internal validity (credibility), external validity (transferability), reliability (dependability), and objectivity (confirmability).

   Credibility (or internal validity) in qualitative studies is largely controlled by the researcher. Because researchers may not know initially what they want to measure, perfect validity is theoretically impossible since it is difficult to know if measurement is appropriate (Henderson 1991). In qualitative studies, internal validity is related to the emerging theory, and findings should be credible if grounded theory corresponds to observations. To improve credibility, qualitative researchers (1) provide quotes and descriptions that support the conclusions; (2) use corroboration and triangulation techniques; (3) document data with extensive field notes; and (4) use **member checks,** or have study participants comment on the conclusions.

   Transferability (or external validity) in qualitative studies is concerned with the degree to which the individuals studied are representative of individuals to which results might be generalized (Henderson 1991). There is much debate over whether qualitative results can or should be generalized, but qualitative researchers tend to think of transferability in terms of *kinds* of people or units that are examined, rather than *number* of people or units studied. Some researchers think of findings as working hypotheses or theoretical frameworks that can be transferred to other studies (Guba and Lincoln 1981). Transferability can be heightened by (1) careful explanations of the research setting and individuals; and (2) providing thick descriptions of data.

Dependability (or reliability) of qualitative data can be thought of as the closeness of fit between what researchers record as data and what actually occurs in the setting (Kirk and Miller 1986; Henderson 1991). There are those qualitative researchers who believe that reliability can be achieved similarly to the way it is achieved in quantitative studies (Goetz and LeCompte 1984). Others suggest that replicability is not important in qualitative studies because variables are not controlled (Marshall and Rossman 1989). There are a number of things that can be done to increase dependability: (1) carefully document the research plan, especially any changes in the plan that occur; (2) triangulate the methods used; (3) triangulate researchers to gather other data interpretations; and (4) document the researcher's role.

Confirmability (or objectivity) suggests that data are factual and reliable. The objectivity of qualitative studies that are factual and that report the differences in information collected in the study can be assessed by other researchers. Confirmability can be increased by (1) being clear about observations in the final report, and (2) providing several explanations for observations (Henderson 1991).

Judging the Merit of a Qualitative Research Article

While qualitative studies were once presented mainly in book format, they are now likely to appear as studies in research journals. A survey of these journals reveals very little standardization in research reports as yet. Style of reporting varies with the type of study and can range from the well-known format of most quantitative studies to "the creation of an evocative form whose meaning is embedded in the shape of what is expressed" (Eisner 1981, 6). Some qualitative research is so lacking in focus that it appears to have no design. Without standardized criteria on which to rely, the reader may have difficulty judging the quality of the study presented. The following questions have been compiled to assist the reader and provide guidance in evaluating the "quality" of a qualitative research article (Goetz and LeCompte 1984; Chilcott 1987; Smith 1987; Lincoln and Guba 1990; Wolcott 1990).

> What are the study's goals? Purpose?
>
> Are the research questions stated?
>
> Why was this particular research setting chosen? How was entry obtained? How long and how regularly was the researcher involved in the setting? Is the setting described in sufficient detail to communicate a concrete picture to the reader?
>
> What is the period of time of the study?
>
> What evidence does the researcher provide for having obtained trust and rapport with the participants?

Is the researcher's role identified (participant observer; observer; interviewer)?

Who actually collected the data?

Does the researcher report the use of a theoretical perspective? If not, can it be inferred?

How were respondents selected (convenience sample [available subjects]; theoretical sample [selected subjects by plan]; snowball sample [subjects named by other subjects])?

Is demographic information on respondents presented?

Is generalizability of the data addressed?

How does the researcher support the accuracy and truthfulness of the report (participant verification; comparable studies from supporting literature; triangulation of methods, data, researchers)?

How was data collection accomplished (note-taking, tape recording, videotape)?

If interviews were used, what kind were they (structured, unstructured)? When during the study did the interviews take place? How is interview material combined with other data in the study?

Are direct quotations from participants used?

How does the researcher account for possible bias (reflective field notes, discussions with interested colleagues)?

What analytic strategies did the researcher use?

Is the researcher using a participant or personal approach to meanings (*etic* = external, perspective of the observer; *emic* = internal, participants' categories)?

How does the researcher support the stated conclusions? Does the researcher present negative evidence?

Does the report generally make sense (orderly, effective, logical)?

The reader should be able to answer the majority of the questions. The credibility of the results in qualitative studies depends in large part on the researcher's ability to demonstrate value and trustworthiness. This is why qualitative reports explicitly "tell" the reader a great deal about data collection methods and research conditions, including decisions to alter strategies, doubts, and concerns. Some recent articles include a paragraph written by one or more participant(s), particularly if they disagree with the researcher's conclusions; this honest difference of opinion is presented to help readers decide for themselves with regard to the study's credibility (Lincoln 1991).

Uses and Applications of Qualitative Data

Researchers in HHP conduct qualitative studies for a variety of reasons and audiences. An increasing number of qualitative studies have been conducted for purposes of making practical decisions about and improvements in programs, curricula, and practices. Program evaluation research has increasingly involved a qualitative component.

Participant interviews and observations can add richly illustrative information to heighten understanding of the evaluation report. Qualitative methods can provide unique and valuable data about the motivations of participants, their adherence to health and fitness regimens, and their reasons for low participation rates in health promotion and adult fitness regimens, or, alternatively, high adoption rates by others. For example, Steckler, Eng, and Goodman (1991) combined quantitative and qualitative evaluation strategies to evaluate a health education workshop on combating childhood communicable diseases in Nigeria. Using focus groups and participant observation, they were able to improve the workshop's content and methods, and the program has been disseminated to other countries. Howe (1988) reported on older women's adoption of an exercise program for senior adults, identifying barriers and other influences on the decision to adopt the activity. Henderson and Bialeschki (1987) used participant observation to evaluate the perceptions of individuals who participated in a "women's week" experience and described aspects that made the experience a success.

Qualitative research is also useful in pedagogy, the evaluation of curricula and teaching. Ennis and Chepyator-Thomson (1990) used qualitative methods to examine the learning styles of field-dependent children within a movement curriculum. Their observations enabled them to recommend changes in teaching styles to help field-dependent children function more analytically. A large curriculum evaluation project used naturalistic methods to explain results obtained quantitatively (McLaughlin et al. 1992). A randomized control trial of a high blood pressure curriculum for sixth graders revealed that comparable families diffuse information about hypertension differently. A qualitative investigation revealed profiles of "high transfer of information" and "low transfer of information" families, as well as typologies of the children and parenting styles, enabling changes to be made in the curriculum. Maatz-Majestic and Tapp (1992) used qualitative methods to explore strategies used by college students to avoid problems associated with alcohol and to study their definitions of responsible use. Health educators can use this information to develop more effective prevention strategies, because the study points out the need for specific and targeted messages in teaching about responsible decision making in the use of alcohol.

Qualitative methods can be used as a preliminary step to questionnaire or survey instrument design. Interviews with a sample of the survey population one wishes to study can provide insights into the meanings of such concepts as health, wellness, fitness, or leisure, thus enabling the construction of more reliable and valid instruments. Additionally, when researchers wish to study the continuum of behaviors of a population and little is known about a phenomenon, qualitative interviews can help reveal these many behaviors. In a study of self-care behaviors and multiple sclerosis, the researchers wanted to survey persons with multiple sclerosis regarding coping strategies, but the self-care actions that people took to manage symptoms, reduce depression, and promote well-being had not been systematically studied. Qualitative interviews with a sample of respondents uncovered a variety of behaviors for the management of multiple sclerosis and resulted in an inventory with items grounded in the perspectives and experiences of the population of interest (McLaughlin and Sliepcevich 1985). Qualitative research has always included basic work, and its explanatory powers ensure its application to programmatic, curricular, and action research.

Summary

The purpose of this chapter has been to present an overview of the process of qualitative research. Obviously, qualitative methods are not equally easy for all to use; it will be particularly appealing to those who enjoy interviewing and interacting with others. The best way to become a better qualitative researcher is to practice, and many universities now offer courses in qualitative design and research. Qualitative methods offer exciting options for HHP researchers asking questions about complex human issues in programs, behavior, and curricula.

Formative Evaluation of Objectives

Objective 1   Define qualitative research and its most frequently used synonyms, such as ethnography, naturalistic inquiry, and field research.

1. Are there any differences among the four terms—qualitative research, ethnography, naturalistic inquiry, and field research?
2. Which terms are used most frequently in your experience?

Objective 2   Outline differences between qualitative and quantitative studies:

1. List the major differences between qualitative research and quantitative research regarding the following:
   a) form of the data
   b) sample size
   c) focus of the research
   d) role of the researcher
   e) study design characteristics
   f) researcher's involvement with subjects
   g) generalizability of findings
2. Upon what major consideration does the decision to use quantitative or qualitative methods depend?

Objective 3   Identify major theoretical frameworks in qualitative research.

1. What is the importance of "interpretation" to the theory of symbolic interaction?

2. What are the goals and strengths and weaknesses of phenomenology?

3. How are interview questions derived in phenomenology?

4. Define grounded theory, and describe the final goal of this theory.

5. Compare and contrast critical theory and feminist theory.

Objective 4 Outline the general process for conceptualizing a qualitative study, framing the research question, collecting and analyzing data, and writing up a research report.

1. Why does one's original research outline often end up being a tentative plan in qualitative research?

2. Where does the qualitative researcher get ideas for study?

3. Give an example of a typical qualitative research question.

4. Compare and contrast the following data collection strategies:
   a) direct observation
   b) focused interviewing
   c) document analysis
   d) photograph and video analysis

5. Ask a qualitative researcher how he or she used triangulation in his/her study. What is the advantage of triangulation?

6. If you are planning a qualitative study at a fitness center in a corporate workplace, what are some things you could do to assure and maintain good field relationships?

7. What is meant by data "saturation?"

8. What is the major task of the author when writing a qualitative research paper? How does it differ from a quantitative research paper?

Objective 5 Describe the features of trustworthiness of qualitative data, including credibility, transferability, dependability, and confirmability.

1. Define "trustworthiness." What is your opinion of comparing quantitative and qualitative studies in terms of rigor?

2. What can one do to increase the credibility, transferability, dependability, and confirmability of qualitative studies?

Objective 6   Identify questions that can be used to evaluate the quality of a qualitative research article.

1. Use the list of questions to evaluate a given qualitative research article.

2. Why is there so much emphasis on research conditions, data collection strategies, and analysis in qualitative research articles?

III

DATA ANALYSIS

part

Data are the measures, scores, and other information collected in a research study. Usually, the term *data* is used to refer to the scores of the subjects for a variable, although it is not uncommon to have multiple data sets because information was collected on multiple variables. Researchers draw their conclusions based on the data. Presented in chapters 10 and 11 of Part III are a variety of commonly used data analysis techniques. It will be useful to be aware of what techniques are available in selecting the most appropriate one for use in your research. Knowledge of these techniques will also make the research literature easier to understand. These techniques typically require some mathematical calculation.

There are three distinct steps in data analysis: (1) select the technique appropriate for the data and the research questions; (2) apply the technique or calculate using the technique; and (3) interpret the result of the technique. Step 2 is often quite difficult when a large amount of data is involved or the analysis technique is complex. Thus, step 2 is best accomplished with the aid of the computer. A computer package will be frequently referenced in chapters 10 and 11, and no calculational formulas or computational examples will be presented in these chapters unless they help the reader understand the data analysis technique. Using the computer for step 2 takes nothing away from the researcher in terms of decision making but is of great benefit in terms of the time saved and the accuracy of the result. An excellent reference on interpreting statistics is Huck, Cormier, and Bounds (1974).

In most research studies, a population is identified, a sample is drawn from the population, the research study is conducted on the sample, and the results for the sample are inferred to the population. Thus, sample information **(statistics)** are used to estimate population information **(parameters).** For example, the mean, or arithmetic average, for a sample is a statistic used as an estimate of the mean for a population, which is a parameter. All calculated values in chapters 10 and 11 will be called statistics. Statistics can be classified in a number of ways. One classification is the **descriptive** versus **inferential statistic.** A descriptive statistic is used to describe characteristics of a group, while an inferential statistic is used in the process of making an inference from a sample to a population. Some statistics (the mean is one) can be used in either a descriptive or inferential manner. Another classification is the **parametric** versus **nonparametric statistic.** Most of the statistics presented in Part III are parametric. Parametric statistics usually require interval data and a normal distribution (see chapter 10). Nonparametric statistics have neither of these requirements. A third classification is the **univariate** versus **multivariate statistic.** Most of the statistics presented in Part III are univariate. With univariate statistics each subject contributes one score on one variable to the analysis, while with multivariate statistics each subject contributes multiple scores on multiple variables to the analysis. Any statistics book can be consulted on calculating statistics, but Ferguson and Takane (1989) is excellent.

10   Descriptive Data Analysis

Key Words

Central tendency
Coefficient of determination
Continuous scores
Correlation
Correlation coefficient
Curvilinear relationship
Descriptive statistics
Discrete scores
Frequency polygon
Histogram
Inferential statistics
Interval scores
Leptokurtic
Linear relationship
Line of best fit, regression line

Mean
Median
Mode
Multivariate statistic
Negatively skewed curve
Nominal scores
Nonparametric statistic
Normal curve, bell-shaped curve
Ordinal scores
Outlier
Parameters
Parametric statistic
Percentile, percentile rank
Platykurtic
Positively skewed curve

Range
Ratio scores
Rho, Spearman's rho, rank order
    correlation coefficient
Scattergram
Simple frequency distribution
Standard deviation
Standard scores
Statistics
Univariate statistic
Variability
Variance
z score

Objectives

This chapter presents statistical techniques that can be applied to evaluate a set of scores. You should be familiar with them in order to select the appropriate one for a given situation and to understand the research literature.

After reading chapter 10, you should be able to:

1. Select the appropriate statistic(s) for each research situation.
2. Interpret correctly each of the statistics commonly used by researchers.
3. Use the computer to statistically analyze a set of scores.

This chapter covers techniques and statistics commonly used to describe the characteristics and performance of a group and to interpret the scores of individuals within a group. There are many reasons why we analyze data. For a large group, a simple listing of the scores has no meaning to the researcher or the person reading the research report. Only by applying some analysis to the data can it be condensed to a point where it can be meaningful to all interested people in terms of overall performance or characteristics of the group. Also, to make comparisons between groups there must be a single score for each group representing the typical score of the group.

Sometimes it is necessary to describe the performance of an individual within a group. Some data analysis is necessary before the performance of an individual can be compared to the performance of others in the group or to the overall group performance. Before presenting various descriptive data analysis techniques, types of scores, common units of measure, and computer analysis must be discussed, since these elements influence the data analysis.

Types of Scores

Scores can be classified as either continuous or discrete. **Continuous scores,** as most are in HHP, have a potentially infinite number of values allowing variables to be measured with varying degrees of accuracy. Between any two values of a continuous score are countless other values that may be expressed as fractions. For example, 100-yard dash scores are usually recorded to the nearest tenth of a second, but they could be recorded in hundredths or thousandths of a second if timing equipment accurate to that level of precision was available. Body weight accurate to the closest five-pound interval, to the whole pound, or to the half-pound might be recorded depending on how exact the measurement needs to be. **Discrete scores** are limited to a specific number of values and usually are not expressed as fractions. Scores on a throw or shot at a target numbered 5-4-3-2-1-0 are discrete because whole number scores of 5, 4, 3, 2, 1, or 0 are the only ones possible. A score of 4.5 or 1.67 is impossible.

Most continuous scores are rounded off to the nearest unit of measurement when they are recorded. For example, the score of a student who runs the 100-yard dash in 10.57 seconds is recorded as 10.6 because 10.57 is closer to 10.6 than to 10.5. Usually when a number is rounded off to the nearest unit of measurement, it is increased only when the number being dropped is 5 or more. Thus 11.45 is rounded off to 11.5, while 11.44 is recorded as 11.4. A less common method is to round off to the last unit of measure, awarding the next higher score only when that score is actually accomplished. For example, an individual who does eight sit-ups but cannot complete the ninth receives a score of 8.

We can also classify scores as ratio, interval, ordinal, or nominal (Ferguson and Takane 1989). How scores are classified influences what calculations may be performed on the data. **Ratio scores** have a common unit of measurement between each score and a true zero point so that statements about equality of ratios can be made. Length and weight are examples, since one measurement may be expressed as two or three times that of another. **Interval scores** have a common unit of measurement between each score but do not have a true zero point. (A score of 0 as a measure of distance is a true zero, indicating no distance. However, a score of 0 on a knowledge test is not a true zero because it does not indicate a total lack of knowledge; it simply means that the respondent answered none of the questions correctly). Most physical performance scores are either ratio or interval. **Ordinal scores** do not have a common unit of measurement between each score but are ordered in a way that makes it possible to characterize one score as higher than another. Class ranks, for example, are ordinal: If three students receive sit-up scores of 16, 10, and 8, respectively, the first is ranked 1; the next, 2; and the last, 3. Notice that the number of sit-ups necessary to change the class ranks of the second and third students differs. Thus there is not a common unit of measurement between consecutive scores. **Nominal scores** cannot be hierarchically ordered and are mutually exclusive. For example, individuals can be classified by church preference, but we cannot say that one religion is better than another. Gender is another example.

Common Units of Measure

Many scores are recorded in feet and inches or in minutes and seconds. To analyze scores, they must be recorded in a single unit of measurement, usually the smaller one. Thus distances and heights are recorded in inches rather than feet and inches, and times are recorded in seconds rather than minutes and seconds. Recording scores in the smaller unit of measure as they are collected is less time-consuming than translating them into that form later.

Computer Analysis

Score analysis should be accurate and quick. Particularly when a set of scores is large, say fifty or more, computers should be used to ensure both accuracy and speed. Computers are increasingly available in school districts and universities, agencies, and businesses. Each statistical example in this chapter is accompanied by an example of the desktop computer application. Sometimes the output from the desktop computer program will include more information than will have been discussed in the chapter. Do not be concerned if this information is unfamiliar or you do not understand what it means.

Many computer program packages for statistical computations have been developed. Some nationally distributed packages of statistical programs such as SAS, BMDP, and SPSS run on both mainframe and desktop computers. These packages are available on many college campuses. Other packages of statistical programs only run on one type of desktop computer (IBM or MacIntosh). Most computer programs provide similar information for any particular statistical technique. The computer examples in chapters 10 and 11 were generated using a package of statistical programs for a desktop computer because most students, both at present and once they have a job, will have access to desktop computers. Baumgartner and Jackson (1995) include a chapter introducing computers and their use.

Chapters 10 and 11 will reference computer programs from the SYSTAT (1992) package. If you don't have access to and/or familiarity with any other package of computer programs you may decide to use this one. SYSTAT was selected because there is a DOS, Windows, and Mac version of the package so it can be used on most computer operating systems. Also, SYSTAT is quite complete in meeting the needs of the researcher but not as expensive or requiring as large a computer as packages of programs like SAS or SPSS. There is a small version of SYSTAT available called Student SYSTAT (1994) for approximately $30 and a smaller version still called MYSTAT (1994) for around $20. One nice feature is that MYSTAT and SYSTAT operate basically the same so learning how to use one of them prepares a person to use the other one. Another desirable feature is that data entered with another computer program can be used by SYSTAT and data entered using SYSTAT can be used with another computer program. A third nice feature of SYSTAT is that it has graphic capabilities. The manuals that come with the SYSTAT and MYSTAT programs are quite good.

The SYSTAT package of programs requires that the data be entered and then an analysis program selected. Normally after the data are entered they will be saved to disk before any analysis is undertaken. If the data are not saved to disk, when the computer is turned off, the data are lost. If the data ever needs to be reanalyzed because of a mistake in the original analysis or if a different analysis becomes necessary, the data must be entered again. Doing additional analysis on the data happens quite often, and for large amounts of data having to reenter it represents a considerable inconvenience. Thus, when using SYSTAT or some other computer program, it is a good idea to enter and save the data to disk prior to analyzing the data.

All instructions in chapters 10 and 11 concerning how to use the computer assume that the Windows version of SYSTAT is being used. The instructions for other versions of SYSTAT and for MYSTAT are quite similar. Most of the example computer printouts in the book are based on SYSTAT output.

The following steps are used to enter and save data with the Windows version of SYSTAT:

1. Click File on the SYSTAT Main menu.

2. Click New on the drop down menu.

3. Name the variables in the top row of the SYSTAT Worksheet which is displayed.

4. Enter the scores for all the people. All scores of a person are entered in the same row (score—1, score—2, etc.).

5. Click on File in the SYSTAT Worksheet and then click on Save As to save the data.

6. Make sure a formatted floppy disk is in the disk drive. At File Name in the Save A File window type the disk drive letter and file name with a **sys** extension (example—a:datarun.sys) and nothing else.

7. Click on Save.

TABLE 10.1 Knowledge Test Scores for Fifty Subjects				
66*	67	54	63	90
56	56	65	71	82
68	68	76	55	78
47	58	68	78	76
46	68	68	90	62
58	49	62	84	75
75	65	66	72	73
71	75	83	83	64
60	76	65	79	56
68	70	48	77	59

*Number correct

8. The SYSTAT Worksheet is still displayed, so the data can be edited and if necessary corrections saved.

The following steps are used to select the data analysis technique, select the variables and options to be used in analyzing the data, and print the results using the Windows version of SYSTAT:

1. Select the data analysis program by clicking on the required selections.
2. In the menu displayed, click on the variable(s) to be used, click on Add, and when ready for the analysis, click on Ok.
3. To print the results of the analysis, click on File in the SYSTAT Main menu, click on Print in the drop down menu, and then click on Ok in the print window.

Organizing and Graphing Test Scores

Simple Frequency Distributions

The fifty scores in table 10.1 are not very useful in their present form. They become more meaningful if we order the scores to find out how many subjects received each score. To do this, we first find the lowest and highest scores in the table. Now we find the number of subjects who received each score between the lowest (46) and the highest (90).

Once the scores are ordered, it is easy to make up a simple frequency distribution of the results (see columns 1 and 2 of table 10.2). We list the scores in descending order with the best score first. In most cases, the higher scores are better scores, but this is not true when, for example, distance running event times, number

TABLE 10.2 Simple Frequency Distribution of Knowledge Test Scores of Fifty Subjects in Table 10.1

SCORE	FREQ.	CUM. F	PERCENT	CUM. %
90	2	50	4.00	100.00
84	1	48	2.00	96.00
83	2	47	4.00	94.00
82	1	45	2.00	90.00
79	1	44	2.00	88.00
78	2	43	4.00	86.00
77	1	41	2.00	82.00
76	3	40	6.00	80.00
75	3	37	6.00	74.00
73	1	34	2.00	68.00
72	1	33	2.00	66.00
71	2	32	4.00	64.00
70	1	30	2.00	60.00
68	6	29	12.00	58.00
67	1	23	2.00	46.00
66	2	22	4.00	44.00
65	3	20	6.00	40.00
64	1	17	2.00	34.00
63	1	16	2.00	32.00
62	2	15	4.00	30.00
60	1	13	2.00	26.00
59	1	12	2.00	24.00
58	2	11	4.00	22.00
56	3	9	6.00	18.00
55	1	6	2.00	12.00
54	1	5	2.00	10.00
49	1	4	2.00	8.00
48	1	3	2.00	6.00
47	1	2	2.00	4.00
46	1	1	2.00	2.00

of accidents, or number of errors are being measured. A **simple frequency distribution** of times from a distance running event would list the lower scores first.

From a simple frequency distribution we can determine the range of scores at a glance, as well as the most frequently received score and the number of subjects who received each score. For example, from table 10.2 we can see that the scores ranged from 90 down to 46, that the most frequently received score was 68, and that scores had a frequency of 3 or less in all cases but one.

Where the number of scores is large, forming a simple frequency distribution is time-consuming without a computer. Using a computer, scores can be entered and analyzed with any one of a number of programs. Most statistical packages for mainframe and desktop computers include a frequency count program.

The frequency count program in SYSTAT is one such program. The following steps are used to obtain frequency counts with SYSTAT:

1. Click on STATS under SYSTAT Main and then click on Tables.
2. Click on Tabulate if it is displayed and then click on List Format and Sort Categories.
3. Now follow the steps presented earlier for doing the analysis and printing the results.

The output from SYSTAT for the data in table 10.1 is presented in table 10.2. From table 10.2 it can be seen that test scores ranged from 46 to 90, and six subjects scored 68.

Some researchers use a frequency count program to screen their data for extreme scores or incorrect scores before conducting any more complex analysis. It is a wise thing to do because scores do get incorrectly recorded and entered into the computer.

Grouping Scores for Graphing

The scores and their frequencies in table 10.2 could be presented in the form of a graph that shows the general shape of a score distribution. Based on the shape of a score distribution decisions are made about how to interpret the performance of the group measured. If there are many different scores, the graph is usually formed by grouping like scores together. In grouping a set of scores, we try to form about fifteen groupings by dividing the difference between the largest and smallest scores by 15, and rounding off the result to the nearest whole number if necessary.

$$\text{interval size} = (\text{largest score} - \text{smallest score}) \div 15.$$

The interval size tells us how many scores to group together. Design the first grouping to contain the best score. Table 10.3 is a grouping of the data in table 10.2 using an interval size of three.

Figure 10.1 is a graph of the data in table 10.3. Test scores, in intervals of three (only midpoints are plotted), are listed along the horizontal axis with low scores on the left to high scores on the right. The frequency is listed on the vertical axis starting with 0 and increasing upward. A dot above each score indicates its frequency. For example, the dot above score 66 is opposite the frequency value 6, indicating that six

TABLE 10.3 Grouping of the Knowledge Test Scores in Table 10.2

GROUPING	FREQUENCY
89–91	2
86–88	0
83–85	3
80–82	1
77–79	4
74–76	6
71–73	4
68–70	7
65–67	6
62–64	4
59–61	2
56–58	5
53–55	2
50–52	0
47–49	3
44–46	1

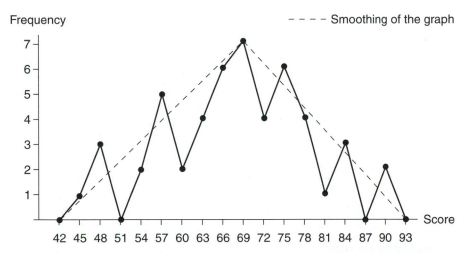

Frequency   – – – – Smoothing of the graph

Score

FIGURE 10.1
Graph of the knowledge test scores in table 10.3.

subjects received scores in the grouping 65–67. By connecting the dots with straight lines, we complete the graph, forming an angled figure called a **frequency polygon.**

   Smoothing out the frequency polygon creates a curve that, by its shape, tells us the nature of the distribution. In figure 10.1, the smoothing out is indicated by the

FIGURE 10.2
A normal curve.

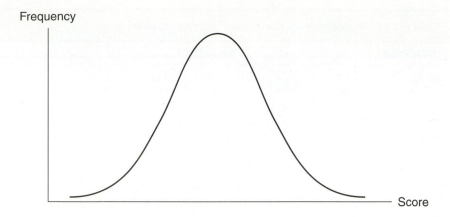

broken line. If that line resembles the curve in figure 10.2, the graph is called a **normal curve** or **bell-shaped curve.** The normal curve is often used as a model. If the graph of the data resembles the normal curve (data are normally distributed) one decision is made, but if the graph does not resemble the normal curve a different decision is made.

When a smoothed graph has a long, low tail on the left, indicating that few subjects received low scores, it is called a **negatively skewed curve.** When the tail of the curve is on the right, the curve is called **positively skewed.** A curve is called **leptokurtic** when it is more sharply peaked than a normal curve and **platykurtic** when it is less sharply peaked (fig. 10.3). Leptokurtic curves are characteristic of extremely homogeneous groups. Platykurtic curves are characteristic of heterogeneous groups.

A computer can be utilized to form a graph. An option of most computer programs is any number of groupings and several different types of graphs. Another type of graph that is quite common is a **histogram.** Again, the frequencies for the intervals are plotted and bars are constructed at the height of the frequency running the full length of the interval. A histogram for the data in table 10.3 is presented in figure 10.4. Several types of graphs can be obtained with SYSTAT by clicking on GRAPH under SYSTAT Main, clicking on Density, clicking on the type of graph desired, and then following the steps presented earlier for doing the analysis and printing the results. Other types of graphs and how to construct graphs are presented in most basic statistics books, such as Ferguson and Takane (1989).

Descriptive Values

Once a large set of scores has been collected, certain descriptive values can be calculated; these values will summarize or condense the set of scores and give it meaning. Descriptive values are used by researchers primarily to describe the performance of a group or compare its performance with that of another group.

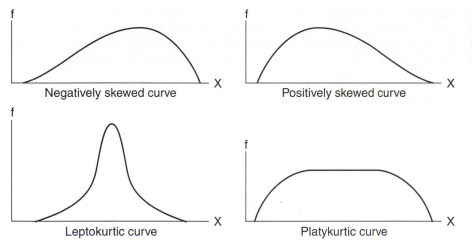

FIGURE 10.3
Negatively skewed, positively skewed, leptokurtic, and platykurtic curves.

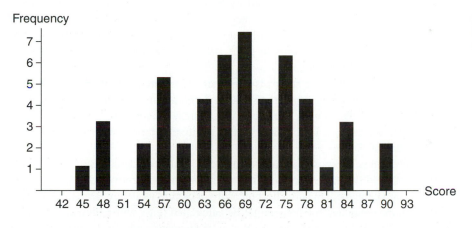

FIGURE 10.4
Histogram for table 10.3 data.

Measures of Central Tendency

One type of descriptive value is the measure of **central tendency,** which indicates those points at which scores tend to be concentrated. There are three measures of central tendency: the mode, the median, and the mean.

Mode.   The **mode** is the score most frequently received, and it is used with nominal data. In table 10.2 the mode is 68: More subjects received a score of 68 than any other one score in the set. It is possible to have several modes if a number of scores tie for most frequent. The mode is not a stable measure because the addition or deletion of a single score can change its value considerably. Unless the data are nominal or the most frequent score is desired, other measures of central tendency are more appropriate.

Median.   The **median** is the middle score; half the scores fall above the median and half below. It requires data that are at least ordinal. It cannot be calculated unless the scores are listed in order from best to worst. For example, the median score for the nine numbers 4, 3, 1, 4, 10, 7, 7, 8, and 6 is 6 since it is the middle score.

$$10, 8, 7, 7, 6, 4, 4, 3, 1$$
$$\uparrow \text{ Median}$$

Notice that the value of the median is affected only by the position, not the value, of each score. If, in the example above, the scores were 10, 8, 7, 7, 6, 3, 2, 1, and 0, the median would still be 6. This characteristic of the median is sometimes a limitation.

When scores are listed in a simple frequency distribution, we can obtain a value of the median by a computational formula. This value of the median is usually a fractional number.

Mean.   The **mean** is ordinarily the most appropriate measure of central tendency for interval or ratio data. It is affected by both the value and the position of each score. The mean ($\bar{x}$) is the sum of the scores divided by the number of scores. Notice that the scores need not be ordered hierarchically to calculate the mean. For example, the mean for the scores in table 10.1 is 67.78, the sum of the randomly ordered scores divided by 50.

When the graph of the scores is a normal curve, the mode, median, and mean are equal. When the graph is positively skewed, the mean is larger than the median; when it is negatively skewed, the mean is less than the median. For example, the graph for the scores 2, 3, 1, 4, 1, 8, and 10 is positively skewed with a mean of 4.14 and a median of 3.

The mean is the most common measure of central tendency. But when scores are quite skewed or lack a common interval between consecutive scores (e.g., with ordinal scores), the median is the best measure of central tendency. The mode is used only when the mean and median cannot be calculated (e.g., with nominal scores) or when the only information wanted is the most frequent score (e.g., most common uniform size, most frequent error).

Measures of Variability

A second type of descriptive value is the measure of **variability,** which describes the data in terms of their spread or heterogeneity. For example, consider these scores for two groups:

Group 1	Group 2
9	5
1	6
5	4

For both groups, the mean and median are 5. If you simply report that the mean and median for both groups are identical without showing the data, another person could conclude that the two groups have equal or similar ability. This is not true: Group 2 is more homogeneous in performance than is group 1. A measure of variability is the descriptive term that indicates this difference in the spread, or heterogeneity, of the data. There are two such measures: the range and the standard deviation.

Range.   The **range** is the easiest measure of variability to obtain and is the one used when the measure of central tendency is the mode or median. The range is the difference between the highest and lowest score. For example, the range for the data in table 10.2 is 44 (90 − 46). The range is neither a precise nor stable measure because it depends on only two scores and is affected by a change in either of them. For example, the range for the data in table 10.2 would have been 38 (84 − 46) if the subjects who scored 90 had instead scored 84 or less.

Standard Deviation.   The **standard deviation** is the measure of variability used with the mean. It indicates the amount that all the scores differ from the mean. The more the scores differ from the mean, the larger the standard deviation. The minimum value of the standard deviation is 0, indicating that all scores were the same value. Presented below is a formula illustrating how the standard deviation is defined.

$$s = \sqrt{\frac{\Sigma\,(x - \bar{x})^2}{n - 1}}$$

In the formula, s is the standard deviation, x is a score, $\bar{x}$ is the mean, n is the number of scores, and Σ is a summation sign. There is a much easier formula than this one for calculating s.

If the data are normally distributed, few if any scores will be more than three standard deviations away from the mean. For example, if the mean is 60 and the standard deviation 10, the lowest score might be around 30 ($\bar{x} - 3s = 60 - 30$) and the highest score might be around 90. Often, when a score is more than three standard deviations from the mean it is called an **outlier** and may be removed from the data. The researcher is concerned that the outlier score is not correct or the subject did not belong in the group.

The mean, standard deviation, and other useful statistics can be obtained with SYSTAT by clicking on STATS under SYSTAT Main, clicking on Stats, clicking on Statistics, selecting the statistics you desire (Note: Click on All and get all the statistics the program provides), and then following the steps presented earlier for doing the analysis and printing the results. The output from SYSTAT (all the statistics provided) for the data in table 10.1 is presented in table 10.4.

Variance.   A third measure of variability is the **variance.** It is not a descriptive statistic like the range or standard deviation, but rather, a useful statistic in certain

TABLE 10.4 All the Statistics Output from SYSTAT for the Data in Table 10.1

VARIABLE	SCORE
N of Cases	50
Minimum	46.000
Maximum	90.000
Range	44.000
Mean	67.780
Variance	115.277
Standard Dev	10.737
Std. Error	1.518
Skewness (G1)	−0.056
Kurtosis (G2)	−0.471
Sum	3389.000
C.V.	0.158
Median	68.000

other statistical procedures and interpretations of statistics that will be discussed later. The variance is the square of the standard deviation. If, for example, the standard deviation is 4, the variance is 16.

Measuring Group Position

Percentile Ranks and Percentiles

Sometimes a researcher needs to indicate the position or rank of subjects within a group based on their test scores. This can be accomplished by the use of **percentile ranks** and **percentiles.** Although their calculations differ, their interpretations are basically the same, so the two terms are used interchangeably in the literature. Both statistics indicate the percentage of subjects below a particular score. Thus, if a researcher reports that the percentile rank (PR) for a score of 28 is 60, this indicates that 60 percent of the subjects scored below the score of 28. However, the researcher might report that a subject with a score of 28 scored at the 60th percentile (P). Percentile ranks and percentiles are often calculated when developing norms.

One disadvantage of percentile ranks is that they are ordinal scores. There is no common unit of measure between consecutive percentile rank values because they are position measures. Thus, it is inappropriate to add, subtract, multiply, or divide percentile rank values. Another disadvantage of percentile ranks is that small changes in score values near the mean result in large changes in percentile ranks. Baumgartner and Jackson (1995) present a detailed coverage of percentile ranks and percentiles.

Percentiles and percentile ranks computer programs are available but they are not common in packages of statistical programs like SYSTAT. Some researchers use the CUM. % values presented in table 10.2 as an estimate of percentile ranks. Computer programs usually assume that a large score is good. When this is not true (score is number of auto accidents), subtract the percentile rank of each subject from 100 to get the correct value.

Standard Scores

Researchers use **standard scores** when they have data on subjects from several different tests, and they want all the data in the same unit of measurement. An example of this is the sit-up, mile-run, skin-fold, and sit-and-reach tests common to many fitness batteries. Test scores for a test are converted to standard scores by the formula

$$z = (x - \bar{x})/s$$

where z is a standard score, x is a test score, $\bar{x}$ is the mean for the test, and s is the standard deviation for the test. Thus, for each test, test scores are converted to z **scores** by using the formula. Once all test scores are converted to z scores, the researcher can obtain the sum of the z scores for each subject or determine on which test the subject scored best.

A z score indicates how many standard deviations a test score is from the mean. Thus, a z score of 1.5 indicates the test score was 1.5 standard deviations above the mean. Typically z scores are between -3.0 and 3.0 and are fractional. The mean z score is 0, and the standard deviation for a distribution of z scores is 1.0.

Computer programs to obtain z scores are usually available, although SYSTAT does not have one. Most packages of statistical programs have a transformation feature that could be used to calculate new scores (like z scores) using scores already entered into the computer. To accomplish this, first enter the scores into the computer, then obtain the mean and standard deviation for the scores using the computer, and finally, using the transformation feature, calculate z scores. Using SYSTAT click on Editor in the SYSTAT Worksheet, click on Math, and then fill in the boxes. Also, the SYSTAT Data manual shows a procedure for obtaining z scores using the Standardize command. The z scores for the data in table 10.1 are presented in table 10.5.

There is another standard score called a T score, which physical education teachers often use in preference to z scores. Baumgartner and Jackson (1995) discuss T scores in detail.

Determining Relationships between Scores

There are many situations in which researchers would like to know the relationship between scores on two different tests (e.g., the relationship between beliefs about the importance of leisure time pursuits and leisure time practices). Sometimes the major

TABLE 10.5	z Scores for the Data in Table 10.1				
CASE	SCORE	z-SCORE	CASE	SCORE	z-SCORE
1	66	−0.166	26	62	−0.538
2	56	−1.097	27	66	−0.166
3	68	0.020	28	83	1.418
4	47	−1.935	29	65	−0.259
5	46	−2.029	30	48	−1.842
6	58	−0.911	31	63	−0.445
7	75	0.672	32	71	0.300
8	71	0.300	33	55	−1.190
9	60	−0.725	34	78	0.952
10	68	0.020	35	90	2.070
11	67	−0.073	36	84	1.511
12	56	−1.097	37	72	0.393
13	68	0.020	38	83	1.418
14	58	−0.911	39	79	1.045
15	68	0.020	40	77	0.859
16	49	−1.749	41	90	2.070
17	65	−0.259	42	82	1.324
18	75	0.672	43	78	0.952
19	76	0.766	44	76	0.766
20	70	0.207	45	62	−0.538
21	54	−1.283	46	75	0.672
22	65	−0.259	47	73	0.486
23	76	0.766	48	64	−0.352
24	68	0.020	49	56	−1.097
25	68	0.020	50	59	−0.818

Mean   = 67.78
Std Dev = 10.74

objective of the research is to determine relationships, but in other studies it may be a minor objective. To determine if there is a relationship between two variables every subject must be measured on each variable. There are two different techniques to determine score relationships: a graphing technique and a mathematical technique called correlation.

The graphing technique is not as precise as the mathematical technique, but prior to computers it was easier and quicker. Many of the terms used in the mathematical technique come from the graphing technique. Presently, with the availability of computers, many researchers are using the graphing technique initially to check

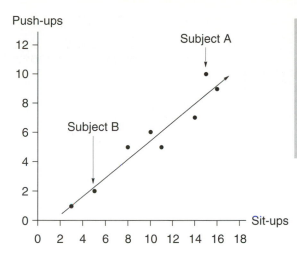

Subject	Sit-ups	Push-ups
A	15	10
B	5	2
C	11	5
D	10	6
E	14	7
F	3	1
G	16	9
H	8	5

FIGURE 10.5
Graph of a positive relationship between scores.

some of the assumptions underlying the mathematical technique and as a way to graphically show the relationship. They then use the mathematical technique to obtain a value that precisely indicates the amount of relationship between the two variables.

The Graphing Technique

To graph a relationship, the computer develops a coordinate system with values of one variable listed along the horizontal axis and values of the other variable listed along the vertical axis. It plots a point for each subject above his/her score on the horizontal axis and opposite his/her score on the vertical axis, as shown in figure 10.5. The graph that results is called a **scattergram.**

The point plotted for subject A is at the intersection of sit-up score 15 and push-up score 10, the scores the subject received on the two tests. The straight line—the **line of best fit** or the **regression line**—represents the trend in the data, in this case that subjects with large sit-up scores have large push-up scores, and vice versa. When large scores on one measure are associated with large scores on the other measure, the relationship is positive. When large scores on one measure are associated with small scores on the other measure, the relationship is negative (fig. 10.6).

The closer the plotted points to the trend line, the higher or larger the relationship. The maximum relationship occurs when all plotted points are on the trend line. When the plotted points resemble a circle, making it impossible to draw a trend line, no linear relationship exists between the two measures being graphed (fig. 10.7).

Computer programs contain scattergram graphic programs that facilitate plotting data. An example of a computer-generated graph using SYSTAT and the data in figure 10.5 is presented in figure 10.8. To obtain a scattergram using SYSTAT, click on GRAPH under SYSTAT Main, then click on the little triangle in the Plot square, then follow the steps presented earlier for doing the analysis and printing the results.

FIGURE 10.6
Graph of a negative
relationship between
scores.

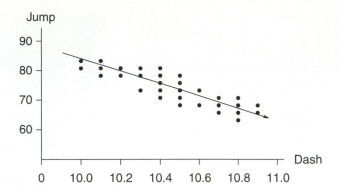

FIGURE 10.7
Graph of no relationship
between scores.

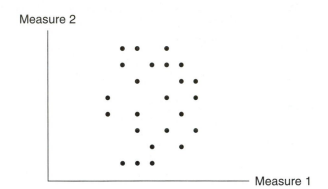

The Correlation Technique

Correlation is a mathematical technique for determining the relationship between two sets of scores. The formula was developed by Karl Pearson to determine the degree of relationship between two sets of measures (called *X* measures and *Y* measures).

A **correlation coefficient** (r) has two characteristics, direction and strength. Direction of the relationship is indicated by whether the correlation coefficient is positive or negative, as indicated under the graphing technique. Strength of the relationship is indicated by how close the r is to 1, the maximum value possible. A correlation of 1 ($r = 1$) shows a perfect positive relationship, indicating that an increase in scores on one measure is accompanied by an increase in scores on the second measure. A perfect negative relationship ($r = -1$) indicates that an increase in scores on one measure is accompanied by a decrease in scores on the second. (Notice that a correlation of -1 is just as strong as a correlation of 1). Perfect relationships are rare, but any such relationship that does exist is exactly described by a

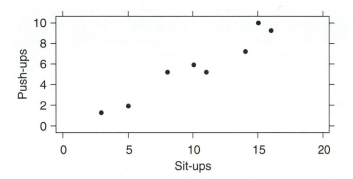

FIGURE 10.8
Computer-generated
scattergram of the data in
table 10.8.

TABLE 10.6 Examples of Perfect Relationships

SUBJECT	HEIGHT	WEIGHT	SUBJECT	100-YARD DASH	PULL-UPS
A	60	130	A	10.6	14
B	52	122	B	10.6	14
C	75	145	C	11.2	8
D	66	136	D	11.7	3
E	70	140	E	10.5	15
	$r = 1$			$r = -1$	
	Exact formula: weight = height + 70			Exact formula: dash = 12 − .1 (pull-ups)	

mathematical formula. An example of a perfect positive and a perfect negative relationship is shown in table 10.6. When the correlation coefficient is 0 ($r = 0$), there is
no linear relationship between the two sets of scores.

Because the relationship between two sets of scores is seldom perfect, the
majority of correlation coefficients are fractions (e.g., .93, −.85). The closer the correlation coefficient is to 1 or −1, the stronger the relationship. When the relationship
is not perfect, the scores on one measure only tend to change with a change in the
scores on the other measure. Look, for example, at table 10.7. The correlation
between height and weight is not perfect: Subject C, whose height is 75 inches, is
not heavier than Subject E, whose height is only 70 inches.

When the scores for the two sets of scores are ranks, a correlation coefficient
called **rho** or **Spearman's rho** or the **rank order correlation coefficient** may be
calculated. The formula is just a simplification of the Pearson correlation formula
and will produce the same result when applied to the two sets of ranks, provided that
no tied ranks exist. Rho is commonly included in computer statistical programs.

TABLE 10.7 Example of an Imperfect Correlation		
SUBJECT	**HEIGHT**	**WEIGHT**
A	60	130
B	52	125
C	75	145
D	66	136
E	70	150
	$r = .91$	

Interpreting the Correlation Coefficient. A high correlation between two measures does not usually indicate a cause-and-effect-relationship. The perfect height and weight relationship in table 10.6, for example, does not indicate that an increase in weight *causes* an increase in height. Also, the degree of relationship between two sets of measures does not increase at the same rate as does the correlation coefficient. The true indicator of the degree of relationship is the **coefficient of determination**—the amount of variability (variance) in one measure that is explained by the other measure. The coefficient of determination is the square of the correlation coefficient (r^2). For example, the square of the correlation coefficient in table 10.7 is .83 ($.91^2$), meaning that 83 percent of the variability in height scores is due to the individuals having different weight scores.

Thus, when one correlation coefficient is twice as large as another, the larger coefficient really explains four times the amount of variation that the smaller coefficient explains. For example, when the r between height and weight is .80 and the r between strength and athletic ability is .40, the r^2 for height and weight is $.80^2$, or 64 percent, and the r^2 for strength and athletic ability is $.40^2$, or 16 percent.

Remember: When you interpret a correlation coefficient, there are no absolute standards for labeling a given r as "good" or "poor"; only the relationship you want or expect determines the quality of a given r. For example, a correlation coefficient of .67 between leg strength and distance run scores for males might lead you to expect a similar correlation coefficient in comparing leg strength and distance run scores for females. If the relationship between the females' scores were only .45, you might label that correlation coefficient "poor" because you expected it to be as high as that of the males.

There are two reasons why correlation coefficients can be negative: (1) opposite scoring scales and (2) true negative relationships. When a measure on which a small score is a better score is correlated with a measure on which a larger score is a better score, the correlation coefficient probably will be negative. Consider, for example, the relationship between scores on a speed event like the 50-yard dash and a nonspeed event like the high jump. Usually, the best jumpers are the best runners, but the correlation is negative because the scoring scales are reversed. Two measures

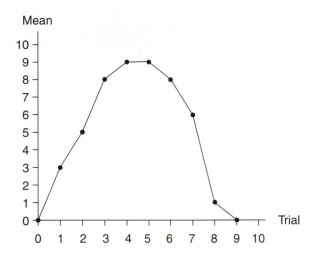

Practice trial	Group mean
1	3
2	5
3	8
4	9
5	9
6	8
7	6
8	1

FIGURE 10.9
Example of a curvilinear relationship between group performance and practice trials within a day when learning a new skill.

can be negatively related as well. We would expect, for example, a negative correlation between body weight and measures involving support or motion of the body (e.g., pull-ups).

The Question of Accuracy. In calculating r we assume that the relationship between the two sets of scores is basically linear. A **linear relationship** is best shown graphically by a straight line, as is the trend line in figure 10.5. However, a relationship between two sets of scores may be best represented by a curved line, indicating a **curvilinear relationship.** If a relationship is truly curvilinear, the correlation coefficient will underestimate the relationship. For example, r could equal 0 even when a definite curvilinear relationship exists. Learning curves and fatigue curves are typically curvilinear. An example of a curvilinear relationship is presented in figure 10.9.

Although we need not assume when calculating r that the graph of each of the two sets of scores is a normal curve, we do assume that the two graphs resemble each other. If they are dissimilar, the correlation coefficient will underestimate the relationship between the scores. Considerable differences in the two graphs are occasionally found, usually when the number of people tested is small. For this reason, the correlation coefficient ideally should be calculated using the scores of several hundred people.

Other factors also affect the correlation coefficient. One is the reliability of the scores; low reliability reduces the correlation coefficient. Another factor is the range in the scores; the correlation coefficient will be smaller for a homogeneous group than for a heterogeneous group. Ferguson and Takane (1989) suggest that, generally, the range in scores increases as the size of the group tested increases. Certainly, the measurements or test scores for small groups exhibit a greater tendency than those of large groups to be either more homogeneous or more heterogeneous

TABLE 10.8 Individual Physical Characteristic Data of 40 Subjects

SUBJECT	SEX	AGE	HEIGHT	WEIGHT	SUBJECT	SEX	AGE	HEIGHT	WEIGHT
1	0	6	123.0	22.5	21	1	7	122.7	23.8
2	0	6	115.0	24.9	22	1	7	132.9	33.9
3	0	6	115.0	22.7	23	1	7	128.8	28.3
4	0	6	121.5	24.3	24	1	7	133.6	30.2
5	0	6	116.5	19.7	25	0	8	136.0	31.8
6	1	6	119.6	21.9	26	0	8	129.0	26.8
7	0	7	124.6	24.5	27	1	8	128.2	27.6
8	0	7	111.8	19.3	28	1	8	131.1	28.8
9	0	7	120.3	19.8	29	1	8	139.1	31.1
10	0	7	119.0	21.3	30	1	8	124.1	25.4
11	0	7	119.5	21.3	31	1	9	137.1	34.8
12	0	7	132.0	26.9	32	1	9	134.6	31.9
13	0	7	122.5	22.7	33	1	9	137.6	29.8
14	0	7	128.5	31.6	34	1	9	140.1	34.4
15	0	7	119.5	21.3	35	1	9	140.2	32.3
16	1	7	126.0	24.3	36	1	9	149.9	36.6
17	1	7	132.2	29.3	37	0	10	140.5	29.0
18	1	7	136.8	28.9	38	0	10	131.5	29.6
19	1	7	125.8	25.5	39	0	10	146.4	35.5
20	1	7	116.9	22.6	40	0	10	136.5	28.1

Sex: 0 = Female, 1 = Male
Age: In years
Height: In centimeters
Weight: In kilograms

TABLE 10.9 Correlations Among All Variables for the Data in Table 10.8

	SEX	AGE	HEIGHT	WEIGHT
SEX	1.00			
AGE	0.13	1.00		
HEIGHT	0.36	0.77	1.00	
WEIGHT	0.41	0.67	0.91	1.00

than is typical for the group measured and the test administered. This is another reason to calculate the correlation coefficient for only large groups. Ferguson and Takane (1989) and Walker and Lev (1969) cover this subject in greater detail.

When the group tested is large or when the researcher wants the correlation between all possible pairings of more than two variables (sex, age, height, weight, etc.), a computer is the most efficient way to generate the correlation coefficients. Programs for calculating correlation coefficients are commonly found in statistical packages for computers. In SYSTAT, correlations are obtained by clicking on STATS under SYSTAT Main, clicking on Corr, clicking on Pearson, and selecting the variables to be correlated. Before clicking on Ok to do the analysis, click on Listwise deletion (Listwise deletion is not using the scores of a subject who has any missing scores. Pairwise deletion is not using the scores of a subject who has missing scores on the two variables being correlated.).

The correlations for the data in table 10.8 are presented in table 10.9 using SYSTAT. The correlations between any two variables are found by finding the value listed in the cell formed by the row and column of the two variables. For example, the correlation between height and weight is .91.

Summary

The importance of selecting the appropriate statistic for the situation and interpreting it correctly has been stressed in this chapter. This ability to choose and interpret statistical measures is of consequence for both a researcher and a person reading research journals. A variety of descriptive statistics were presented and the student will need a thorough understanding of these statistical techniques in order to fully grasp the material in chapter 11.

Finally, the student should have some ability to use the computer and have practiced using some package of statistical programs by the time this chapter has been covered. This skill is assumed in the next chapter and should prove valuable in the future as well.

Formative Evaluation of Objectives

Objective 1   Select the appropriate statistic(s) for each research situation.

1. In each situation below, what statistic(s) are needed?
   a) Describe the characteristics or scores of a group.
   b) Determine if the scores of a group are normally distributed.
   c) Allow scores from tests differing in unit of measurement to be combined into a total score.
   d) Determine how much the performance of a group changed from the pretest to the posttest.

e) Identify the degree of relationship between the scores of a group on two different tests.

Objective 2 Interpret correctly each of the statistics commonly used by researchers.

1. In each situation below, how is the statistic reported correctly interpreted?

a) The median score for the group is 11.6.
b) The mean score for the group is 7.5.
c) The standard deviation for the scores of the group is 6.6.
d) Subject 17 has a percentile rank of 53 based on her score of 16.
e) The correlation between IQ scores and knowledge test scores is .77.
f) Number of mistakes on a job proficiency test correlated −.35 with scores on a job knowledge test.

Objective 3 Use the computer to statistically analyze a set of scores.

1. In terms of the statistical package of computer programs available to you, answer the following questions.

a) What is the procedure followed in analyzing the data no matter what program in the statistical package is used?
b) What program in the statistical package provides descriptive statistics (e.g., mean, standard deviation)?
c) What program in the statistical package provides all possible correlations between the variables when scores on three or more variables are collected on each subject?

Inferential Data Analysis

11

Key Words

Alpha level
Analysis of covariance (ANCOVA)
Analysis of variance (ANOVA)
Beta (ß)
Cell
Correlation
Covariate
Critical region
Critical value
Cross validation
Degrees of freedom
Expected frequency
Experiment-wise error rate
Factorial design
Matched pairs
Mean square (MS)
Multiple prediction
Multivariate tests
Nonparametric
Nonsignificant

Null hypothesis
Observed frequency
One-group *t* test
One-way ANOVA
One-way (goodness of fit) chi-square test
Parametric
Per-comparison error rate
Polynomial regression
Prediction
Random blocks ANOVA
Real difference
Regression
Repeated measures
Repeated measures ANOVA
Research hypothesis
Sampling error
Significant
Simple effects tests
Simple prediction

Slope
Standard error of prediction
Statistical hypothesis
Statistical power
Sums of squares (SS)
Two dependent groups *t* test
Two-dimensional ANOVA
Two group comparisons, multiple comparisons, *a posteriori* comparisons
Two independent groups *t* test
Two-way ANOVA
Two-way (contingency table) chi-square test
Type I error
Type II error
Univariate tests
Variate
Y-intercept

Objectives

This chapter presents statistical tests that researchers commonly use in analyzing their data. You should be familiar with them in order to select the appropriate one(s) in your research and to understand the research of others as reported in research journals.

After reading chapter 11, you should be able to:

1. Identify the different research designs and statistical tests commonly used.

2. Understand the five-step hypothesis-testing procedure and how it is reported in research journals.

3. Understand and evaluate common statistical tests when they are used in the research literature.

The data analysis techniques discussed in this chapter are those most commonly used by researchers to analyze their data. These are the techniques you are most likely to use as a researcher and to see in the research literature as a consumer of research. Not all data analysis techniques available can be discussed in this context. On occasion you will need to use techniques or will see techniques in the literature that have not been discussed in this chapter. Hopefully, what you learn here will provide you with the foundation you will need to put these additional techniques to work.

No statistical training is assumed in order to understand the material in this chapter. The material presented should prepare you to understand the statistical information presented in the research literature. This chapter is not a comprehensive coverage of each statistical technique as would be found in a statistics book, so some of you may want to consult a statistics book. Others may want to skip some of the more advanced topics (e.g., two-way ANOVA). Ferguson and Takane (1989) is an excellent statistics book covering most of the statistical techniques presented. Selected statistics books are referenced throughout the chapter.

Inference

A researcher typically identifies or defines a population to which the findings of the research are to apply, states a research hypothesis about the population, selects a sample(s) from the population using random sampling procedures, conducts the research study on the sample(s), and finally, infers the results of the study to the population (see steps in research, chapters 2 and 5).

Example: The researcher wants to determine which of three teaching methods (A, B, or C) is the best way to teach rope skipping to third-grade boys. The researcher defines the population as third-grade boys in Georgia. The research hypothesis is that teaching method A is superior to the other two methods. The researcher selects three samples of fifty subjects each from the population using random sampling procedures. The study is conducted by teaching a different method of skipping rope to each sample and administering a rope-skipping test to all subjects. After analyzing the rope-skipping data, the researcher finds that method B is the superior teaching method. The researcher infers this finding to the population by stating that the research hypothesis is false and method B is the superior method for teaching third-grade boys in Georgia.

Let us examine this example further. The rope-skipping test has 20 points possible. The mean rope-skipping test scores for groups A, B, and C are 10.5, 15.9, and 12.1, respectively. In regard to the differences in the means, one position the researcher could take is that any difference indicates that the teaching methods are not equally effective and that teaching method B is the superior method. This position however, ignores the possibility of **sampling error** which may have partially or totally caused the differences among the groups in mean score. Sampling error occurs when a sample is not 100 percent representative of the population. Blommers and Forsyth (1983) define sampling error as the difference between the value of a population parameter and that of the corresponding sample statistic. Therefore, the differences among groups A, B, and C in mean score could be due to sampling error. Essentially, all samples should have started the experiment with the same mean, but due to sampling error the sample means differed. This could be what caused the differences at the end of the experiment, rather than any differences in the effectiveness of the three treatments. As a result, the differences among the sample means may be a **real difference** due to the treatments not being equally effective, or the differences may be due to sampling error.

If the differences among the means in the rope-skipping example are large, it is reasonable to conclude the differences are real and the treatments are not equally effective. However, if the differences among the means are small, they may well be due to sampling error. The question becomes, Are the differences among the sample means (10.5, 15.9, 12.1) large enough to indicate a real difference? Posing this question to a group of people, some would say yes and some would say no, but many would say they could not tell. The researcher needs a standard procedure to follow in reaching such a decision. Standardization increases the likelihood that researchers following the procedure will reach the same conclusion. Agreement among researchers in this situation is desirable.

Hypothesis-Testing Procedure

Hypothesis testing involves a five-step procedure that researchers use to decide whether to accept or reject the research hypothesis based on the information collected on the sample(s) in the research studies. Though they may execute these steps, researchers may not report all five in their written report or journal article. This five-step procedure, which can be used in a variety of situations, is explained below. Following this explanation, a number of different research designs are presented showing how the hypothesis-testing procedure is used.

Step 1: State the Hypotheses

A researcher starts out with a statement concerning what may be the situation at the population level. If the research involves multiple groups, the statement is that the groups are equal in terms of the measure of interest in the research. Since this is a statement of no or null difference, this statement is called the **null hypothesis** and is indicated using the symbol H_0. This is the **statistical hypothesis,** and it does not have to agree with the **research hypothesis.** In the rope-skipping example, the research hypothesis is that method A is superior, but the null hypothesis is that all three methods are equally good. At least one, and often two, alternate hypotheses symbolized by H_1 and H_2 must be stated to provide a hypothesis to accept if H_0 is rejected.

Step 2: Select the Probability Level

The difference between the population statement in the null hypothesis and what is found in the sample(s) in the research studies is due either to the null hypothesis being false or to sampling error. To make an objective decision, the researcher will conduct a statistical test at the fourth step of the five-step hypothesis-testing procedure. The results of the statistical test provide the probability of the sample finding occurring if the null hypothesis is true. If the probability is small, the null hypothesis is rejected and the difference is considered to be real. Otherwise, the null hypothesis is accepted and the difference is considered to be due to sampling error. In step 2 the researcher selects some probability level that warrants rejection of the null hypothesis. This probability level is called the **alpha level** (α) and is usually specified as .05 or .01.

Step 3: Consult the Statistical Table

Most researchers examine the appropriate statistical table to find the value that the statistical test of the sample would need to equal or exceed in order to reject the null hypothesis at the chosen alpha level. Many computer programs provide a probability value (p) for the value of the statistical test selected in step 4. In this case, the researcher rejects the null hypothesis if the p value is less than or equal to the alpha level.

Step 4: Conduct the Statistical Test

In this step the statistical test is calculated. The statistical test may be calculated by hand or by using a computer.

Step 5: Accept or Reject the Null Hypothesis

In the final step, the decision is made either to accept or to reject the null hypothesis. If the value of the statistical test is greater than the table value or if the p value for the value of the statistical test is less than the alpha level, the null hypothesis is rejected. If the opposite is true, the null hypothesis is accepted.

Accepting the null hypothesis does not prove it is true, only that it is plausible. The null hypothesis could be false by such a small amount that the statistical test did not detect it (e.g., H_0: $\mu = 10$ when really $\mu = 10.03$). So, some researchers use the terms *fail to reject* and *reject* rather than *accept* and *reject*. A statement in the research literature that the statistical test was **significant** indicates that the value of the statistical test warranted rejection of the null hypothesis. More specifically, it indicates that the difference between the null hypothesis population statement and what was found in the sample(s) in the research seems to be a real difference and not due to sampling error. Therefore, a statement that the statistical test was **nonsignificant** indicates that the null hypothesis was retained, and any differences were attributed to sampling error.

The five-step hypothesis-testing procedure is applied in the examples that follow. Each uses a different research design and statistical test. Some additional explanation of the steps in the research process is provided along with the examples. The most extensive explanation of the steps occurs in the first example. The presentation of the five-step hypothesis-testing procedure in subsequent examples is abbreviated to save space. Since the same five-step procedure is followed in each example, make sure you understand the one-group t test example well before venturing on to other examples. The t test and analysis of variance (ANOVA) examples generally apply to situations in experimental research (chapter 5) while the chi-square test examples usually apply to situations in descriptive research (chapter 6).

One-Group t Test

A researcher believes the mean percentage of body fat for a population of male workers is 18 percent. To test this hypothesis, the researcher randomly selects a sample of forty-one men from the population and measures their percentage of body fat.

Step 1: The researcher's hypothesis is that the mean percentage of body fat is 18, so the null hypothesis is that the population mean (μ) is 18 (H_0: $\mu = 18$). As alternatives to this hypothesis, the researcher thought it possible that the mean could be less than 18 (H_1: $\mu < 18$) or greater than 18 (H_2: $\mu > 18$).

Step 2: An alpha level of .05 is selected.

Step 3: A **one-group t test** will be the statistical test, and the sample size is 41. The researcher uses the t tables to find that in order to reject the null hypothesis at an alpha level of .05, the value of the t test has to be at least ± 2.021. Step 3 is not needed if a microcomputer program is used because a p value is calculated and can be compared to the selected alpha level in step 2 (.05 in this case).

Step 4: The researcher calculates the mean for the body fat measurements and calculates the t test.

$$\bar{x} = 16.50$$

$$t = \frac{\bar{x} - \mu}{SE} = \frac{16.50 - 18}{SE} = -3.85, \text{ where SE is the standard error}$$

(calculated by using a formula presented in a statistics book or by the computer program).

Step 5: Since the calculated value of t (-3.85) at step 4 is less than the tabled value of t (-2.021) at step 3, the researcher concludes that the difference between the null hypothesis value (18 percent) at step 1 and the sample value (16.50 percent) at step 4 is real and not due to sampling error. The researcher rejects the null hypothesis and accepts the most likely alternate hypothesis, which in this case is H_1. The population mean is less than 18 percent, since the sample mean is less than 18 percent.

Summary of Example

At step 3 when the researcher used the t tables (see appendix A) to identify the t value needed for rejecting the null hypothesis, the **degrees of freedom** and the alpha level had to be lined up to find the t value. The degrees of freedom for this t test was ($n - 1$) where n is the sample size. Because there are two alternate hypotheses, the researcher uses the alpha level under a two-tailed test. For a two-tailed test this value is always interpreted as both plus and minus. If there is only the one alternate hypothesis, the alpha level under the one-tailed test is used; the value read from the table is interpreted as plus if the alternate hypothesis is greater than (H_1: $\mu >$) and minus if the alternate hypothesis is less than (H_1: $\mu <$). The tabled value is sometimes called the **critical value.** All values at or beyond the critical value are in the **critical region.** If the value of the statistical test used at step 4 is equal to or greater than the tabled value found at step 3 (in the critical region), the difference and the statistical test are called significant (the difference is considered to be real), and the null hypothesis is rejected at step 5. If the value of the statistical test is not equal to or greater than the table value, the difference and statistical test are called nonsignificant (the difference is considered to be due to sampling error), and the null hypothesis is accepted.

At step 4, the larger the difference between the hypothesized population mean (18) and the sample mean (16.50), the larger the value of t. Also, the standard error (SE) is an indication of the amount of sampling error.

This one-group t test just studied is one of three t tests available. Fortunately, most computer packages of statistical programs contain all three t tests. In SYSTAT, the t test for one group is obtained by adding a column to the data file that contains a constant value equal to the population mean and using the two dependent groups t test. Thus, when entering the data shown in table 11.1, each subject has a first aid test score and a constant score of 10 corresponding to the hypothesized population mean. To obtain the t test with SYSTAT, click on STATS under SYSTAT Main, click on Stats, click on t test, put both the first aid test score and the constant score in the Add box, and finally click on Ok. The sample mean is not provided in the printout, so run another program to get it (see chapter 10).

The scores of three groups on a first aid test are presented in table 11.1. The scores of group A are analyzed using SYSTAT to test the null hypothesis that the population mean equals 10 (H_0: $\mu = 10$). The t test output is presented in table 11.2. Notice that the computer provides a probability value (p value—.025, in our example) so that it is not necessary to look up the table value.

TABLE 11.1 Scores for Three Groups on a First Aid Test		
GROUP A	**GROUP B**	**GROUP C**
12	7	13
15	10	14
10	11	10
11	8	9
9	9	12
14	10	11
12	12	11
13	9	15

TABLE 11.2 Output for the One-Group *t* Test of Group A in Table 11.1	
Cases	8
Sample Mean	12.00
Mean Difference	2.00
t	2.83
df	7
Prob	.025

Two Independent Groups *t* Test

The **two independent groups *t* test** is used either when two samples are drawn from the same population and each is administered a different treatment or when a sample is drawn from each of two populations. In the first case, two samples of seventy-five each are drawn from a population of female college freshmen and each sample is taught by a different method. After the treatments (methods) are administered, each sample represents a different population: a population of freshmen who have received or will in the future receive the particular treatment. In the second case, two samples of forty are drawn, one from a population of athletes and one from a population of nonathletes. Both samples represent different populations; the question is whether there is a difference between the two samples in mean performance as an indication of a difference at the population level.

The *t* test for two independent groups can be obtained with SYSTAT. The data of groups A and B in table 11.1 are used to demonstrate this analysis and the five-step hypothesis-testing procedure. When entering the data into the computer each subject must have two scores: one identifying group membership and the other being the score of the subject. An example of this for the first two scores in group A and then group B in table 11.1 is shown below.

CASE	ID	SCORE	
1	1	12	ID was the name the researcher used to identify
2	1	15	group membership (1 = A group, 2 = B group)
3	2	7	and SCORE was the name the researcher used
4	2	10	for the score of a subject.

To conduct the t test using SYSTAT, click on STATS under SYSTAT Main, click on Stats, click on t test, put the data variable (SCORE in the example) in the Add box and the group identification variable (ID in the example) in the Group box, and finally click on Ok.

Step 1: H_0: $\mu_A - \mu_B = 0$ (hypothesis that population means are equal)

H_1: $\mu_A - \mu_B > 0$ (hypothesis that A population mean is greater)

H_2: $\mu_A - \mu_B < 0$ (hypothesis that B population mean is greater)

Step 2: Alpha = .05

Step 3: The t test table critical value is based on degrees of freedom equal to ($n_1 + n_2 - 2$) where n_1 is the sample size for group A and n_2 is for group B. The degrees of freedom is 14 (or $8 + 8 - 2$). The table value for an alpha of .05 under a two-tailed test and degrees of freedom 14 is ± 2.145.

Step 4: The scores of each group are analyzed and the t test calculated.

$$t = \frac{\bar{x}_A - \bar{x}_B}{SE}$$

The results of the computer analysis are presented in table 11.3.

Step 5: The calculated t value from step 4 is compared with the table t value at step 3 or the computer p value with the alpha level at step 2.

The computer provided a p value of .015. No matter whether the calculated t value of 2.76 is compared with the table t value of ± 2.145, or the p value of .015 is compared with the alpha level (.05) in step 2, the difference between the means for A and B groups is significant and the null hypothesis (H_0) is rejected in favor of H_1 because the t value is positive and group A has the larger mean.

Two Dependent Groups t Test

One example of the **two dependent groups t test** is a **repeated measures** design, and the other example is a **matched pairs** design. In either case there are two columns of scores and some degree of correlation or dependency between them. With the repeated measures design, a population is defined from which a sample is

TABLE 11.3 Output for the Two Independent Groups *t* Test for Groups A and B
in Table 11.1

ITEM	GROUP A	GROUP B
n	8	8
Mean	12.00	9.50
Standard Deviation	2.00	1.60
t-Value	2.76	
df	14	
Prob	.015	

drawn using random sampling procedures. Subjects are tested initially, an experimental treatment is administered, and the subjects finally retested. Usually, the same test is administered both before and after the treatment so the research situation is called a test-retest design or pretest-posttest design. With paper-and-pencil tests, one form of the test (form A) could be administered at pretest and form B of the test could be administered at posttest. The purpose of this research design is to determine if an experimental treatment is effective.

The research question could also be investigated using two independent groups, with one group receiving the experimental treatment (experimental group) and the other receiving no treatment (control group). The repeated measures design is more efficient and precise than the two independent groups design because all subjects receive the treatment and act as their own control. The experimental research chapter describes the repeated measures design as having numerous internal and external validity problems; however, this design is commonly used.

With the matched pairs design, a population is defined and some measure(s) is collected on each member of the population that the researcher feels must be controlled in the research study. The researcher wants the two groups involved in this design to start the experiment basically equal in terms of the measure(s) collected. Subjects are paired on this measure(s), with one subject from each pair randomly assigned to each of the two groups. Each group receives a different treatment, so there may be one experimental group and one control group, or there may be two experimental groups. After the groups receive the treatments, they are measured and the data are analyzed to determine if the groups seem equal in mean performance.

Example: The population is college freshmen at a large university. Two different methods of teaching a large lecture class are going to be compared. A gender score and IQ score are obtained for each of the 600 members of the population. For two students to be paired, they have to be of the same gender and have IQ scores that differ by no more than 5. One hundred pairs are formed. One subject from each pair is randomly assigned to each teaching method. Subjects are taught by their assigned teaching method for fifteen weeks. After that, all subjects take a knowledge test. The data are analyzed to determine if the two teaching methods seem to be equally effective.

The matched pairs design is an alternative to the two independent groups design but is more precise in that the two groups start the experiment equal on at least the measure(s) used for forming pairs. Loss of subjects can be a problem with the matched pairs design because some members of the population cannot be paired, and during the experiment, if one member of a pair is lost from the experiment, the other member of the pair must be removed from the study.

The t test is the same for the repeated measures design and matched pairs design.

$$t = \frac{\bar{x}_I - \bar{x}_F}{SE}$$ for repeated measures where $\bar{x}_F$ is the mean for the final scores

or

$$t = \frac{\bar{x}_1 - \bar{x}_2}{SE}$$ for matched pairs where $\bar{x}_2$ is the mean for group 2,

with degrees of freedom equal to $n - 1$, where n is the number of subjects for a repeated measures design or the number of pairs for a matched pairs design. An example of the five-step hypothesis-testing procedure with a repeated measures design is presented below.

Suppose eight subjects are selected and initially (I) measured for number of mistakes made when juggling a ball. The subjects are then taught to juggle and finally (F) measured. Let us say that, in table 11.1, the group A scores are the initial scores and the group B scores are the final scores. To determine if the subjects improved in juggling ability as a result of the juggling instruction, a t test for dependent groups is conducted.

Step 1: H_0: $\mu_I - \mu_F = 0$ (hypothesis that final and initial means are equal at
H_1: $\mu_I - \mu_F < 0$ the population level)

Step 2: Alpha = .05

Step 3: Find the t test table value with degrees of freedom equal to $n - 1$, where n is the number of subjects. In this example, the degrees of freedom is 7 ($8 - 1$) and the tabled t value is -1.895 for an alpha of .05 in a one-tailed test.

Step 4: Analyze the initial and final data, and calculate the t test.

$$t = \frac{\bar{x}_I - \bar{x}_F}{SE}$$

The repeated measures t test can be obtained with SYSTAT. The data are entered in pairs by subject with the initial and final score for subject 1 (12, 7) entered first, followed by the initial and final score for subject 2 (15, 10), and each of the remaining subjects. To conduct the t test using SYSTAT follow the same procedure

TABLE 11.4	Output for the Repeated Measures *t* Test Treating the A and B Group Data in Table 11.1 as Repeated Measures	
ITEM	SCORE 1	SCORE 2
Cases	8	8
Mean	12.00	9.50
Std. Dev.	2.00	1.60
Mean Difference	2.50	
t	2.89	
df	7	
Prob	.023	

as for the two independent groups *t* test except put both the scores of the subjects in the Add box. Since the means and standard deviations are not provided in the print-out, after running the repeated measures *t* test run the program that provides means and standard deviations (discussed in chapter 10). The printout of this analysis is presented in table 11.4.

Step 5: Because the *p* value in table 11.4 is less than the .05 alpha level selected at step 2, the difference between the initial and final means is significant and the null hypothesis is rejected. Notice that the calculated *t* exceeds the tabled *t*, and the same conclusion is drawn. Also notice that because the measured variable is number of mistakes, the final mean of 9.50 is superior to the initial mean of 12.00. Therefore, the researcher concludes that the treatment is effective.

Decision on Alternate Hypotheses and Alpha Level

Before considering other research designs and statistical tests, selection of alternate hypotheses and the alpha level must be explained in greater detail. With the five-step hypothesis-testing procedure at least one, and often two, alternate hypotheses are stated. Usually two alternate hypotheses are stated because the null hypothesis and the two alternate hypotheses cover all possibilities. The researcher believes that if the null hypothesis is false it could be in either direction, and the researcher is interested in both alternatives. For example, all possibilities are covered in the situation where H_0: mean IQ is 100; H_1: mean IQ is less than 100; and H_2: mean IQ is greater than 100. The researcher may have decided that the teaching method to be used will depend on which hypothesis is accepted. However, in situations where the researcher knows there is only one alternative to the null hypothesis or only one alternative is of interest to the researcher, only one alternative hypothesis is stated. For example, in a repeated measures design the researcher usually knows that the treatment will either have no effect or a positive effect; the treatment will not make the subjects worse.

Another example is situations where a traditional method is being compared with a new method. Only if the new method is superior to the traditional method will the researcher recommend a change in method.

It is important to remember that the number of alternate hypotheses determines whether the statistical test is one-tailed or two-tailed. If there are two alternate hypotheses, the statistical test is two-tailed. Notice in the *t* tables that for any degrees of freedom and alpha level, the value for a one-tailed test is smaller than for a two-tailed test. The smaller the table value, the easier it is to reject the null hypothesis. Thus, acceptance or rejection of the null hypothesis may be dependent on the number of alternate hypotheses.

While examining the *t* table, notice that for any degrees of freedom, the smaller the alpha level, the larger the table value. Selection of the alpha level also influences the acceptance or rejection of the null hypothesis. Traditionally researchers have used an alpha level of .05 unless there were reasons for selecting a different value. The second most commonly used alpha level is .01. Using an alpha level of .01 rather than .05 makes it more difficult to reject the null hypothesis, meaning the smaller the alpha level, the larger the difference must be between what is hypothesized at the population level and what is found at the sample level. In situations where rejecting the null hypothesis has major implications, researchers tend to use alpha levels of .01 or even .001. For example, if rejecting the null hypothesis means that an effective traditional drug is going to be replaced by a new drug, the researcher might use an alpha level of .01 or .001 because the researcher wants to be particularly confident that the new drug is superior to the effective traditional drug.

A diagram of the four possible outcomes of a research study is presented in figure 11.1. In any research study, the null hypothesis is either true or false, but the researcher never knows for sure which is correct. Based on the statistical test, the researcher either accepts or rejects the null hypothesis. If the null hypothesis really is true, and based on the statistical test the researcher accepts it, this is a good decision. However, if the researcher rejects a null hypothesis that is really true this is called a **type I error.** A type I error is defined as rejecting a true null hypothesis. The probability of making a type I error is equal to the alpha level. Therefore, the researcher usually selects the alpha level based on the seriousness of a type I error. Researchers always use small alpha levels as a way of protecting themselves against making a type I error.

If the null hypothesis really is false, and based on the statistical test the researcher rejects it, this is also a good decision. But if the researcher did not reject a false null hypothesis, this is called a **type II error** and is symbolized by **beta (β)**. A type II error is defined either as accepting a false null hypothesis or not rejecting a false null hypothesis. Many things can influence the probability of making a type II error. The larger the alpha level, the smaller the probability of making a type II error. Since the alpha level also affects the probability of a type I error, most researchers do not try to influence the probability of a type II error with the alpha selection. The larger the sample size, the smaller the probability of a type II error,

Decision

		Accept	**Reject**
True		Good decision	Type I error
H$_0$			
False		Type II error	Good decision

FIGURE 11.1
Four possible outcomes in
a research study.

and sample size is often something the researcher can control. The more false the null hypothesis, the less likely a type II error will occur. This is not something the researcher controls, but it should be kept in mind when small differences are found in a research study.

The term **statistical power** is commonly found in the research literature. Statistical power is the probability of not making a type II error, so power is the probability of rejecting a false null hypothesis. Power equals one minus beta $(1 - \beta)$. One-tailed tests have more statistical power than two-tailed tests, and a two dependent groups design has more statistical power than a two independent groups design. Everything that decreases the probability of making a type II error, increases statistical power.

Analysis of Variance

Many research problems or questions involve more than two treatment groups. In these situations, **analysis of variance (ANOVA)** is used to analyze the data. Actually, ANOVA can also be used when there are just two treatment groups, so in this situation it could be used rather than a t test. There are many different ANOVA designs. An overview of the technique should help in understanding each design.

Using the ANOVA technique, the total variability in a set of scores is divided into two or more components. These variability values are called **sums of squares (SS).** A degrees of freedom value (df) is obtained for both the total variability value and each of the component values. The sum of squares value for each component is divided by its degrees of freedom value to obtain a **mean square (MS) value.** The ratio of two mean square values is an F statistic, which is used to test the null hypothesis. The F test is conducted at step 4 of the five-step hypothesis-testing procedure.

One-Way ANOVA

One-way ANOVA is an extension of the two independent groups design already discussed, but typically involves statistical analysis of three or more independent groups. Ferguson and Takane (1989) refer to this test as a one-way ANOVA because each score only has one classification (group membership). The placement of the score in the group has no effect on the data analysis. Actually, a one-way ANOVA can be used with two or more independent groups, so it could be used in place of the *t* test for two independent groups. The null hypothesis being tested is that the populations represented by the groups (samples) are equal in mean performance. The one alternate hypothesis is that the population means are not equal.

Some explanation of the one-way ANOVA is necessary to understand how the technique is used and how to interpret the output from the computer analysis. Also, a few symbols are necessary in order to develop formulas for determining degrees of freedom.

Two or more independent groups each receive a different treatment. The number of groups will be represented symbolically by K, and the total number of scores by N. For the data in table 11.1, $K = 3$ and $N = 24$. All the scores in all the groups are combined into one set of scores and the mean is calculated. The variability of the scores from this mean is the total variability for the set of scores and is called the sum of squares total (SS_T). The sum of squares total is divided into sum of squares among groups (SS_A) and sum of squares within groups (SS_W).

$$SS_T = SS_A + SS_W$$

Group means are calculated; if these group means are not equal, the sum of squares among groups is greater than zero. Thus, SS_A is an indication of differences among the groups. The sum of squares within groups is an indication of how much the scores in the groups differ from their group mean. Thus, if in any groups all scores are not the same value, SS_W will be greater than zero.

Each sum of squares has a degrees of freedom value. The degrees of freedom for total (df_T) is divided into a degrees of freedom among (df_A) and within (df_W) groups.

$$df_T = df_A + df_W,$$
$$\text{where } df_T = N - 1, df_A = K - 1, df_W = N - K.$$

Applied to the data in table 11.1:

$$df_T = 24 - 1 = 23$$
$$df_A = 3 - 1 = 2$$
$$df_W = 23 - 3 = 20$$

The sums of squares values for among and within groups are divided by their degrees of freedom to provide mean square (MS) values and an F statistic is calculated from the two mean square values:

$$MS_A = \frac{SS_A}{df_A}, MS_W = \frac{SS_W}{df_W}, F = \frac{MS_A}{MS_W}$$

Any F statistic is represented by two degrees of freedom values in the F table. The first degrees of freedom value is for the numerator and the second degrees of freedom value is for the denominator of the F statistic. The numerator degrees of freedom is df_A and the denominator degrees of freedom is df_W. So,

TABLE 11.5 Output for the One-Way ANOVA for the Data in Table 11.1

SOURCE	SS	DF	MS	F-RATIO	P
Among	31.75	2	15.88	4.45	.024
Within	74.88	21	3.57		
Total	106.63	23			

GROUP	N	MEAN			
A	8	12.00			
B	8	9.50			
C	8	11.88			

$$F = \frac{MS_A}{MS_W}$$ has degrees of freedom equal to $(K - 1)$ and $(N - K)$.

The F table is presented in appendix B. The first degrees of freedom value is read across the top of the table, and the second degrees of freedom value is read down the left side of the table. Two table values appear where the line down from the first degrees of freedom value and across from the second degrees of freedom value intersect. The larger value is the F value needed for significance at the .01 alpha level, and the other level is for the .05 alpha level. If the degrees of freedom is 2 and 24, the table values are 3.40 for alpha equals .05 and 5.61 for alpha equals .01.

An example of the five-step hypothesis-testing procedure using the data in table 11.1 follows:

Step 1: H_0: $\mu_A = \mu_B = \mu_C$ (the three population means are equal)
        H_1: $\mu_A \neq \mu_B \neq \mu_C$ (the three population means are not equal)

Step 2: Alpha = .05

Step 3: Find the critical value in the F test table with degrees of freedom $(K - 1)$ and $(N - K)$ at the alpha level selected. In this example, the degrees of freedom are 2 and 21 so the table value is 3.47 for alpha equals .05.

Step 4: Analyze the data using a one-way ANOVA. In SYSTAT, one-way ANOVA is conducted by clicking on MGLH, and then clicking on Means Model. As in the t test for two independent groups, when the data are entered, there must be a variable identifying group membership and a score for each subject. At Means Model in MGLH, the Dependent variable is the data variable and the Category variable is the variable identifying group membership. Select the Mean option to get group means. Click on Ok when ready to analyze the data. Applied to the data from table 11.1, the one-way ANOVA output is presented in table 11.5. The statistical test is the F ratio, and it can be seen that the F ratio is 4.45 and the p value of the F ratio is .024.

Step 5: Since the p value of .024 is less than the alpha level of .05, a researcher concludes that there is a significant difference among the group means and accepts the alternate hypothesis. The same decision is made if the F ratio of 4.45 is compared with the table value of 3.47 in step 3.

Repeated Measures ANOVA

The **repeated measures ANOVA** design is an extension of the t test for two dependent groups design, using repeated measurement of subjects. Each subject is measured on two or more occasions. If there are only two measures for each subject, the repeated measures ANOVA design is an alternative to the t test for dependent groups design. However, if there are more than two measures for each subject, the repeated measures ANOVA design must be used. The repeated measures ANOVA design is also referred to as a one-way ANOVA with repeated measures. The null hypothesis being tested is that, at the population level, the means for the repeated measures are equal. The alternate hypothesis is that the means are not equal.

Suppose a group of subjects is drawn from a population using random sampling procedures. Before the experimental treatment is administered the subjects are initially tested. The experimental treatment is then administered for nine weeks, and every three weeks the subjects are tested. The data layout for this study is presented in table 11.6.

The data layout is two-dimensional since each score has two classifiers—a row designation (subject) and a column designation (repeated measure). The score of 10 for subject A must be placed in the Initial Test column of the row for subject A (each row-column intersection is called a **cell**) or it is in the wrong cell. Notice in the one-way ANOVA previously discussed, that each score had only the single classification of group membership.

Again, some symbolism is needed to develop degrees of freedom formulas. The total number of scores is N, the number of repeated measures is K, and the number of subjects is n. In table 11.6, $N = 32$, $K = 4$, and $n = 8$. In this ANOVA design, sum of squares total (SS_T) is partitioned into the following components: sum of squares subjects (SS_S); sum of squares repeated measures (SS_M); and sum of squares interaction (SS_I).

$$SS_T = SS_S + SS_M + SS_I$$

The minimum value for each of the sum of squares values is zero. The SS_T is greater than zero if all N scores are not the same. The SS_S is greater than zero if subjects differ in mean score across repeated measures. The SS_M is greater than zero if the means for repeated measures are not equal. The SS_I is greater than zero if all subjects did not follow the same scoring pattern across the repeated measures. In table 11.6, SS_I is greater than zero because the scores for subject A increased by three, then by two, then by one from test to test, but the other subjects demonstrated different patterns. Each of these terms has a degrees of freedom (df) value.

TABLE 11.6 Repeated Measures ANOVA Example Data				
SUBJECTS	INITIAL TEST	3-WEEK TEST	6-WEEK TEST	9-WEEK TEST
A	10	13	15	16
B	5	9	10	13
C	11	12	12	13
D	6	9	12	14
E	6	8	10	12
F	5	6	10	13
G	8	10	11	13
H	9	11	13	14

$$df_T = df_S + df_M + df_I$$

The formulas for the degrees of freedom are as follows:

$$df_T = N - 1 \qquad df_S = n - 1 \qquad df_M = K - 1 \qquad df_I = (n - 1)(K - 1)$$

In table 11.6, $df_T = 32 - 1 = 31$, $df_S = 8 - 1 = 7$, $df_M = 4 - 1 = 3$, and $df_I = (8 - 1)(4 - 1) = 21$.

Mean square values are obtained for subjects, for repeated measures, and for interaction components. The statistical hypothesis being tested is that the means for the repeated measures are equal. To form the F statistic the mean square value indicating the differences among the means for the repeated measures (MS_M) becomes the numerator, and the mean square value indicating sampling error (MS_I) becomes the denominator. The F test takes this form:

$$F = \frac{MS_M}{MS_I}, \qquad \begin{array}{l} \text{with } K - 1 \text{ degrees of freedom and} \\ (n - 1)(K - 1) \text{ degrees of freedom} \end{array}$$

An example of the five-step hypothesis-testing procedure is presented using the data in table 11.6.

Step 1: H_0: $\mu_{initial} = \mu_3 = \mu_6 = \mu_9$
H_1: $\mu_{initial} \neq \mu_3 \neq \mu_6 \neq \mu_9$

Step 2: Alpha = .05

Step 3: Find the table value of F with degrees of freedom $K - 1$ and $(n - 1)(K - 1)$ at the .05 alpha level. The value of F with degrees of freedom 3 and 21 at the .05 alpha level is 3.07.

TABLE 11.7 Output for the Repeated Measures ANOVA for the Data in Table 11.6

SOURCE	SS	DF	MS	F-RATIO	P
Between Subj.	82.47	7	11.78	1.56	.195
Treatments	158.34	3	52.78	48.39	.000
Error	22.91	21	1.09		
Total	263.72	31	8.51		

	Treatment	Mean	Std. Dev.
	Initial	7.50	2.33
	3-week	9.75	2.25
	6-week	11.63	1.77
	9-week	13.50	1.20

Step 4: This repeated measures ANOVA design is not possible on SYSTAT, so another statistical package of computer programs was used to analyze the data in table 11.6. The output from the computer is presented in table 11.7. The repeated measures F value for treatments is 48.39, which is greater than the table value of F at step 3. The p value of .000 for treatments is less than the alpha level at step 2. Using either indicator, the calculated F value for treatments is significant. The mean and standard deviation is provided for each treatment as part of the output. The F value for subjects is not of interest in this analysis.

Labels for the sources or components in the ANOVA vary among statistics books and computer programs. Knowing what to expect in the ANOVA summary table helps the reader interpret the labels. In table 11.7 the error source is the interaction source. Other computer programs may label the interaction source as *residual* or as *ST* to suggest a subject (S) by treatment (T) interaction.

Step 5: Based on step 4, conclude that H_0 is false; accept H_1 that the treatment means are not equal.

Random Blocks ANOVA

Earlier in this chapter, a matched pairs *t* test design was presented. In this design pairs are formed by pairing two subjects. Then, using random procedures, one subject from each pair is assigned to one group, and the other subject is assigned to a second group. The **random blocks ANOVA** design is an extension of the matched pairs *t* test when there are three or more groups, and is the same as the matched pairs *t* test when there are two groups. In the random blocks design, subjects similar in terms of a variable(s) are placed together in what is called a *block,* rather than a *pair*

TABLE 11.8 Example Data Layout for a Random Blocks ANOVA Design					
BLOCK	**GROUP 1**	**GROUP 2**	**GROUP 3**	• • •	**GROUP K**
1	X	X	X	• • •	X
2	X	X	X	• • •	X
3	X	X	X	• • •	X
•	•	•	•		•
•	•	•	•		•
•	•	•	•		•
n	X	X	X	• • •	X

as in the *t* test. The number of subjects in each block is equal to the number of treatment groups in the research study. The procedures used in the matched pairs *t* test might serve as a helpful reference for this design.

After subjects are assigned to groups, each group receives a different treatment, and at the end of the study the data are collected. The random block design has all the advantages and disadvantages of the matched pairs *t* test.

Table 11.8 is an example data layout for a random blocks design. Notice that the same notation is used in this design as is used for the repeated measures ANOVA design. In fact, blocks are like subjects, treatment groups are like repeated measures, and the hypothesis tested is that the group means are equal. Thus, the analysis for the random blocks design is the same as the analysis for the repeated measures ANOVA design.

Two-Way ANOVA, Multiple Scores per Cell

Two-way ANOVA is a term used by Ferguson and Takane (1989) and some other authors of statistics books and computer programs. A variety of other terms referring to the same design are commonly found in statistics books and the research literature, as well. In a two-way ANOVA design, each score has a row and a column classifier.

The two ANOVA designs previously discussed involved just one score per cell. Three examples of two-way ANOVA designs with multiple scores in each cell are presented next. The data analysis is the same in all three examples. In each example, it is possible to test several statistical hypotheses that require different *F* tests. An explanation of the data analysis follows each example.

The first example is a random blocks design with more than one score per cell. This is the same as the previous random blocks design except that enough subjects are placed in each block to have multiple scores per cell. For example, if there are five treatment groups, the number of subjects in each block has to be ten, fifteen, or some other multiple of five. The statistical hypothesis is always that the treatment

TABLE 11.9 Example Data Layout for a Factorial ANOVA (Gender × Treatment)			
	TREATMENT GROUP		
GENDER	**A**	**B**	**C**
Female	2, 1, 3, 2, 3	6, 3, 4, 5, 6	5, 4, 7, 6, 8
Male	4, 3, 2, 3, 1	4, 5, 7, 6, 8	10, 9, 10, 8, 11

groups are equal in mean score; additional statistical hypotheses of interest are tested in certain situations.

The second example is referred to as **factorial design.** In this two-way data layout, the rows represent some classification of the subjects (e.g., gender, age, school grade), the columns identify the treatment group, and there are multiple subjects in each cell. In table 11.9, subjects are classified by gender with five females and five males randomly assigned to each treatment group. Data are collected at the end of the research study after the groups experienced the treatments. The analysis for this example design could be referred to as a **two-dimensional ANOVA** or a 2 × 3 (Gender × Treatment) ANOVA. Gender has two levels and treatment has three levels because there are two classifications of gender and three treatment groups.

In this example, the researcher is interested in testing the statistical hypothesis that the treatment group (column) means are equal. The row variable may be a dimension if the researcher wants to test a second statistical hypothesis that the row means are equal. Or, it is possible that this hypothesis is not of interest to the researcher, so the row variable is a dimension used to gain experimental control as discussed in the experimental research chapter. In the table 11.9 example, gender as a dimension will be a source in the ANOVA summary table. If gender is not a dimension, the design is a one-way ANOVA with three treatment groups, gender is not a source in the ANOVA summary table, and any differences between the genders in mean score are put into the "within" component of the one-way ANOVA. Since in the one-way ANOVA, $F = MS_{among}/MS_{within}$, putting the gender difference into the within component will decrease the value of the F test and increase the chances of making a type II error.

A third statistical hypothesis can be tested in this example: no interaction between the row variable and the column variable. In terms of table 11.9, this hypothesis states that any differences in the effectiveness of the treatments are the same for both genders. The no interaction hypothesis will be discussed later in the chapter.

The third example is also a factorial design, but rows are levels of one treatment, columns are levels of a second treatment, and there are multiple subjects in each cell. It is commonly used because it is a combination of two treatments. For example, in table 11.10 treatment A, is the number of days per week people participated in an adult fitness program (A1 = 1 day, A2 = 3 days); treatment B, is how

TABLE 11.10 Example Data Layout for a Factorial ANOVA (Days × Minutes)			
TREATMENT	**B1**	**B2**	**B3**
A1	12, 10, 9, 11, 10	10, 11, 9, 10, 11	10, 9, 8, 7, 8
A2	14, 12, 13, 15, 12	8, 9, 10, 9, 11	6, 7, 5, 6, 4

Note: A1 = 1 day/week; A2 = 3 days/week; B1 = 15 minutes/day; B2 = 30 minutes/day; B3 = 45 minutes/day.

many minutes per participation day people participated (B1 = 15 minutes, B2 = 30 minutes, B3 = 45 minutes). Five subjects are randomly assigned to receive each treatment combination. For example, the A1B1 group participated 1 day a week, 15 minutes a day. The experimental period is six months. At the end of that period, all subjects are tested on a fitness test where a low score reflects high fitness.

Three null hypotheses are usually tested in this ANOVA design. The first hypothesis is that there is no interaction between the row and column variables. If there is no interaction, the difference between any two column means is the same for each row, and vice versa. If there is no interaction effect, the difference between the A1B1 and A1B2 cell means is the same as the difference between the A2B1 and A2B2 cell means. The second hypothesis is that the row means are equal. If the hypothesis is true, the A1 and A2 row means are equal. The third hypothesis is that the column means are equal. If the hypothesis is true, the B1, B2, and B3 column means are equal.

The particular symbols used to represent two-way ANOVA designs with multiple scores per cell apply to all three of the example designs that have been presented. The symbol C represents the number of columns in the design; the number of rows in the design is R. The number of scores in each cell is represented by n; the total number of scores in the whole design is represented by N, which is equal to CRn (columns × rows × cell size). In table 11.10, $C = 3$, $R = 2$, $n = 5$, and $N = 30$.

In the two-way ANOVA design with multiple scores per cell, the sum of squares total (SS_T) is partitioned into a sum of squares columns (SS_C), a sum of squares rows (SS_R), a sum of squares interaction (SS_I), and a sum of squares within (SS_W):

$$SS_T = SS_C + SS_R + SS_I + SS_W$$

The minimum value for each of these sum of squares is zero. The SS_T is greater than zero if all N scores are not equal. The SS_C is greater than zero if the means for the columns are unequal. The greater the inequality among the columns, the larger SS_C. Likewise, the more the row means differ, the larger is SS_R. There will be no interaction ($SS_I = 0$) if the pattern of differences among column means is the same for each row, and vice versa. Finally, SS_W will equal zero if for each cell all scores in the cell are the same value.

Each of these sum of squares values has an associated degrees of freedom value. So,

$$df_T = df_C + df_R + df_I + df_W, \text{ where}$$
$$df_T = N - 1,$$
$$df_C = C - 1,$$
$$df_R = R - 1,$$
$$df_I = (C - 1)(R - 1),$$
$$df_W = (C)(R)(n - 1).$$

As always, each of the parts of SS_T is divided by its degrees of freedom (df) to produce a mean square (MS) value. So,

$$MS_C = SS_C/df_C,$$
$$MS_R = SS_R/df_R,$$
$$MS_I = SS_I/df_I,$$
$$MS_W = SS_W/df_W.$$

These mean square values are used to form the F tests for the various statistical hypotheses. All three potential hypotheses are presented below; although a researcher might not test a hypothesis if it is not of interest.

Typically the first hypothesis tested is one of no interaction. The alternate hypothesis (H_1) is one of interaction. The hypothesis is tested with $F = MS_I/MS_W$ with degrees of freedom $(C - 1)(R - 1)$ and $(C)(R)(n - 1)$. A significant F value could affect how subsequent F tests are calculated and/or how the overall data analysis is conducted. Discussion of this issue is left to books such as Winer, Brown, and Michels (1991), Maxwell and Delaney (1990), Keppel (1991), and other experimental design books.

A second hypothesis tested is that the column means are equal. The alternate hypothesis is that the column means are not equal. This test is usually with $F = MS_C/MS_W$ and degrees of freedom $(C - 1)$ and $(C)(R)(n - 1)$. Occasionally, the denominator is not MS_W; this will alter the second degrees of freedom value. Remember, for any F test the first degrees of freedom value is for the numerator and the second degrees of freedom value is for the denominator. In the F test just presented, the numerator will always be MS_C. Notice that the numerator of any F test corresponds to the hypothesis being tested. The hypothesis in the last example dealt with the column means, so the numerator of the F test was MS_C.

A third hypothesis tested is that the row means are equal. The alternate hypothesis is the row means are not equal. This hypothesis is seldom tested in a random blocks design. The F test is normally $F = MS_R/MS_W$ with degrees of freedom $(R - 1)$ and $(C)(R)(n - 1)$.

The following is an example of the data analysis for a factorial design using the data in table 11.10. Remember, this data is fitness test scores, so small scores are better than large scores.

Step 1: A. First hypothesis tested is that there is no interaction between rows and columns.

$$H_0: \mu_I = 0 \text{ (mean interaction } [\mu_I] = 0)$$
$$H_1: \mu_I \neq 0 \text{ (mean interaction } > 0)$$

B. Second hypothesis tested is that the row means are equal.

$$H_0: \mu_1 = \mu_2 \text{ (row means are equal)}$$
$$H_1: \mu_1 \neq \mu_2$$

C. Third hypothesis tested is that the column means are equal.

$$H_0: \mu_1 = \mu_2 = \mu_3 \text{ (column means are equal)}$$
$$H_1: \mu_1 \neq \mu_2 \neq \mu_3$$

Step 2: Alpha = .05

Step 3: Find the table value for each of the three hypotheses stated in step 1 for the alpha level stated in step 2.

A. $F(2,24) = 3.40$ (for testing interaction) (F with 2 and 24 degrees of freedom = 3.40)

B. $F(1,24) = 4.26$ (for testing row means)

C. $F(2,24) = 3.40$ (for testing column means)

Step 4: A factorial ANOVA is conducted on the data in table 11.10 using SYSTAT. In entering the data there is a variable for treatment A, treatment B, and the score of a subject. To obtain the analysis click on STATS under SYSTAT Main, click on MGLH, click on Fully Factorial ANOVA. The Dependent variable is the data variable and the Factors variable is the variable used to form the rows and columns in the factorial ANOVA. Select the Means option. Finally, click on Ok. The output of the data analysis is presented in table 11.11. Notice that a summary of the ANOVA, row means, column means, and cell means are provided in this output.

Based on table 11.11, there is a significant interaction effect. This is determined either by noting that the F ratio for the interaction effect from the computer (15.89) exceeds the tabled F (3.40) or noting that the significance value (p value) for the interaction effect from the computer (.000) is less than the alpha level (.05) specified in step 2. Figure 11.2 is a plot of the means that illustrates the significant interaction. The significant interaction can be easily seen in the graph because the lines formed by the cell means are not parallel. For those who exercised only one day per week (A1), 45 minutes of exercise per week is better than 15 or 30 minutes; however, the group that exercised three days per week (A2) improved their fitness by exercising more minutes per day.

Significant interactions are reacted to in many different ways depending on the research situation and the type of interaction that the graph of the means appears to show. A discussion of how to interpret significant interactions is beyond the scope of this book. However, in the factorial design example discussed, the significant interaction might invalidate the F tests on row means and on column means. In this case, **simple effects tests** are conducted. Simple effects tests could be comparing the

TABLE 11.11 Output for the Two-Way ANOVA for the Data in Table 11.10

SOURCE	SS	DF	MS	F-RATIO	P
Rows	0.53	1	0.53	0.42	.523
Columns	116.27	2	58.13	45.89	.000
Rows × Columns	40.27	2	20.13	15.89	.000
Error	30.40	24	1.27		
Total	187.47	29	6.46		

Row	N	Mean
1:	15	9.67
2:	15	9.40

Column	N	Mean
1:	10	11.80
2:	10	9.80
3:	10	7.00

Row/Column	N	Mean
1 and 1	5	10.40
1 and 2	5	10.20
1 and 3	5	8.40
2 and 1	5	13.20
2 and 2	5	9.40
2 and 3	5	5.60

column means for each row or the row means for each column. For example, the test could check for differences among the three column means for row 1 and then for row 2.

As presented in table 11.11, there is not a significant difference between the row means ($F = .42$, $p = .523$). For the difference to be significant, the F value would have to be at least 4.26, or the p value would have to be .05 or smaller.

There is, however, a significant difference among the column means. In table 11.11 the F value for columns is 45.89, which exceeds the table value of 3.40; the p value is .000, which is less than the alpha level of .05. An inspection of the column means shows that the means get progressively smaller as the subjects exercise longer per day.

Step 5: The researcher concludes, based on the findings at step 4, that there is an interaction between number of days per week of exercise (rows) and length of each

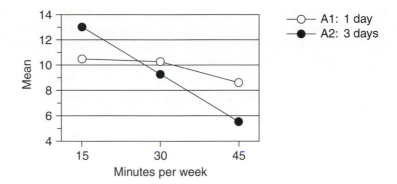

FIGURE 11.2
A plot of the cell means for the data in table 11.10.

exercise session (columns). Also, the researcher concludes that the three lengths of an exercise session (columns) are not equally effective. However, the researcher concludes that the number of days per week of exercise (rows) are equally effective.

Other ANOVA Designs

The ANOVA designs presented are those most often found in the research literature. Many more ANOVA designs are possible and can be found in the research literature. Whole statistics courses are taught on ANOVA designs from texts like Dayton (1970), Keppel (1991), Kirk (1982), Maxwell and Delaney (1990), and Winer, Brown, and Michels (1991). One- and two-way ANOVA designs have been discussed, but three- and four-way ANOVA designs are not uncommon in the research literature. Many computer programs will analyze up to an eight-way ANOVA. However, researchers should be cautious when designing studies that require an ANOVA design larger than a three-way because they are usually complex and the many interaction terms are difficult to interpret.

Assumptions Underlying Statistical Tests

The statisticians who developed the t and F statistical tests based these tests on certain assumptions. Researchers should be aware of these assumptions and try to satisfy them. Failure to at least partially satisfy the assumptions underlying a statistical test invalidates the test. The assumptions underlying statistical tests sometimes vary from test to test. Assumptions underlying each of the statistical tests discussed up to this point are presented in most statistics books. Presented below is a discussion of assumptions common to most of these statistical tests.

First, it is assumed scores are at least interval (see chapter 10). In some situations, and with some data, it may be acceptable to use the statistical tests with ordinal scores.

Random sampling of subjects is assumed when using the statistical tests. In theory, the researcher has access to all members of the population, and from this population one or more samples is randomly selected. Sample size should be a small percentage of population size. However, in many studies the researcher does not have access to all members of the population, and almost all of the accessible members of the population are included in the sample. If random sampling is used for sample selection in such cases, most researchers accept that the random sampling assumption is met.

With the *t* test for two independent groups, one-way ANOVA, and factorial ANOVA, it is assumed that the groups are independent of each other. Groups are independent if the selection and placement of any individual into a particular group has no bearing on what other subjects are selected or placed into that group. The assumption of independence is not totally met in some studies where volunteer subjects are used. For example, a researcher wants to have an experimental group and a control group. If potential subjects are volunteers, ideally some are randomly selected and assigned to the experimental group, some are randomly selected and assigned to the control group, and some are not selected as subjects. However, only sixty people volunteer and five people say they will not participate in the study unless they are in the experimental group. So, the researcher puts the five people in the experimental group, randomly selects twenty-five other people for the experimental group, and places the remaining thirty volunteers in the control group. Basically, the assumption of independence is met.

It is also assumed that scores are normally distributed at the population level (i.e., the graph resembles a normal curve; see chapter 10). The best evidence that this assumption is true is that sample scores are normally distributed. With small sample sizes, scores are often not normally distributed even if scores at the population level are normally distributed. For this reason, a group size of thirty is considered the minimum sample size, and larger sample sizes are recommended. Often researchers have fewer than thirty available subjects for each group, so the groups are smaller. Fortunately, as long as the assumption of normal distribution is basically met, the statistical tests are justified.

In studies using multiple samples, the populations they represent are assumed to be equally variable. The assumption is checked by comparing the samples. If the variance (see chapter 10) for any group equals the variance for the other groups, the assumption is met. As long as the assumption of equal variability is basically met, the application of the statistical test is appropriate.

A researcher can do several things to improve the probability that the assumptions underlying a statistical test are basically met. Be sure that the members of the population available for selection as subjects are truly representative of the population; in most studies this means having a large number of people from which to sample. Large sample sizes are definitely advantageous. With multiple groups, it is recommended that approximately the same number of subjects be included in each group.

Overview of Two-Group Comparisons

Two-group comparisons are sometimes referred to as **multiple comparisons** or *a posteriori* **comparisons.** These techniques are used to compare groups two at a time following a significant F test in ANOVA. Having rejected H_0 that the group means are equal and accepted H_1 that the group means are not equal, the researcher wants to compare pairs of means to determine if they differ significantly. For example, if there are three groups (A, B, and C), this involves comparing A to B, A to C, and B to C.

There are several techniques developed specially for two-group comparisons. It is important for beginning researchers to know something of these techniques in case there is need to use them and in order to have some understanding of their application in the research literature. Some of the techniques commonly used are by Scheffe, Tukey, Duncan, Newman-Keuls, and Bonferroni. Discussion of the techniques can be found in statistics books like Ferguson and Takane (1989), and Winer, Brown, and Michels (1991). Which technique to use is influenced partly by personal preference and partly by the research situation.

Two-group comparison techniques may differ in terms of three important attributes: per-comparison error rate, experiment-wise error rate, and statistical power. Each of these attributes should be considered when selecting a technique for a particular research situation. **Per-comparison error rate** is the probability of making a type I error in a single two-group comparison. **Experiment-wise error rate** is the probability of making a type I error somewhere in all of the two-group comparisons conducted. Statistical power is the probability of not making a type II error in a two-group comparison.

Scheffe's technique, for example, controls type I errors very well, but is lacking in statistical power unless sample sizes are large. Tukey's technique does not control type I errors as well, but has better statistical power than Scheffe.

Two-group comparisons are conducted after a significant F test in any ANOVA design, provided there are three or more levels or groups associated with the F test. For example, if for the data in table 11.10 there is a significant F test for columns, then two-group comparisons are conducted; but a significant F test for rows indicates that the two row means are not equal, making two-group comparison unnecessary.

In statistics books, two-group comparisons are very often discussed after one-way ANOVA, and in packages of statistical computer programs two-group comparisons are often part of the one-way ANOVA program. Further, computer programs may not contain all of the two-group comparison techniques. Thus, using a particular two-group comparison with ANOVA designs other than a one-way may require hand calculation of the two-group comparison. A hand calculation is not difficult with the information provided in the computer printout for the ANOVA conducted to justify the two-group comparisons.

Overview of Analysis of Covariance

Analysis of covariance (ANCOVA) was discussed briefly in the experimental research chapter; it would be helpful to review that material before proceeding. ANCOVA is an alternative to most ANOVA designs, and it is commonly found in the research literature. Basically, ANCOVA statistically adjusts the difference among the group means on the criterion (data) variable to allow for the fact that the groups differ in mean score on some other variable(s) and then applies ANOVA to the adjusted criterion variable. A variable used for adjusting the data is called the **covariate,** and the data variable is called the **variate.** If there is no adjustment in the variate, ANOVA and ANCOVA yield the same results.

One reason for using ANCOVA is to reduce error variance (reflected in the denominator of the F test) in a design. Another reason is to adjust for the inequality of groups at the start of the research study in terms of one or more variables that need to be controlled in the research study.

ANCOVA is more complex than ANOVA in terms of the assumptions underlying its use, data collection, and analysis. Prior to using ANCOVA the researcher should become familiar with the technique by consulting statistics books like Huck, Cormier, and Bounds (1974), Keppel (1991), and Winer, Brown, and Michels (1991). Manuals for packages of statistical computer programs such as SAS (1985), BMDP (1990), and SPSSX (1986) often include good explanations of statistical techniques.

Overview of Nonparametric Tests

All of the statistical tests discussed so far have been **parametric** tests in that interval data and normal distribution of the scores for each population are assumed. This section discusses statistical tests that do not require that these two assumptions be met. **Nonparametric** statistical tests are used when the data are not interval or the data are interval but not normally distributed. For example, small sample sizes per group ($n < 10$) seldom yield data that are normally distributed. An overview of nonparametric statistical tests is presented and then one commonly used test, chi-square, is discussed in detail.

Books devoted entirely to nonparametric statistical tests include Siegel (1956), which is a classic but is out of print; Siegel and Castellan (1988), which is a revision of Siegel; Hollander and Wolfe (1973); and Marascuilo and McSweeney (1977). Nonparametric statistics courses are available at most universities. Many statistics books (e.g., Ferguson and Takane [1989]) have a chapter devoted to the common nonparametric statistical tests. For each of the common parametric statistical tests discussed in this chapter, there is an alternative nonparametric statistical test. Where parametric statistical tests deal with the mean, nonparametric statistical tests deal with the median, ranks, and frequencies. Note that the second-best measure of central tendency is the median, and the mode is based on frequencies. Often, nonparametric statistical tests do not have as much statistical power as parametric statistical tests. However, random sampling is still assumed with nonparametric statistical tests.

The Kruskal-Wallis one-way ANOVA by ranks and the Friedman two-way ANOVA by ranks are two nonparametric statistical tests commonly found in the research literature. Both of these statistical tests can be found in statistical packages for the computer.

The chi-square (χ^2) statistical test is a nonparametric test often used by researchers conducting descriptive research. Most general statistics books discuss the chi-square test. The **one-way (goodness of fit)** and **two-way (contingency table) chi-square tests** are discussed in detail in subsequent paragraphs because of their many uses in research studies.

One-Way Chi-Square

In a research study where a one-way or goodness of fit chi-square test is used to analyze the data, the researcher hypothesizes some distribution for the data of a population. Based on the distribution of sample data, the researcher either accepts or rejects the hypothesis. Again, the five-step hypothesis-testing procedure is used. An example will help to clarify this test.

Suppose a researcher is interested in determining whether freshmen at a university are satisfied with living in a dorm. The population of university freshmen is 6,000. A sample of 1,000 students is selected using random procedures. A four-item questionnaire with five possible answers (strongly agree, agree, neutral, disagree, strongly disagree) per item is sent to the sample. Eight hundred students return the questionnaire. Prior to mailing the questionnaires to the sample, the researcher hypothesizes that the population distribution on items is 10 percent strongly agree, 10 percent strongly disagree, 20 percent agree, 20 percent disagree, and 40 percent neutral. These hypothesized percentages generate the **expected frequency** for each answer, whereas the number of subjects in the sample selecting each answer generates the **observed frequency** for each answer. Presented in table 11.12 are the frequencies of response (observed frequencies) for the sample to each item of the questionnaire. Presented in table 11.13 are the expected frequencies for each answer to the questionnaire in table 11.12. Are the observed frequencies and expected frequencies for a questionnaire item in close enough agreement to accept the hypothesized distribution of responses?

The one-way or goodness of fit chi-square test is used with the five-step hypothesis-testing procedure to determine whether the observed and expected frequencies are in agreement with each other. This chi-square test is called *one-way* because the response of each subject to an item has only one classification—which answer was selected. The *goodness of fit* name comes from the chi-square test as a test of the extent to which the expected and observed frequencies were in agreement.

TABLE 11.12 Frequency of Responses of a Sample ($n = 800$) to a Four-Item Questionnaire About Dorm Conditions

ITEM	STRONGLY AGREE	AGREE	NEUTRAL	DISAGREE	STRONGLY DISAGREE	N
1. Food is great.	50	135	400	200	15	800
2. Roommate is terrible.	70	150	350	170	60	800
3. Public dorm area is a mess.	100	200	325	145	30	800
4. Own room is nice.	20	100	200	300	180	800

TABLE 11.13 Expected Frequencies for Questionnaire Items in Table 11.12 ($n = 800$)

ANSWER	HYPOTHESIZED %	EXPECTED FREQUENCY
Strongly Agree	10	80
Agree	20	160
Neutral	40	320
Disagree	20	160
Strongly Disagree	10	80
Total	100	800

The less the agreement between the expected and observed frequencies for the answers to an item, the larger the chi-square value. If there was perfect agreement, the chi-square value would be zero. The one-way chi-square test has degrees of freedom equal to the number of different responses to an item or number of different observed values of a variable (K) minus one (df $= K - 1$). The tabled values of chi-square are provided in appendix C. Tabled values are positioned where the degrees of freedom row and alpha-level column intersect.

The five-step hypothesis-testing procedure is presented using the responses to item 1 in table 11.12.

Step 1: H_0: Model or distribution of responses is 10%–20%–40%–20%–10%
H_1: Model is not correct

Step 2: Alpha $= .05$

Step 3: Since there are five different answers to the item, the degrees of freedom is 4 (5 − 1). With df $= 4$ and alpha $= .05$, the tabled chi-square value is 9.49.

TABLE 11.14 Output for the One-Way Chi-Square for Item 1 in Table 11.12 and the Expected Values in Table 11.13

Number of Observations			800	
Chi-Square			97.97	
Degrees of Freedom			4	
Significance Level			.000	
Observed Frequencies:				
50	135	400	200	15
Expected Frequencies:				
80.00	160.00	320.00	160.00	80.00

Step 4: Analyze the data item by item. The data for item 1 in table 11.12 is analyzed. SYSTAT can be used to get the observed frequencies but the chi-square value will have to be calculated by hand. Using another statistical package of computer programs the output presented in table 11.14 was obtained. Both the chi-square value and p value indicate significance.

Step 5: The researcher concludes that the hypothesized model is not correct.

Two-Way Chi-Square

In a research study where a two-way or contingency table chi-square test is used to analyze the data, the researcher has hypothesized that, for a population, two variables are independent of each other or uncorrelated. Based on the data of a sample from the population the researcher accepts or rejects the hypothesis. As always, the five-step hypothesis-testing procedure is followed. The following example is an easy way to present this chi-square test.

A questionnaire is sent to a sample of 100 former participants in an industrial fitness program and 30 of them return it. Subjects are asked to indicate their gender, age, and response to each of three items about the fitness program. The data from the questionnaire is presented in table 11.15. The researcher hypothesizes that males and females respond in a similar manner to item 1. This is equivalent to believing that gender and response to item 1 are independent of each other.

The two-way or contingency chi-square test is applied to the data following the five-step hypothesis-testing procedure to determine whether the researcher's belief seems to be true. This chi-square test is called *two-way* because the response of each subject to an item has two classifications on it. In this example, the two classifications are answer selected and gender. If the percent of males and females selecting an answer to an item is the same and this prevails for each answer choice within an item, the chi-square value of the item is zero (e.g., if 15 percent of the males and 15 percent of the females selected strongly disagree, 40 percent of each

TABLE 11.15 Data from a Questionnaire Completed by Former Participants in an Industrial Fitness Program					
SUBJECT	**GENDER**	**AGE**	**I-1**	**I-2**	**I-3**
1	1	2	2	3	2
2	1	3	2	4	2
3	2	2	1	3	2
4	1	1	2	3	1
5	2	3	3	2	3
6	2	1	2	4	3
7	2	2	3	2	1
8	1	2	2	2	2
9	1	1	3	3	3
10	2	2	3	4	3
11	1	3	2	3	3
12	1	2	1	2	1
13	1	1	1	2	3
14	1	2	2	2	3
15	2	3	2	3	2
16	2	2	1	2	2
17	1	3	2	3	3
18	2	3	3	3	2
19	2	3	1	2	2
20	1	1	2	2	3
21	1	2	3	3	3
22	1	3	2	2	1
23	2	1	1	2	1
24	2	1	3	2	1
25	1	3	3	4	3
26	1	1	2	2	2
27	2	3	3	4	3
28	1	2	1	2	1
29	2	3	2	3	1
30	1	3	1	4	1

Gender: 1 = Female, 2 = Male
Age: 1 = 18–25, 2 = 26–39, 3 = 40–60
Item: 1 = Strongly Agree, 2 = Agree, 3 = Disagree, 4 = Strongly Disagree

gender selected disagree, and so forth). In this example, response to the item is independent of gender since both genders responded in the same manner.

With a two-way chi-square test, a two-dimensional table is developed with the rows identifying the levels or values of one variable and the columns identifying the levels of the other variable. The number of subjects in each cell of the two-dimensional table is then determined. The degrees of freedom for the two-way chi-square test is $(n - 1)(K - 1)$ where n = number of rows and K = number of columns in the two-dimensional table. Tabled values of chi-square are provided in appendix C.

The five-step hypothesis-testing procedure is presented using the gender and item 1 (I-1) data from table 11.15.

Step 1: H_0: Gender and I-1 are independent of each other
H_1: Gender and I-1 are dependent

Step 2: Alpha = .05

Step 3: Since gender has two levels or values (1 and 2) and I-1 has three levels (1, 2, and 3), the degrees of freedom is 2 $[(2 - 1)(3 - 1)]$. With df = 2 and alpha = .05, the tabled chi-square value is 5.99.

Step 4: Analyze the data item by item. The data for gender and I-1 in table 11.15 is analyzed using SYSTAT. First, click on DATA under SYSTAT Main, click on Formats, and then under Results to Print select Extended. Second, click on STATS under SYSTAT Main, click on Tables (the Tables screen should be displayed but if Tabulate is displayed click on it and the Tables screen will be displayed). At this point select one variable using Add and one variable using the top By. Note, if both variables are selected using Add, a one-way chi-square frequency count is obtained. Also note, that the following options should be selected to obtain a very complete printout: column and row percents, frequency, percent, print extended statistics, and sort categories. Computer output for this analysis is presented in table 11.16.

First cell frequencies and total frequencies for each row and column are provided in table 11.16. Seventeen females (row code 1) and 13 males answered item 1. Eight subjects strongly agreed (column code 1), 13 subjects agreed, and 9 subjects disagreed with item 1. Ten females agreed (row code 1 and column code 2) with item 1. Then percents of total, row percents, and column percents are provided for each cell. The females who strongly agreed (row code 1 and column code 1) are 13.33 percent of all 30 subjects (percent of total), 23.53 percent of all 17 females (row percents), and 50 percent of all 8 subjects who strongly agreed (column percents). Finally test statistics and coefficients (not introduced in this chapter) are provided. The Pearson Chi-Square is the statistic to use. Neither the chi-square value (4.313) nor p value (.116) indicate significance.

Step 5: Accept H_0 that males and females responded in a similar manner to I-1.

Overview of Multivariate Tests

The statistical tests discussed to this point have been **univariate tests** in that each subject contributed one score to the data analysis, or in the case of repeated measures contributed one score per cell. With **multivariate tests,** each subject contributes multiple scores. So, for example, in the case of a multivariate one-way ANOVA,

TABLE 11.16 Output of the Two-Way Chi-Square for Gender and I-1 in Table 11.15

ROWS = GENDER, COLUMNS = I-1

Frequencies

	1.000	2.000	3.000	Total
1.000	4	10	3	17
2.000	4	3	6	13
Total	8	13	9	30

Percents of Total

	1.000	2.000	3.000	Total	N
1.000	13.33	33.33	10.00	56.67	17.00
2.000	13.33	10.00	20.00	43.33	13.00
Total	26.67	43.33	30.00	100.00	
N	8	13	9	30	

Row Percents

	1.000	2.000	3.000	Total	N
1.000	23.53	58.82	17.65	100.00	17.00
2.000	30.77	23.08	46.15	100.00	13.00
Total	26.67	43.33	30.00	100.00	
N	8	13	9	30	

Column Percents

	1.000	2.000	3.000	Total	N
1.000	50.00	76.92	33.33	56.67	17.00
2.000	50.00	23.08	66.67	43.33	13.00
Total	100.00	100.00	100.00	100.00	
N	8	13	9	30	

Test Statistic	Value	DF	Prob
Pearson Chi-Square	4.313	2	0.116
Likelihood Ratio Chi-Square	4.461	2	0.107

Coefficient	Value	Asymptotic Std Error
Phi	0.379	
Cramer V	0.379	
Contingency	0.355	
Goodman-Kruskal Gamma	0.223	0.295
Kendall Tau-B	0.138	0.184
Stuart Tau-C	0.156	0.209
Spearman Rho	0.146	0.187
Somers D (Column Dependent)	0.158	0.212
Lambda D (Column Dependent)	0.176	0.160
Uncertainty (Column Dependent)	0.069	0.063

each subject contributes a knowledge test score, a physical performance score, and an attitude test score. The purpose of the data analysis is to determine if there is a difference among the groups in terms of a composite score composed of the three test scores.

Books devoted entirely to multivariate statistical tests are available, such as Tabachnick and Fidell (1989), Harris (1985), Stevens (1986), and Tatsuoka (1988). Multivariate statistics courses are offered at most universities. Usually these courses are the third to fourth course in a sequence of statistics courses. For each of the common univariate statistical tests discussed in this chapter there is usually a parallel multivariate statistical test. Multivariate statistical tests that parallel the t test and ANOVA procedures are common in the research literature. Other multivariate techniques often used by researchers are canonical correlation, discriminant analysis, and factor analysis. Discussion of these techniques is beyond the scope of this book.

Multivariate statistical tests can be found in statistical packages for the computer such as SAS (1985), SPSSX (1986), SYSTAT (1992) and BMDP (1990). Use of multivariate statistical tests is common in the research literature.

As a word of caution, multivariate statistical tests are fairly complex, and so some formal training and experience is recommended before using them in a research study. The use and understanding of multivariate statistical tests is usually too much to expect of the typical master's student or doctoral student who have had only minimal statistical training. Just because a researcher collects some data and analyzes it by using a multivariate statistical test on the computer is no guarantee that the output from the computer is good or that the interpretation of the output is correct. There is a saying among computer users that applies here: Garbage in and garbage out. Bad data going into the computer results in bad information coming out of the computer.

Overview of Prediction-Regression Analysis

The terms correlation, regression, and prediction are so closely related in statistics that they are often used interchangeably. **Correlation** refers to the relationship between two variables. When two variables are correlated, it becomes possible to make a prediction. **Regression** is the statistical model used to predict performance on one variable from another. An example is the prediction of percent body fat from skinfold measurements.

Practitioners and researchers are interested in predicting scores that are either difficult or impossible to obtain at a given moment. **Prediction** is estimating a person's score on one measure based on the individual's score on one or more other measures. Although prediction is often imprecise, it is occasionally useful to develop a prediction formula.

Simple Prediction

Simple prediction involves predicting an unknown score (Y) for an individual by using that person's performance (X) on a known measure. To develop a simple prediction, or regression formula, a large number of subjects must be measured, and a score on the independent or predictor variable X and the dependent or predicted variable Y must be obtained for each. Once the formula is developed for any given relationship, only the predictor variable X is needed to predict the performance of an individual on measure Y. An example of simple prediction is predicting college grade point average (Y) with high school grade point average (X). One index of the accuracy of a simple prediction equation is the correlation coefficient (r).

Prediction being a correlational technique, there is a line of best fit or regression line that can be generated (see graphing technique, p. 209). In the case of simple prediction, this is the regression line for the graph of the X variable on the horizontal axis and the Y variable on the vertical axis.

The general form of the simple prediction equation is

$$Y' = bX + c$$

where, Y' is a predicted Y score, b is a constant and represents the slope of the regression line. The **slope** is the rate at which Y changes with change on X. The constant c is called the **Y-intercept** and is the point at which the line crosses the vertical axis. It is the value of Y that corresponds to an X of 0. Sometimes computer programs report the simple prediction equation in terms of slope and Y-intercept.

An individual's predicted score Y' does not equal the actual score Y unless the correlation coefficient used in the formula is perfect—a rare event. Thus, for each individual there is an error of prediction. The standard deviation of this error is called the **standard error of prediction.** The standard error of prediction is another index of the accuracy of a simple prediction equation.

If the prediction formula and standard error seem acceptable, the researcher should check the accuracy of the prediction formula on a second group of individuals similar to the first. This process is called **cross-validation.** If the formula works satisfactorily for the second group, it can be used with confidence to predict score Y for any individual who resembles the individuals used to form and cross-validate the equation. If the formula does not work well for the second group, it is considered to be unique to the group used to form the equation and has little value in predicting performance in other groups.

Multiple Prediction

A prediction formula using a single measure X is usually not very accurate for predicting a person's score on measure Y. **Multiple prediction** (or regression) techniques allow Y scores to be predicted using several X scores (e.g., the prediction of college grade point average based on high school grade point average and SAT scores).

A multiple regression equation has one intercept and one b value for each independent variable. The general form of two- and three-predictor multiple regression equations are

$$Y' = b_1X_1 + b_2X_2 + c \text{ (two-predictor)}$$
$$Y' = b_1X_1 + b_2X_2 + b_3X_3 + c \text{ (three-predictor)}$$

The multiple correlation coefficient R is one index of the accuracy of a multiple prediction equation. The minimum and maximum values of R are 0 and 1, respectively. The percentage of variance in the Y scores explained by the multiple prediction equation is R^2. A second index of the accuracy of a multiple prediction equation is the standard error of prediction. Whole books have been written on multiple regression by Cohen and Cohen (1975) and Pedhazur (1982). Chapters on the topic can be found in the SPSS manual (Nie et al., 1975), Safrit and Wood (1989), and Ferguson and Takane (1989).

Nonlinear Regression

The regression models discussed to this point assume a linear relationship, but this assumption is not the case for all data. For example, when relating age and strength, the relation is linear for the ages of 10 through 17 because the person is growing and gaining muscle mass; for ages 18 through 65, however, the relationship is nonlinear (or is curvilinear) because increasing age through this period is usually accompanied by a loss of strength. As explained earlier, if the relationship is curvilinear, the linear correlation will be lower than the true correlation. Computer programs have what is termed a **polynomial regression** program to compute the curvilinear correlation. Polynomial regression analysis is beyond the scope of this book.

Overview of Testing Correlation Coefficients

Correlation was introduced as a descriptive statistical technique in the previous chapter. As such, the correlation coefficient is usually viewed as an indication of the relationship between two variables for a group. However, it is not uncommon for a researcher to state a hypothesis about the correlation in a population, randomly select a sample from a population, calculate a correlation coefficient for the sample, and based on the sample correlation coefficient, accept or reject the hypothesis. It is common for a researcher to apply the five-step hypothesis-testing procedure to correlation coefficients. The commonly applied statistical tests on correlation coefficients are usually presented in general purpose statistics books like Ferguson and Takane (1989). Less commonly applied statistical tests on correlation coefficients and statistical tests involving multiple prediction or regression are presented in books like Pedhazur (1982). A brief overview of two statistical tests on correlation coefficients is presented because these tests are common in the research literature and will provide a basic understanding of their application.

Situation 1: H_0: The correlation coefficient at the population level is zero. H_1: The correlation coefficient is greater than zero. If the correlation coefficient for the sample is considerably larger than zero, H_0 is rejected. The researcher states that the correlation coefficient is significant, which indicates that the coefficient is significantly greater than zero and did not happen by chance.

Situation 2: H_0: The correlation between two variables is the same for each of two populations. H_1: The correlation coefficients are not equal. If the correlation coefficients for each of the two independent samples differ considerably in value, H_0 is rejected and the researcher concludes that there is a difference between the two correlation coefficients.

Selecting the Statistical Test

Selecting the appropriate statistical test for a given research situation is sometimes difficult for the inexperienced researcher. In terms of the statistical tests discussed in detail in this chapter, figure 11.3 may be helpful in selecting the appropriate statistical test. Starting at the top of the figure, move down the figure selecting options until a statistical test is selected at the bottom of a path of lines. For example, the null hypothesis concerns means (move to YES), there are three independent groups (move to 2 or more groups and then One-way ANOVA), and so the statistical test is a one-way ANOVA.

Summary

A number of different research designs and statistical tests have been presented in this chapter. As a result of studying this chapter the student should understand the concept of inference from a sample to a population, the five-step hypothesis-testing procedure, and the related terminology. The first objective of this chapter is that the student be able to read the statistical analysis section of a research journal article with reasonably good understanding. The second objective is that a student researcher be able to select and execute a statistical analysis of some data with some guidance from a faculty member. If the student understands and is able to work with the research designs and statistical tests presented in this chapter, these two objectives have been met. However, mastery of this chapter certainly does not suggest that the student will understand the statistics presented in all research articles.

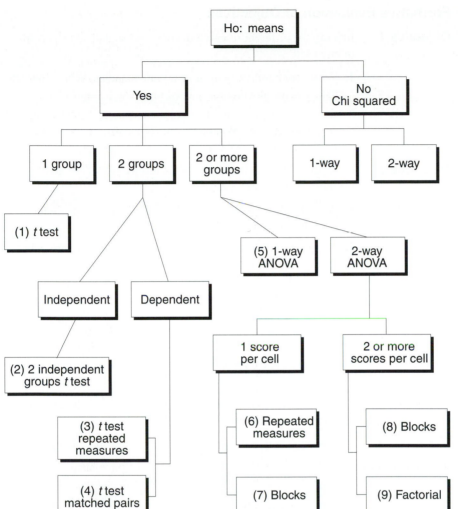

FIGURE 11.3
A chart for selecting the appropriate statistical test.

Formative Evaluation of Objectives

Objective 1   Identify the different research designs and statistical tests commonly used.

1. F tests are commonly used in research studies. What other statistical tests are commonly used in research studies?
2. Research designs could be classified as independent groups or dependent groups. What are some other ways designs might be classified?

Objective 2   Understand the five-step hypothesis-testing procedure and how it is reported in research journals.

1. What are the five steps in the hypothesis-testing procedure and what occurs at each step?
2. In regard to the five-step hypothesis-testing procedure, what is a researcher indicating when he/she says
   a) the difference is significant?
   b) the difference is not significant?
   c) $F(2,57) = 3.17$, $p < .05$?
   d) the hypothesis is rejected at the .01 level?
   e) a type one error may have occurred?
3. What are the commomly used alpha levels and why would a researcher use them or other levels?

Objective 3   Understand and evaluate common statistical tests when they are used in the research literature.

1. In each situation below, what is the table value, the value needed for rejection?
   a) Two tailed t test, alpha $= .05$, df $= 8$.
   b) F test, alpha $= .01$, df $= 3,56$.
   c) Chi-square test, alpha $= .05$, df $= 8$.
2. In each situation below, what statistical test is appropriate?
   a) Each of the two groups received a different experimental treatment.
   b) Each of forty-two subjects was measured at the beginning of the experiment and every two weeks after that for eight weeks.
   c) The gender and response (SA, A, D, SD) to a ten-item questionnaire was determined to see if gender influenced response to the questionnaire.

part

IV

THE RESEARCH REPORT

It is important to note that research is a shared enterprise among members of a professional group. The reports generated through research are perhaps the most common medium for researchers to communicate their findings to each other. Journal articles, master's degree theses, and doctoral dissertations all have the same objective—to disseminate ideas and information. The research procedure and results of an investigation become a record for posterity. The role of the report in the research process is important in that the preparation of a good, detailed report is a mechanism by which researchers can refine their thinking about the research problems they have investigated. In a way, the researcher evaluates the completed work through the research report.

Part IV of this book contains one detailed chapter titled "The Research Report." Covered in this chapter are (1) examples of the elements typically included in a graduate student thesis or dissertation, (2) how to prepare an article for publication, and (3) how to critique a research report.

12 The Research Report

Key Words

Abstract
Checklist for evaluating a research
 paper

Criteria for critiquing an article
Preliminary items
Published article format

Supplementary items
Text
Thesis format

Objectives

The function of a research report is to communicate a set of ideas and facts to those who are interested in the problem area in which the research was undertaken. Reports will differ in how they are treated, but, in general, the writers of the reports tend to follow similar style formats. Students completing research are usually required to follow a style of reporting selected by the faculty of the students' department. The style for published research will follow a format required by the journal to which the report is submitted for publication.

After reading chapter 12, you should be able to:

1. Determine the characteristics of a good research report.
2. Understand the format for a report and the kinds of information required in each division of the report.
3. Differentiate between the style of writing a research report for a thesis or dissertation as opposed to a research report for publication in a journal.
4. Critique and evaluate a research report.

The purpose of the written research report, whether it is in the form of a master's thesis, doctoral dissertation, or journal article, is to convey ideas and facts generated by the research to those who will read the report. To be effective, the information must be communicated in a manner that is clear and easily understood. *Clarity* is fundamental. The reader should not be required to guess how the research was performed or have to make any assumptions about what was found. The reader should hold no doubts or questions about the meaning of any statement included in the report.

Besides clarity, other important characteristics of the report include (1) *organization,* or the logic underlying the order in which the various parts of the report appear and the degree to which the transition between parts is clear and smooth;

(2) *good and correct presentation,* which includes adherence to proper spelling, grammar, diction, punctuation, and the mechanics of a systematic format for presentation of the research material; (3) *completeness,* meaning that the total body of facts should be presented to enhance clarity; and (4) *conciseness,* an elimination of any material if it merely adds unnecessary length to the report rather than adding to its completeness and clarity.

Format of the Report

Graduate students completing a thesis or dissertation are often required by their respective colleges or universities to follow a particular **thesis format** for organizing and presenting the report. If the institution has no established requirement, then the college, school, division, or department of HHP probably will. Various published and standardized formats are frequently used. Some examples are Campbell and Ballou (1978), American Psychological Association (1983), Council of Biology Editors (1972), Gibaldi and Achtert (1980), Turabian (1973), Day (1983), and Locke and Spirduso (1976).

Divisions of a Thesis or Dissertation

Usually, a research report such as a thesis or dissertation, is arranged in three major parts: preliminary items, the text or body of the report, and supplementary items.

Preliminary Items

The **preliminary items** usually included are the title page, acceptance page, acknowledgments, table of contents, list of tables, list of figures, and abstract. Example 12.1 provides samples of these items completed by former students at Indiana University.

The Text

The **text,** or body, of the thesis for most descriptive and experimental studies usually consists of five chapters. The first three chapters (introduction, review of related literature, and procedures for collecting data) are discussed in detail in chapter 2 of this book under the topic, "Developing the Research Proposal." The inclusions in these first three chapters are summarized.

Chapter 4, covering the analysis of data, and chapter 5, which includes the summary, findings, conclusions, implementations, and recommendations, make up the remainder of the body of the thesis or dissertation. These chapters are discussed in some detail, and several examples for illustrating their content are included at the end of this chapter.

EXAMPLE 12.1A
Title Page
From J. K. Clark, *Two curricular settings of a HIV education unit related to secondary school students' HIV knowledge and attitude.* Doctoral dissertation, 1991. Reprinted by permission of Jeff K. Clark.

TWO CURRICULAR SETTINGS OF A HIV EDUCATION UNIT RELATED TO SECONDARY SCHOOL STUDENTS' HIV KNOWLEDGE AND ATTITUDE

by
Jeffrey K. Clark

Submitted in partial fulfillment of the requirements
for the Doctor of Health and Safety Degree
in the School of Health, Physical
Education, and Recreation
Indiana University

July 1991

Accepted by the faculty of the School of Health, Physical Education, and Recreation, Indiana University, in partial fulfillment of the requirements for the Doctor of Physical Education degree.

_____
Director of Thesis

Doctoral Committee: _____
Chairperson

_____

_____

_____

EXAMPLE 12.1B
Acceptance Page
From J. K. Clark, _Two curricular settings of a HIV education unit related to secondary school students' HIV knowledge and attitude._ Doctoral dissertation, 1991. Reprinted by permission of Jeff K. Clark.

EXAMPLE 12.1C
Acknowledgments Page

Acknowledgments

     The author wishes to express his gratitude to Dr. _____ , Dr. _____ , and Dr. _____ for their assistance and guidance in this investigation. The author is especially indebted to Dr. _____ whose help and encouragement was invaluable to the completion of this study.

     Special thanks is offered to the author's new young friends and their teachers who provided their time and energy so generously during the data-collection process.

B. J.

Table of Contents

LIST OF TABLES vi

LIST OF FIGURES viii

Chapter

1. INTRODUCTION 1
   Statement of the Problem 1
   Purpose of the Study 2
   Need for the Study 2
   Delimitations 4
   Limitations 5
   Assumptions 5
   Hypotheses 6
   Definitions 7

2. REVIEW OF RELATED LITERATURE 10
   Description of the Field Hockey Drive 10
   Summary of the Description of the Field Hockey Drive 23
   Parameter Measurement Technique 24
   Summary 27

3. EXPERIMENTAL PROCEDURES 29
   General Procedures 30
   Cinematographic Techniques 32
   Kinematic Analysis of Filmed Data 35
   Data Analysis Procedure 35

4. ANALYSIS AND DISCUSSION OF DATA 39
   Processing the Data and Presentation of Findings 39
   Discussion of the Findings 62

5. SUMMARY, FINDINGS, CONCLUSIONS,
   IMPLEMENTATIONS AND RECOMMENDATIONS 62
   Summary 62
   Findings 63
   Conclusions 67
   Implementations 67
   Recommendations 68

EXAMPLE 12.1D
Table of Contents
J. L. Hendrick, *Biomechanical analysis of selected parameters in the field hockey drive.* Master degree thesis, 1981. Reprinted by permission of Joy L. Hendrick.

EXAMPLE 12.1D
Concluded

REFERENCES 70

APPENDIXES

    A.   SUBJECT INFORMATION 75

    B.   FILMING RECORD SHEET 76

(Hendricks, 1981)

EXAMPLE 12.1E
List of Tables
From R. J. Ogletree, *Selected factors related to help-seeking behavior in college women victims of sexual coercion.* Doctoral dissertation, 1991. Reprinted by permission of Roberta J. Ogletree.

List of Tables

Table		Page
1.	Sample Characteristics	47
2.	Sample Characteristics by Victimization Classification	49
3.	Test-Retest Item Agreement Percentages	52
4.	Number and Percent of Women Responding to Each Sexual Coercion Question	53
5.	Source of Help-Seeking for Victims	55
6.	How Soon After the Incident Victims Sought Help	56
7.	Means and Standard Deviations for the Data Used to Test the Null Hypothesis	57
8.	ANOVA Summary Table—Assertiveness	57
9.	ANOVA Summary Table—Self-Esteem	58
10.	ANOVA Summary Table—Sex Role Stereotype Acceptance	59
11.	Discriminant Analysis Summary Table	60

(Ogletree, 1991)

List of Figures

Figure   Page

1. Force Plate Mounted in a Specially Constructed
    Cement Pit 67

2. Electrical Equipment Utilized in the Filming Procedures 71

3. Locam 16mm High Speed Motion Picture and
    Hercules Quick-Set Heavy Duty Tripod 73

4. Two Banks of Color-Tran Mini Brute Floodlights 74

5. Diagram of the Experimental Arrangements in the
    Soccer Instep Kick Study 75

6. Vanguard Projector Motion Analyzer and Scriptographic
    Digitizing Surface 81

7. A Wang-Modified IBM Electric Typewriter, A Wang
    Programmable Calculator and Wang Cassette Tape Drives 82

8. Method of Measuring Body Angles 87

9. Strain Elements Location of the Force Platform in the
    Soccer Instep Kick Study 89

10. Bell and Howell Recording Oscillograph with Amplifier 91

11. Force Platform Connected with Recording Oscillograph
    with Amplifier and Pre-Amplifier Used for Recording of
    Kinetic Parameters 94

12. Equipment Used for Calculation of Kinetic Data 97

13. Angles Calculated in Three Phases of the Soccer
    Instep Kick 121

14. Sample Oscillographic Recording of Forces Generated by
    the Kicker During the Action of the Soccer Instep Kick 159

15. Force Platform Calibration Curve (Z) 210

Abo-Abdo (1981)

EXAMPLE 12.1F
List of Figures
From H. E. Abo Abdo,
*Kinematic and kinetic analysis
of the soccer instep kick.*
Doctoral dissertation, 1981.
Reprinted by permission of
H. E. Abo Abdo.

EXAMPLE 12.1G
Abstract
From M. E. Collins, *Body figure perceptions and preferences among preadolescent children.* Doctoral dissertation, 1989. Reprinted by permission of M. E. Collins.

Body Figure Perceptions and Preferences Among Preadolescent Children

(Dissertation Abstract)
Mary Elizabeth Collins, H.S.D.
Indiana University

Chairperson:

Problem

The problem of the study was to determine and compare body figure perceptions and preferences among male and female preadolescent children, grades one through three, in Indiana.

Procedures

This study was a cross-sectional survey of 1,118 first, second, and third grade, black and white children in Indiana. Subjects attended seven elementary schools in two public school corporations, selected purposely to represent a broad range of school/community settings. A pictorial instrument consisting of four sets of figure drawings was developed, reviewed, and modified for this study. The pictorial instrument was pilot-tested and examined for test-retest reliability, criterion-related validity, and face validity. Subjects indicated perceptions of their own body figures and preferences for ideal figures in children and adults. Analyses of variance and t-tests were used to test hypotheses related to differences in figure selections by gender, grade, race, and school/community setting.

Findings

A total of 1,118 children completed the survey. The representative sample consisted of male (51%) and female (49%), black (26%) and white (74%), and first (32%), second (33%), and third (35%) grade children. Acceptable levels of reliability and validity were demonstrated for the pictorial instrument, with accuracy of pictorial self-selection increasing around age nine, particularly among females. Males and females selected similar current figures as self. Though males selected slightly thinner figures as ideal, females chose ideal figure significantly thinner than males selected. Females' ideal figure selections not only were thinner than their perceptions of their current figures but also thinner than figures boys selected as ideal for girls. In addition, females selected thinner ideal adult figures than males selected. Blacks chose heavier figures than whites; however, preferences for thinner figures occurred among females of both races.

EXAMPLE 12.1G
Concluded

Conclusions

Preadolescent females demonstrated a preference for thinness similar to that reported with adult and adolescent females. Preference for thinner figures occurred across all levels of weight, age, race, and school/community setting. These results suggest that the onset of disparate figure perceptions and expectations regarding thinness among females may be evident as early as six and seven years of age.

(Collins, 1989)

Summary of Chapters 1–5

Chapter 1 Introduction

Statement of the Problem: A clear and definitive statement of what was studied.

Purpose of the Study: A brief statement of why the study was done; a reason for the research or the potential uses for or contribution to be made by the results.

Need for the Study (Significance of the Study, Justification for the Study): An elaboration of the purpose, validating and establishing the importance of the problem.

Delimitations: The scope of the study as identified by including information on what subjects and variables were studied and what instrumentation was used; the methods and techniques incorporated; and the time and duration of the study.

Limitations: An indication of the inherent weaknesses in the study; factors that could not be controlled adequately and could have affected the results.

Assumptions: The particular facts taken for granted about the behaviors, conditions, methods, measures, and relationships inherent in the study.

Hypotheses: Predictions of the eventual outcome of the study.

Definition of Terms: A list of the terminology essential to consistent interpretation of the various concepts surrounding the problem being studied.

Chapter 2 Review of Related Literature

A reporting chapter of previous investigations related to the problem being studied. Theoretical formulations from other studies, the major issues of methodology, instrumentation, and interpretation, and background information are presented. A well-organized chapter that shows how the present study may differ from previous ones, and at the same time add to their contributions. Knowledge gaps in the problem area are noted. Through a review of the literature, a theoretical basis and justification for the present study is formed.

Chapter 3 Procedures for Collecting Data

A systematic and careful plan for attacking the problem. The procedures, methods, and techniques are detailed in a step-by-step set of instructions for conducting the study. The topics frequently included are selection of subjects, instrumentation, design of the study, administrative procedures for collecting the data, and treatment of the data.

Chapter 4 Analysis of Data

This is the reporting chapter of the thesis or dissertation in which the researcher (1) presents the data and (2) discusses and interprets those data. This chapter should begin with an opening paragraph that restates the problem and tells how the chapter is organized (example 12.2). Following that paragraph will be several sections in which the data analysis and/or findings will be reported. Typical items that need to be included are the following indices: (1) What is in the chapter (examples 12.2 and 12.3)? (2) How were the raw data scored or into what values were they converted for the analysis (example 12.4)? (3) How was the reliability of each of the measurements determined and what were the results? (4) How were the data analyzed and what were the results of the analysis (examples 12.5 and 12.6)?

EXAMPLE 12.2
An Opening Paragraph
From T. L. Visker,
Self-consciousness and physical self-efficacy in relationship to exercise adherence. Doctoral dissertation, 1986. Reprinted by permission of Tom L. Visker.

The problem of the study was to determine if the psychological factors of self-consciousness and physical self-efficacy discriminate between female adults who adhere to exercise programs and female adults who do not adhere to exercise programs. Included in the study was an attempt to identify the reasons exercise adherers give for continuing an exercise program and the reasons exercise non-adherers give for discontinuing exercise programs. The analysis of the data is presented in this chapter according to the following topics: (1) data-gathering instrument distribution, (2) demographic data, (3) chi-square analysis, (4) discriminant analysis data, (5) multiple regression data, (6) reasons for continuing or discontinuing an exercise program, and (7) discussion of findings.

(Visker, 1986)

The problem of the study was to determine what, if any, relationship existed between success as an intercollegiate defensive tackle and reaction time in a simulated open skill situation, movement time in a simulated open skill situation, five-yard sprint time, 40-yard sprint time, height, weight, and percent of body fat. The purpose of the study was to develop a system and procedures for accurately determining from objectively secured data the potential of a prospective football player to perform successfully as an intercollegiate defensive tackle.

Seven null hypotheses stating an equality of group means across three groups of subjects were tested. The hypotheses are:

1. There is no relationship between reaction time in a simulated open skill situation and success as an intercollegiate defensive tackle.

2. There is no relationship between movement time in a simulated open skill situation and success as an intercollegiate defensive tackle.

3. There is no relationship between five-yard sprint time and success as an intercollegiate defensive tackle.

4. There is no relationship between 40-yard sprint time and success as an intercollegiate defensive tackle.

5. There is no relationship between height and success as an intercollegiate defensive tackle.

6. There is no relationship between weight and success as an intercollegiate defensive tackle.

7. There is no relationship between percent of body fat and success as an intercollegiate defensive tackle.

Success groups were determined by the following classifications: first team tackles, successful; second team tackles, less successful; and third team tackles, least successful. First team, second team, and third team designations were based on the opinions of the separate coaching staffs taken immediately before the first game of the 1987 season.

Data on the variables were collected at seven colleges during 1987 pre-season football practices. Raw scores of the three groups (Appendix D) were compared by the utilization of a stepwise multiple discriminant analysis computer program (S.P.S.S. subprogram Discriminant). An additional analysis was performed by comparing just the data of the first team tackles with the data of the third team tackles. Differences in group means were accepted as significant at the .05 level.

(Sells, 1977)

EXAMPLE 12.3
Sample Research
Problem and Hypotheses
From T. D. Sells, *Selected movement and anthropometric variables of football defensive tackles.* Doctoral dissertation, 1977. Reprinted by permission of Thomas D. Sells.

EXAMPLE 12.4
Data Reporting Table for
Response Rate Data

From T. L. Visker,
*Self-consciousness and
physical self-efficacy in
relationship to exercise
adherence.* Doctoral
dissertation, 1986.
Reprinted by permission of
Tom L. Visker.

Data-Gathering Instrument Distribution

The population of prospective subjects for the study consisted of 337 females who were enrolled in physical fitness classes at the Monroe County, Indiana, YMCA during the spring of 1985. Each of the 337 females was sent a letter in which they were asked to participate in the study. Each person was asked to return a postcard to the investigator regarding her intention to participate or not participate in the study. The results of this mailing are presented in Table 1.

TABLE 1 Letter Response Rate

	FIRST MAILING	SECOND MAILING	TOTAL
Letters Sent	350	196	546
Postcards Returned	141	139	280
Percent	40	71	83*
Postcards Not Returned	196	57	70
Percent	56	29	21*
Number Agreed to Participate	116	82	198
Percent	82	59	71**
Number Declined to Participate	25	57	82
Percent	18	41	29**
Invalid Addresses	13	0	13
Percent	4	0	4*

*of the 337 valid addresses
**of the 280 postcards returned

The initial mailing yielded a return of 141 postcards (40 percent). Of those subjects who returned the postcard, 116 (82 percent) agreed to participate in the study and 25 (18 percent) declined to participate in the study. There were 13 subjects (4 percent) for whom no valid address could be found. The number of prospective subjects who did not return a postcard was 196 (56 percent).

A second mailing of 196 letters yielded a return of 139 postcards (71 percent). Of those who returned the postcard after this mailing, 82 (59 percent) agreed to participate and 57 (41 percent) declined to participate in the study. Fifty-seven (29 percent) of those to whom a second letter was sent failed to return the postcard.

(Visker, 1986)

Chi-Square Analysis

The chi-square test of association was used to test the hypothesis that there is no difference between exercise adherers and exercise non-adherers in terms of the type of fitness class attended, the highest educational degree earned, or the marital status of the subjects. This test was used since none of the parameters was known; the results of its application are presented in Tables 5 through 7.

TABLE 5 Chi-Square Test of Association for Fitness Class Attended of Exercise Adherers and Non-Adherers

CLASS	CLASSIFICATION		TOTAL
	Adherer	Non-Adherer	
Aerobics Plus	31	8	39
Percent	27	16	23
Aquaerobics	7	9	16
Percent	6	18	10
Fitness Fantasia	47	22	69
Percent	40	43	41
Fit-for-Life	29	11	40
Percent	25	22	24
General Aerobics	3	1	4
Percent	3	2	2
Group Total	117	51	168
Percent	70	30	

Chi-square value = 7.146
Chi-square required at .05 level of significance = 9.45

The chi-square value for the fitness classes was determined to be 7.146. A value of 9.45 was required for statistical significance at the .05 level with four degrees of freedom. Since the chi-square value for fitness classes was non-significant, the null hypothesis that there is no significant difference between exercise adherers and non-adherers in fitness class attended was accepted.

(Visker, 1986)

EXAMPLE 12.5
Data Reporting Table for Analysis: Chi-Square Analysis

From T. L. Visker, *Self-consciousness and physical self-efficacy in relationship to exercise adherence.* Doctoral dissertation, 1986. Reprinted by permission of Tom L. Visker.

EXAMPLE 12.6
Data Reporting Table for
Analysis: *F* Test

From T. D. Sells, *Selected
movement and anthropometric
variables of football defensive
tackles.* Doctoral dissertation,
1977. Reprinted by permission
of Thomas D. Sells.

The F-tests from the one-way analysis of variance of the difference between means of the first, second, and third team defensive tackles are presented in Table 2.

TABLE 2 One-Way Analysis of Variance of the Difference Between Means and the Level of Significance of Difference of the Means of the First Team, Second Team, and Third Team Defensive Tackles

VARIABLE	F-TEST	SIGNIFICANCE LEVEL*
Reaction	.2474	.7821
Movement time	1.8428	.1723
Five-yard sprint	1.7168	.1933
40-yard sprint	1.3740	.2654
Height	2.0586	.1416
Weight	.5299	.5929
Percent body fat	.0743	.9285

*Degrees of freedom = 2 and 38.

The significance of the separate F-tests based on the one-way analysis of variance of difference in group means did not reach the .05 level in the initial phase of the data analysis. At that point in the analysis, the null hypotheses stating an equality of group means across the three success groups could not be rejected for any of the variables.

(Sells, 1977)

Note that the emphasis in this section is usually on *reporting only,* with no editorializing, discussion, or interpretation included. The standard procedure is to introduce a table containing data, present the table, and point out the significant findings in the table. The report of all of the data and findings should be followed by a detailed discussion and interpretation of the findings. This final section of the chapter should be labeled "Discussion of Findings." Here are some questions and thoughts concerning this section:

a. Are there any explanations for any of the findings? If so, these thoughts should be shared with the reader.

b. Do some findings defy explanation? Are some really surprising? If so, what are they? Speculate why these particular results may have come about in this way.

    c. In answering the questions posed in a and b above, the element of hindsight in the procedure sometimes enters the discussion. The hindsight may be clear to the researcher, but not to the reader; so share that hindsight with the reader.

    d. Are the findings consistent with findings in similar studies? Do the findings differ?

This part of the research report is often difficult to accomplish, but a feeling of satisfaction accompanies its completion. For an excellent example illustrating how some researchers have incorporated the information included in the comments made above, see example 12.7.

Chapter 5 Summary, Findings, Conclusions, Implementations, and Recommendations

This is the final and, typically, the shortest chapter in a thesis or dissertation. A summary of the study and the general conclusions and recommendations resulting from the research should be placed in this chapter. Only material mentioned earlier in the report may be included in the summary.

In the summary, the problem should be restated, a general overview of the sources of data and the methods used should be provided, and the *more important* findings should be listed. For this reporting of the findings, brief statements will suffice rather than repeating the details already discussed.

General conclusions drawn from the findings should be presented in the same order as the findings on which they are based. In sampling studies, conclusions are population statements as are the hypotheses stated at the beginning of the research. The conclusions should be definitive and bring the study to an end. Conclusions should not be repetitions or summaries of findings but should answer this question: The data (finding) says this, so what does this tell me as to the conclusion that is warranted? Conclusions beyond the data obtained (i.e., the findings) should not be made. In stating the conclusions, avoid the use of "hedging" words such as "It seems as though . . ." or "It appears that . . ." The data tell the researcher what is or is not, and the conclusion statements should reflect such definitiveness. The distinction between a finding and the conclusion should be made abundantly clear.

The implementations section should indicate how the researcher envisions the findings being applied. How can the findings be used in a practical situation, or in what ways would the findings make a contribution? Could the findings also apply to a research setting? If so, how could they be implemented?

The recommendation section should appear last in the chapter, and the recommendations may be of more than one type. The researcher may recommend that certain specified action be taken in light of the findings; that further study be made of the problem using either the same data or a different sample; or that a study be made of a related problem or of the same problem in greater detail or after a certain length of time has elapsed. A typical chapter 5 of a research report is illustrated in example 12.8.

EXAMPLE 12.7

Discussion of Findings

From T. L. Visker, *Self-consciousness and physical self-efficacy in relationship to exercise adherence.* Doctoral dissertation, 1986. Reprinted by permission of Tom L. Visker.

Discussion of Findings

The consistency in determining the significant contribution of perceived physical ability in the study was similar to the findings of other studies using perceived physical ability as a variable. Snyder and Spreitzer (1984), Spreitzer and Snyder (1983), and Snyder and Spreitzer (1981) found significant correlations between perceived athletic ability and involvement in vigorous physical activities. The finding of the present study reiterates the position that the higher an individual perceives her physical abilities to be, the more likely she will be to stay with an exercise program.

The findings of the study also supported Sonstroem's Physical Activity Model (1978, 1976, 1974). Sonstroem theorized that as one's estimation of physical ability increases, so will one's attraction to physical activity, which will result in an increase in physical activity. In the present study, the subjects who scored higher in perceived physical ability also were engaged in more minutes per week of vigorous physical activity than subjects who scored lower in perceived physical ability.

Since the data of the study were analyzed using multivariate correlational techniques, it would be inappropriate to suggest that a woman's perception of her physical abilities caused her to adhere to or discontinue an exercise program. All that can be inferred from this finding is that a significant positive relationship does exist between a woman's perceived physical ability and the likelihood that she will continue with an exercise program.

The lack of scientific inquiry into reasons for adhering to a program of exercise makes it difficult to draw parallels to other investigations. However, several of the reasons given for adhering to an exercise program have been investigated in other studies. Many of the reasons address the situational factors in which the exercise program is carried out. This alone provides credence to Dishman's (1984) conceptual model for exercise adherence which posits that whether a person stays with an exercise program or not is determined by an interaction between the exerciser and his or her environment. Specifically, the social reason of exercising with others has been found to be significant in other studies. Heinzelman and Bagley (1970) found that 90 percent of the subjects in their investigation preferred to exercise with others. Massie and Shepard (1971) found that exercise adherence was higher for subjects who exercised as a group than for subjects who exercised alone.

Exercise and mental health have been the subject of many research investigations (Sach, 1984; Folkins and Sime, 1981; and Morgan, 1981). It has consistently been shown that regular vigorous physical activity will enhance

EXAMPLE 12.7
Concluded

one's mental health. The frequency of the response of enhancing mental health found in this investigation is consistent with that found in other studies.

The exercise environment was also cited as a reason for adhering to an exercise program. One factor in the exercise environment which was specifically mentioned was the use of music. The use of music in an exercise setting is a dissociative technique which focuses the exerciser's attention away from the discomfort of exercise, resulting in more enjoyable exercise bouts. Martin, et al. (1984) found dissociative intervention strategy to be effective in increasing exercise adherence.

Several studies have investigated the reasons individuals give for discontinuing exercise programs (Lee and Owen, 1985; Andrew, et al. 1981; Boothby, Tungatt and Townsend, 1981). Two of the reasons exercise non-adherers cited in the present study are consistent with earlier findings. Perhaps the most frequent reason given for discontinuing an exercise program is lack of time. The frequency of this reason in the present study is parallel to studies by Boothby, Tungatt and Townsend (1981); Gettman, Pollock and Ward, (1983); and Lee and Owen (1985).

The distance traveled to the exercise setting was also cited as a reason for dropping out of an exercise program. While the frequency of this response is not as high as the response of lack of time, this response is consistent with other studies (Lee and Owen, 1985; Andrew and Parker, 1979; and Morgan, 1977).

Because the present investigation was composed entirely of women, some of the reasons given for adhering to or discontinuing an exercise program were unique to this investigation. Many of these reasons deal with traditional female roles. For example, some of the reasons given for adhering to an exercise program are the availability of babysitting services, reversing the effects of childbirth, and a child's nap schedule. The reasons given for discontinuing an exercise program are even more to the point. The demands of children and pregnancy-childbirth were two of the more frequent responses given. However, the fact that the response of demands of employment was one of the most frequent responses given for discontinuing an exercise program is, perhaps, an indication of the changing nature of women's roles in society.

(Visker, 1986)

It is important to note that chapters 2, 3, and 4 always begin with an opening paragraph identifying what part of the problem is discussed in the chapter and indicating how the chapter is organized. Only in chapter 2 is a summary mandated. Each chapter is to start on a new page.

References

The body of the text is always followed by an alphabetized list of references. It should be presented in accordance with whatever style format is required by the student's college or university or academic unit. With a relatively short list of sources to be referenced, different types of literary pieces may be incorporated. However, if the list of sources is quite long, they may be grouped according to type, such as books, documents, manuscripts, newspapers, pamphlets, and periodicals. The usual convention is to include only those sources that were referenced in footnotes appearing in the text. Occasionally, it may be necessary to include a source that was not footnoted, but the usual caution is not to pad the list of references. Presented in example 12.9 is an example of a reference list using the APA format.

Supplementary Items

The appendixes serve as the repository for **supplementary items** that are unnecessary for inclusion in the body of the text, but can be used by the reader to clarify various aspects of the thesis or research report. They provide additional specific information if the reader desires it. Typically, appendixes will include the following types of items:

1. Copies of the verbal instruments (e.g., questionnaires, interview guides)
2. Instructions to subjects on how to engage in physical performance tests (e.g., fitness, skill tests)
3. Letters and similar documents
4. Human subject consent forms
5. Raw data from both a pilot study and the actual study
6. Diagrams of electrical circuits of test instruments
7. Tables from related research
8. Supplementary reference lists
9. Credentials of the members of a jury of experts or committee of authorities
10. Interview and other data collection schedules
11. Legal codes

All such materials should be clearly labeled and lettered for quick and easy reference. Each appendix should bear a descriptive title of what is included.

Summary

The problem of the study was to determine if the psychological factors of self-consciousness and physical self-efficacy discriminate between female adults who adhere to exercise programs and female adults who do not adhere to exercise programs. Included in the study was an attempt to identify the reasons exercise adherers give for continuing an exercise program and the reasons exercise non-adherers give for discontinuing an exercise program.

The subjects of the study were 168 females who had enrolled in physical fitness classes at the Monroe County YMCA, Bloomington, Indiana, during the spring of 1985. All subjects completed a survey instrument consisting of the self-consciousness scale, the physical self-efficacy scale, and questions designed to determine demographic data and exercise habits. The data for the study were collected during the months of May and June, 1986.

The data were analyzed using four statistical techniques. Chi-square test of association was used to test the differences in fitness class attended, education level, and marital status between exercise adherers and non-adherers. Discriminant analysis was used to determine if the independent variables of private self-consciousness, public self-consciousness, social anxiety, self-consciousness, perceived physical ability, physical self-presentation confidence, physical self-efficacy, age, and income could significantly predict the dependent variables of group membership (exercise adherer or non-adherer). Multiple regression analysis was used to determine if the independent variables of the study could significantly predict the number of minutes per week spent in vigorous physical activity. Finally, a frequency distribution of the reasons exercise adherers gave for continuing an exercise program and the reasons exercise non-adherers gave for discontinuing an exercise program was done. The Statistical Package for the Social Sciences (SPSS) was used for all statistical analysis except the frequency distributions.

Findings

The analysis of the data revealed the following significant findings:

1. The independent variables of private self-consciousness, public self-consciousness, social anxiety, self-consciousness, perceived physical ability, physical self-presentation confidence, physical self-efficacy, age, and income significantly predicted group membership as an exercise adherer or non-adherer.

EXAMPLE 12.8
Sample of a Chapter 5
From T. L. Visker, *Self-consciousness and physical self-efficacy in relationship to exercise adherence.* Doctoral dissertation, 1986. Reprinted by permission of Tom L. Visker.

EXAMPLE 12.8
Continued

2. The independent variables of perceived physical ability and physical self-efficacy accounted for most of the function which discriminated between exercise adherers and non-adherers.

3. The optimal linear combination of the independent variables of private self-consciousness, public self-consciousness, social anxiety, self-consciousness, perceived physical ability, physical self-presentation confidence, physical self-efficacy, age, education level, marital status, and income, taken altogether, significantly predicted the number of minutes per week spent in vigorous physical activity.

4. By itself, only perceived physical ability significantly predicted the number of minutes per week spent in vigorous physical activity.

5. The most frequent reasons given by exercise adherers for continuing an exercise program were to maintain health, social, enhance mental health, relieve stress, and appearance.

6. The most frequent reasons given by exercise non-adherers for discontinuing an exercise program were lack of time, demands of employment, schedule conflicts, demands of children, and illness or injury.

Conclusions

Within the limitations of the study the following conclusions are warranted:

1. Significant psychological differences exist between female exercise adherers and non-adherers.

2. Females who adhere to a program of exercise perceive their physical abilities at a higher level than do females who discontinue a program of physical exercise.

3. Self-consciousness is not an important factor in the psychological differences between female exercise adherers and non-adherers.

4. Females who have a higher perception of their physical abilities exercise more than do females who have a lower perception of their physical abilities.

EXAMPLE 12.8
Continued

Implementations

The findings of the study may be implemented into either a professional practice situation or a research setting in the following ways:

1. The significance of perceived physical ability to discriminate between female exercise adherers and non-adherers should be considered in developing psychological profiles of exercise adherers and non-adherers. The use of these profiles may help to predict those who will continue an exercise program and those who will be inclined to drop out.

2. Adherence to an exercise program could be enhanced by the use of intervention strategies designed to increase the participants' perception of their physical ability. Programs involving the use of progression in skills and intensity of training could increase one's self-perception of physical ability and thereby increase the likelihood of an individual continuing in those exercise programs.

3. If exercise adherence is one of the major goals in physical activity programs, the enhancement of one's self-perceived physical abilities should be a major concern in elementary and secondary physical education programs. Exposure to a variety of skills will increase the likelihood of finding an activity in which the skills can be mastered, thus increasing the chance for regular life-long participation in that activity.

Recommendations for Further Study

The following recommendations are made for further research in the area of exercise adherence:

1. The present study should be replicated using both male and female participants.

2. The relationship of self-consciousness and physical self-efficacy to exercise adherence should be examined in an experimental type of study. This would permit more control in the variable of exercise adherence since it would not rely on the subject's truthfulness regarding their exercise habits.

3. A study should be conducted to determine the cause and effect relationship between perceived physical ability and exercise adherence.

EXAMPLE 12.8
Concluded

4. Additional studies identifying other psychological variables which could be related to exercise adherence are needed.

5. The present investigation should be replicated in other communities to gain a large cross-section of the adult population from which data can be obtained.

6. The psychological variables of self-consciousness and physical self-efficacy related to exercise adherence should be investigated in a non-structured exercise program setting.

7. Additional studies identifying reasons exercise adherers give for continuing an exercise program are needed to corroborate the findings of the present study.

(Visker, 1986)

References

Cetron, M. J., & Rocha, W. (1987). Travel tomorrow: The hospitable future. *Futurist, 21*(4), (INFOTRAC 87–23310), 29–34.

Coates, J. F. (1989). Looking ahead: Travel marketing challenges of the next 25 years. *Travel and Tourism Executive Report, 1/2,* 1.

Cornish, E. (1986). Future free time: How will people use it?. *Parks and Recreation, 5,* 57–59.

Davidson, T. L. (1984). Marketing travel in an emerging economy. *Journal of Travel Research, 22*(4), (INFOTRAC 84–15674), 38–39.

Dillman, D. A. (1978). *Mail and telephone surveys: The total design method.* New York: John Wiley & Sons, 44.

Fesenmaier, D. R. (1987). *Development of a market assistance program for tourist businesses along the Texas gulf coast.* Proposal for Texas A&M University Sea Grant College Program. College Station, Texas: Department of Recreation and Parks, Texas A&M University.

Fesenmaier, D. R. (1988). *A framework for tourism evaluation in Fredericksburg, Texas.* Unpublished report to the city of Fredericksburg, Texas.

Fesenmaier, D. R. (1989). *An assessment of information needs: Indiana convention and visitors bureaus.* Indiana University report. Bloomington, IN: Tourism Resource Center.

Gartrell, R. B. (1988). *Destination marketing for convention and visitors bureaus.* Dubuque, IA: Kendall/Hunt, 6–11.

Gee, C. Y. & Makens, J. C. (1985). The tourism board: Doing it right. *Cornell H.R.A. Quarterly, 11,* 25–33.

Glass, G. V., & Hopkins, K. D. (1984). *Statistical methods in education and psychology.* Englewood Cliffs, NJ: Prentice-Hall, 2.

Gunn, G. V. (1983). U.S. tourism policy development. *Journal of Physical Education, Recreation, and Dance, 4,* 10, 33.

Honomichi, J. (1984). Tourism industry big on research. *Advertising Age, 55,*(79), 24, 28.

(Pena, 1990)

EXAMPLE 12.9
References in APA Style

Abstract

Example 12.1G on page 268 is a sample of an **abstract** for a doctoral dissertation (Collins, 1989). Most institutions require an abstract varying in length from 250 to 350 words. The abstract is one of the preliminary items of the thesis or dissertation. A second abstract of 200 words, not affixed to the dissertation, is also required for publication in *Completed Research in Health, Physical Education, and Recreation.* Most research journals also require an abstract when researchers submit an article for publication. Though the length requirement varies among the journals, 150 to 175 words is typical. The researcher should use all of whatever abstract length is allowed, because the more that can be reported to the reader, the greater is the chance for good understanding of the research.

An abstract must be concise but should include enough detail to enable the reader to determine whether or not the entire research report, article, thesis, or dissertation needs to be read. The abstract should be brief and contain the overall essence of the information included in the larger work. The reader should be able to glean from the abstract all of the main ideas of the original research investigation.

An appropriate abstract will usually include comments concerning each of the following elements:

1. The *problem* that was investigated, including the rationale from which the problem was developed.
2. The *methods* by which the data for the problem were collected. Included here will be an identification of the variables studied, the procedure used in carrying out the research and collecting the data, and a discussion of how the data were analyzed.
3. A brief report of the *findings* resulting from the study. These results are usually not given in tables, figures, and graphs due to the limitations placed on the length of an abstract.
4. The *conclusions* made by the researcher based upon the findings. If room in the abstract exists, it could also include the researcher's interpretation of the possible implementation of the results or recommendations for further research in the problem area.

Thesis Format versus Published Article Format

On the foregoing pages, the format for a thesis or dissertation was described in some detail. The major difference between a thesis or dissertation and a research report is the length of the document. Researchers who publish articles are delimited by the established publishing criteria of particular journals in the amount of detail they can submit. A 6- to 8-page article, as prescribed by a specific publication, cannot possibly include all of the information contained in a 150-page thesis or dissertation. The **published article format** typically requires these items:

Title
Author
Organizational affiliation
Problem (sometimes called the introduction and includes some references to the
    related literature)
Procedures or methods
Results or findings
Brief discussion
Conclusions
Recommendations
References

The style in which the published article is written also will be determined by whatever style manual is followed by the journal. Quite frequently, the style will be different from that found in a thesis or dissertation. Capitalization may differ, as will punctuation, the spelling of numbers, and abbreviations.

Theses or dissertations written by graduate students are considered "final" manuscripts. They usually have a long life span and will be read and referred to over a long time. A journal manuscript tends to be a "copy" manuscript that, in turn, becomes a typeset article. Copy manuscripts have a relatively short life. They are read by reviewers, editors, and typeset experts. The original content can sometimes be changed dramatically as a result of the publication process.

Students who complete a thesis or dissertation are encouraged to publish one or more articles derived from the document. Preparation of an article entails transposing selected thesis content to journal material according to the publishing restrictions of the journal in which the article will appear. This is not a particularly difficult task, although some people find it to be a laborious chore. Some confuse transposition with creating a whole new document. Students who write a thesis under one format are sometimes confused in following the guidelines imposed by the journal format requirements.

In recent years, some professionals in the fields of HHP have advocated having students write their theses and dissertations in the form required by those respective journals in which the students hope to publish the articles based on their research. This would result in documents of 20 to 30 pages in length and containing only the essential information from the literature, procedures, and results sections. The more detailed information from the other thesis sections would become part of appendixes. The underlying idea is to make it quicker and easier for the student to create a journal article for publication from a document written to fulfill a degree requirement. Whether or not the movement away from the traditional thesis format will become large scale is yet to be seen.

Preparing a Manuscript

Before Writing

Prior to starting to prepare a manuscript for publication, the researcher should do several things. One, the researcher needs to select the journal to which the manuscript will be submitted. Two, the researcher needs to examine articles published in that journal to get a general idea of the format used and needs to read the guidelines for submitting manuscripts to the journal. Guidelines are published in the journal. Select the journal primarily on its orientation and type of subscriber. Some journals are geared primarily toward researchers; others are more for practitioners. Some journals are highly specialized, while others are for a general audience. There is no use in submitting a manuscript to a journal that does not publish the type of research described in the manuscript. Also, the researcher should try to determine the manuscript acceptance rate of the journal. Acceptance rates vary from 10 percent for very prestigious and specialized research journals to as high as 70 percent for practical, general-audience state association journals.

By looking at articles in the selected journal, the researcher may discover a useful model to follow. Certainly the researcher will be able to determine whether an abstract is required as part of the manuscript, what organization and major headings are required in the manuscript, and the typical length of a manuscript based on the length of articles in the journal.

During Writing

Any manuscript starts with the title of the research study. The title needs to be short yet represent the research well and stimulate a person to read the entire article. If an abstract is required, that element appears next in the manuscript; it should be one to three paragraphs long. The abstract will contain the statement of purpose for the study, description of subjects, major procedures, major results, and conclusions.

The manuscript for most published articles begins with an introduction and brief review of the most important related literature. Somewhere, wherever appropriate, there should be a statement of the purpose of the study. This part of the manuscript is typically three to six paragraphs.

Next in a manuscript is a procedures or methods section. Typically included in this section are descriptions of subjects, how the research was conducted, data collection techniques, and data collection procedures. The content and length of this section is dependent on the type of research conducted and the complexity of describing how the research was conducted. Tables and figures in this section are commonly used to clearly and economically present information. Not every small point concerning the conduct of the research can be presented, or the manuscript could not be kept to a reasonable length.

A results section follows the procedures section. This section usually makes up a relatively large portion of the manuscript because it includes all of the major data analysis and findings of the research study. Much of this information is presented in text form; however, the use of tables and figures is also common. The recommended organization when using tables and figures is to introduce a table or figure, present it, and then discuss it. This is not always possible, but the recommendation is a good rule of thumb. The discussion following the table or figure may be just a short sentence with the extensive discussion in a later section, or it may be quite extensive. The decision to present major discussion in this section or in a later section is left to the researcher. Probably the majority of researchers place the extensive discussion in the next section.

The discussion and conclusions section are where the results previously reported are discussed at length and conclusions based on the results are stated. This part of the manuscript is usually of considerable length, also. The discussion may include comments on each finding followed by a discussion of all the findings as a whole. However, if each finding was discussed at length when introduced in the results section, then the discussion is reserved for the findings as a whole. Often included in the discussion of findings is a comparison of how the findings agree with those in the literature cited at the beginning of the manuscript. Usually, in the discussion are statements concerning the importance and application of the findings. No matter how the discussion is structured, the conclusions follow it. Anytime the research involves a population from which one or more samples were drawn, conclusions consist of statements concerning what the researcher thinks is true at the population level based on the findings from the samples used in the study.

The last section in a manuscript is a list of references. Included in the list are all sources cited in the manuscript. The length of this section is dependent on the number of sources cited. Normally, it is not a lengthy section and will contain from three to fifteen listings.

After Writing

After writing the first draft of the manuscript considerable time must be spent proofing it. Attention to correctness of manuscript form, correctness of content, economy and clarity of presentation, and correctness of spelling and grammar are important. The more prestigious the journal where the manuscript will be submitted, the more important becomes the proofreading.

The spell check and grammar check options on most word processing computer programs are often quite helpful in revising the manuscript. However, they do not catch all problems and the final responsibility for correctness rests with the writer. Spell check will not catch words left out, the wrong word, confusing sentences, or misspelled words which are the correct spelling of another word (example 12.10).

EXAMPLE 12.10
Examples of spelling and writing problems not easily detected

Wrong Word

Knew vs New	Week vs Weak	Grate vs Great
Break vs Brake	Know vs No	Bare vs Bear
To vs Too vs Two	Disc vs Disk	

Typo

Sex vs Six	Bowl vs Bowel	At vs It vs If
On vs One	Public vs Pubic	Super vs Supper

Sentences

Their (there) is a desert (dessert) meating (meeting) of the PDQ committee to discuss the pour (poor) condition if (of) letters and packages arriving on (in) the male (mail) room.

For those of you who have children and don't know it, we have a nursery in the building.

We are pleased to announce the birth of Polly Ester Smith, the sin (son) of Mr. and Mrs. Doyle Lee Smith.

Today we are taking a collection to defray the cost of the new carpet. All of you wishing to do something on the new carpet may do so at this time.

When the manuscript is ready to be submitted to a journal, send the required number of copies and the necessary cover sheet containing the author name(s) and contact information. If there are multiple authors, names are listed in order from major contribution to minor contribution to the research and manuscript. Major contributions would include such items as developing the problem, formulating hypotheses, setting up the design, selecting the data analysis procedures, interpreting the findings, and writing the majority of the report. Quite frequently students and faculty colleagues will be listed as authors because they participated in one or more of the phases of the research project stated above, but played minor roles compared to that of the lead researcher. If all authors contributed equally, they are listed in alphabetical order. It is unethical to send the manuscript to more than one journal at a time. If the manuscript is rejected, then it is appropriate to send it to another journal. Multiple, but different, manuscripts describing a research study are acceptable. For example, one manuscript may be submitted to an applied or practitioner journal and another to a research journal.

All manuscripts submitted to a journal are evaluated by two to four reviewers or associate editors for the journal. This evaluation takes one to three months. After the manuscript has been evaluated, the journal editor sends copies of the reviews to the author indicating whether the manuscript is accepted, needs revision, or is rejected. Authors should expect that the manuscript will not be acceptable in the form submitted. Thus, when the reviews are returned, revise the manuscript and return it to the original journal, or send it to another journal.

Critique of an Article

Criteria

The **criteria for critiquing an article** are the same criteria a researcher could apply to a manuscript being developed. Most research books and guides contain a list of criteria for evaluating an article or other research publication. These lists differ to some degree but are generally similar. The majority of the criteria on these lists usually apply to any article or research publication, particularly ones based on experimental research. Due to the variety of research conducted, no article or research publication should be expected to fulfill all the criteria on any list.

Isaac and Michael (1981) present an excellent checklist for evaluating an article (example 12.11). They also provide a lengthy checklist for items that might be included in a research proposal and a long list of criteria for evaluating a research report, article, or thesis. The checklist for a research proposal is arranged by the typical chapters of a dissertation: (1) the problem, (2) review of related literature, (3) methodology of procedures, (4) findings (analysis and evaluation), and (5) summary, conclusions, and recommendations. Criteria for evaluation of a research report, article, or thesis are arranged under the title of the article or report, the problem, design and methodology (procedures), presentation and analysis of data, and summary and conclusions.

The authors of this book had an unreferenced list of criteria for evaluating research in health, physical education, and recreation. It is organized similar to the ones previously mentioned with major headings: (1) problem, (2) report, (3) procedures, methods, and techniques, (4) data, and (5) analysis and interpretation of the findings. A **checklist for evaluating a research paper,** similar in organization to those previously presented, appears in example 12.12.

Article Critique

Articles in journals associated with well-qualified manuscript reviewers will have few if any faults, since any faults in the manuscript either caused it to be rejected or were corrected before it was published. Also, keep in mind that all researchers and manuscript reviewers have their own ideas concerning how research should be conducted and what are the most important evaluation criteria. Readers of an article often see certain things they think could be improved, but these may just be opinions. It is always easier to criticize the research of others than to conduct the research yourself.

EXAMPLE 12.11

Checklist for Evaluating an Article—Form for the Evaluation of an Article[1,2]

Form for the Evaluation of an Article on page 156 in Isaac, J. and Michael, W. B. (1981), *Handbook in Research and Evaluation* EdITS Publishers, San Diego, CA. Reproduced with permission.

CHARACTERISTIC	COMPLETELY INDEPENDENT (1)	POOR (2)	MEDIOCRE (3)	GOOD (4)	EXCELLENT (5)
1. Problem is clearly stated					
2. Hypotheses are clearly stated					
3. Problem is significant					
4. Assumptions are clearly stated					
5. Limitations of the study are stated					
6. Important terms are defined					
7. Relationship of the problem to previous research is made clear					
8. Research design is described fully					
9. Research design is appropriate for the solution of the problem					
10. Research design is free of specific weaknesses					
11. Population and sample are described					
12. Method of sampling is appropriate					
13. Data-gathering methods or procedures are described					
14. Data-gathering methods or procedures are appropriate to the solution of the problem					
15. Data-gathering methods or procedures are utilized correctly					
16. Validity and reliability of the evidence gathered are established					
17. Appropriate methods are selected to analyze the data					
18. Methods utilized in analyzing the data are applied correctly					
19. Results of the analysis are presented clearly					
20. Conclusions are clearly stated					
21. Conclusions are substantiated by the evidence presented					
22. Generalizations are confined to the population from which the sample was drawn					
23. Report is clearly written					
24. Report is logically organized					
25. Tone of the report displays an unbiased, impartial scientific attitude.					

1. Wandt, Edwin, California State College, Los Angeles
2. Not all of these twenty-five criteria or characteristics are appropriate in the evaluation of a given article.

EXAMPLE 12.12
Checklist for Evaluating
a Research Paper

An Outline of a Checklist for a Research Paper

Because of the wide diversity of types of research projects as well as the multitude of approaches that may very well be taken with any single problem, it is not possible to present either an outline or a checklist that would be appropriate for all cases. Nevertheless, the researcher should be able to answer the questions listed below. Obviously, if a question does not apply, it should be disregarded. Those that do apply should merit positive answers by the investigator.

I.   The Problem

1. Does the statement of the problem meet the criteria of being:
   (a) stated in a few sentences?
   (b) clearly stated in both theoretical and operational terms?
   (c) firmly based on a stated theory and/or problem?
   (d) clear on the definitions of the variables that are to be studied?
   (e) based on variable hypotheses?

2. Has the problem been delimited in such a fashion that it can be pursued realistically?

3. Has an important problem been selected, the study of which will make a worthwhile contribution to education?

II.   The Review of Relevant Literature

1. Is it apparent that an adequate job was done in sampling the relevant literature on the topic?

2. Were references drawn from recent literature?

3. Is a wide variety of sources represented?

4. Are cited references either quoted sufficiently or interpreted accurately?

5. Have references been organized by topic and/or by date of publication?

III.   Design, Procedure, and Method

1. Is the design appropriate to the problem?

2. Was the population studied clearly specified?

3. Were sampling procedures clearly specified and the total sample adequate?

EXAMPLE 12.12
Continued

4. If a control group was involved, was it selected from same population?

5. Were the various treatments (including control) assigned at random?

6. Were appropriate statistical procedures selected and the level of significance selected in advance?

7. Were the reliability and validity of the data-gathering instruments and procedures established and reported?

8. Are the limitations of the study acknowledged?

9. Were the treatments and/or methods of data collection described so clearly and completely that an independent investigator could replicate the study?

10. Were extraneous sources of error either held constant or randomized among subjects of all groups?

11. Was the response from the sampled population equal to 80 percent or more?

12. Are the characteristics of the respondents clearly representative of the sample?

IV.   **Analysis of the Data**

1. Are the data clearly presented?

2. Is appropriate use made of charts, tables, figures, descriptions, and/or historical narratives?

3. Were all possible comparisons of the data made and reported?

4. Were the statistical assumptions necessary for valid tests of the hypothesis satisfied?

V.   **Interpretation of the Findings and Conclusion**

1. Are generalizations confined to the population from which the sample was drawn?

2. Do the conclusions of the study meet the criteria of being:

    (a) consistent with the obtained results?

    (b) relevant to the problem?

    (c) based on the data?

    (d) justified by the data?

    (e) constructive and free from bias?

    (f) not "stretched" to support a bias?

EXAMPLE 12.12
Concluded

3. Are implications given for both education practice and for further research ?

VI.   **Summary**

1. Is a concise summary given of the problem, design, methodology, findings, interpretation, and conclusions?

2. Does the reading of this section alone present an accurate overall picture of the study?

VII.   **Bibliography**

1. Are complete references presented for all sources read or referred to in conjunction with the study?

VIII.   **Appendix**

1. Are samples present of all questionnaires, lists, interview forms, letters, and so forth used in the study?

2. Are such materials clearly labeled and lettered for quick and easy reference?

Earlier in this chapter, the seven parts of a manuscript were discussed starting with the title and ending with the references. These seven parts are now discussed from the standpoint of reading and understanding the article. Keep in mind that many articles are written assuming the reader has had at least one graduate-level course in the general area of the research. Further, there are certain terms unique to research writing. Thus, do not be too discouraged if you do not understand all research articles.

If the title of the article does not interest you, it is doubtful you will read further. If you do read the abstract, look for the statement of the purpose for the research study, the subjects and methods used in the study, and the major findings and conclusions.

In the introduction and review of related literature section, look for why the research was needed, a review of articles bearing on the conduct of the study, and a statement of purpose for the study. After reading the procedures and methods section, you should have a good understanding of the type and number of subjects involved and the procedures and methods used in the study. Further, you should feel that the study was well conducted. If you do not feel the study was well conducted, there may be no reason to read further.

Most readers of a research article falling within their area of expertise can understand the information up to the results section. The results section may be difficult to understand if your statistical knowledge is limited or if quite advanced statistical techniques are used. To the best of your ability, determine if the appropriate statistical techniques were correctly applied and, more importantly whether the results have been accurately stated. The discussion and conclusions section is based on the results of the study. If you do not fully understand the results section, you may have to accept some of the discussions and conclusions not knowing whether they are totally correct; worse yet, you may not understand them. Even if you do not fully understand the results or discussion and conclusions sections, you may find some comfort in the fact that the reviewers of the manuscript found their presentation acceptable. However, the danger remains that, due to lack of knowledge, you may misinterpret the information set forth in these two sections.

The reference section may be of particular interest to you if you want to evaluate the quality of the books and journals cited in the literature review. Also, the references may be valuable to your own research study.

Summary

The function of the written research report is to convey the results of the research effort. Clarity is a fundamental requirement of the report; the reader of the report should not have to make any assumptions as to what was done in the research and what was found. A typical format for the report has been presented, but this may be modified according to the particular requirements of the student's college, school, division, or department. Information regarding the difference between a thesis format and a published-article format has been presented. The preparation of an article for publication, as well as the critiquing of an article, are detailed. As in the previous chapters, examples are presented to assist the student in understanding the research concepts inherent in a written report.

Formative Evaluation of Objectives

Objective 1   Determine the characteristics of a good research report.

1. Identify the characteristics of a good research report.
2. Why is effective writing so important in research reporting?

Objective 2   Understand the format for a report and the kinds of information required in each division of the report.

1. Identify the divisions of a typical research report.
2. Select a completed study and determine whether the content of each division of the report is appropriate.

Objective 3   Differentiate between the style of writing a research report for a thesis or dissertation as opposed to a research report for publication in a journal.

1. Select some completed research and analyze the style of writing in terms of desirable writing standards.

Objective 4   Critique and evaluate a research report.

1. What is the goal for the abstract of a study?

2. Select a completed research report and critique and evaluate it in terms of how well it communicates the research to you and whether any important information has been omitted.

References

Books

American Psychological Association. (1983). *Publication manual of the American Psychological Association.* Washington, DC: Author.

Arkin, H., and Colton, R. R. (1963). *Tables for statisticians* (2d ed.). New York: Barnes & Noble.

Ary, D., Jacobs, L. C., and Razeveih, A. (1972). *Introduction to research in education.* New York: Holt, Rinehart & Winston.

Babbie, E. (1990). *Survey research methods.* Belmont, CA: Wadsworth.

Babbie, E. (1992). *The practice of social research* (6th ed.). Belmont, CA: Wadsworth.

Baumgartner, T. A., and Jackson, A. S. (1995). *Measurement for evaluation in physical education and exercise science* (5th ed.). Madison, WI: Brown & Benchmark.

Becker, H. (1970). *Sociological works: Methods and substance.* Chicago: Aldine.

Best, J. W. (1981). *Research in education* (4th ed.). Englewood Cliffs, NJ: Prentice-Hall.

Best, J. W., and Kahn, J. V. (1989). *Research in education* (6th ed.). Englewood Cliffs, NJ: Prentice-Hall.

Blommers, P. J., and Forsyth, R. A. (1983). *Elementary statistical methods.* Lanham, MD: University Press of America.

Blumer, H. (1969). *Symbolic interactionism: Perspective and method.* Englewood Cliffs, NJ: Prentice-Hall.

Bogdan, R., and Biklen, S. (1992). *Qualitative research for education.* Boston: Allyn & Bacon.

Bookwalter, C. W., and Bookwalter, K. W. (1959). Library techniques. In M. G. Scott (Ed.), *Research methods in health, physical education, and recreation* (pp. 20–38). Washington, DC: American Association for Health, Physical Education, and Recreation.

Borg, W. R. (1987). *Applying educational research: A practical guide for teachers* (2d ed.). New York: Longman.

Burgess, R. G. (Ed.). (1982). *Field research: A source book and field manual.* New York: Allen & Unwin.

Campbell, D., and Stanley, J. (1963). *Experimental and quasi-experimental designs for research.* Chicago: Rand McNally.

Campbell, W. G., and Ballou, S. V. (1978). *Form and style: Theses, reports, term papers.* Boston: Houghton Mifflin.

Cohen, J., and Cohen, P. (1975). *Applied multiple regression/correlation analysis for the behavioral sciences.* New York: Wiley.

Cook, T. D., and Campbell, D. T. (1979). *Quasi-experimentation: Design and analysis issues for field settings.* Boston: Houghton Mifflin.

Cook, T. D., and Reichardt, C. S. (Eds.). (1979). *Qualitative and quantitative methods in evaluation research.* Beverly Hills, CA: Sage.

Council of Biology Editors, Committee on Form and Style. (1972). *CBE style manual.* (3d ed.). Washington, DC: American Institute of Biological Sciences.

Day, R. A. (1983). *How to write and publish a scientific paper* (2d ed.). Philadelphia: ISI.

Dayton, C. M. (1970). *The design of educational experiments.* New York: McGraw-Hill.

Denzin, N. (1978). *The research act.* New York: McGraw-Hill.

Dillman, D. A. (1978). *Mail and telephone surveys: The total design method.* New York: John Wiley & Sons.

Dixon, W. J., Brown, M. B., Engelman, L., and Jenrich, R. I. (1990). *BMDP software manual.* Berkeley, CA: University of California Press.

Ferguson, G. A., and Takane, Y. (1989). *Statistical analysis in psychology and education* (6th ed.). New York: McGraw-Hill.

Fox, D. J. (1969). *The research process in education.* New York: Holt, Rinehart & Winston.

Geertz, C. (1973). *The interpretation of cultures.* New York: Basic Books.

Gibaldi, J., and Achtert, W. S. (1980). *MLA handbook: For writers of research papers, theses, and dissertations.* New York: Modern Language Association.

Glaser, B. (1978). *Theoretical sensitivity: Advances in the methodology of grounded theory.* Mill Valley, CA: Sociology Press.

Glaser, B., and Strauss, A. (1967). *The discovery of grounded theory: Strategies for qualitative research.* Chicago: Aldine.

Goetz, J., and LeCompte, M. (1984). *Ethnography and qualitative design in educational research.* Orlando, FL: Academic Press.

Good, C. V. (1972). *Essentials of educational research.* New York: Appleton-Century-Crofts.

Gorden, R. (1975). *Interviewing: Strategy, techniques, and tactics.* Homewood, IL: Dorsey.

Green, L., and Lewis, F. M. (1986). *Measurement and evaluation in health education and health promotion.* Mountain View, CA: Mayfield.

Griffin, P. (1983). Gymnastics is a girl's thing: Student participation and interaction patterns in a middle school gymnastic's unit. In T. J. Templin and J. K. Olson (Eds.), *Teaching in physical education* (pp. 71–85). Champaign, IL: Human Kinetics.

Guba, E., and Lincoln, Y. (1981). *Effective evaluation.* San Francisco: Jossey-Bass.

Harrington, W. (1986). Physical education versus athletics: A teacher's perception of who controls the gymnasium. In B. Mergen (Ed.), *Cultural dimensions of play, games, and sport* (pp. 169–173). Champaign, IL: Human Kinetics.

Harris, R. J. (1985). *A primer of multivariate statistics.* Orlando, FL: Academic Press.

Henderson, K. A. (1991). *Dimensions of choice: A qualitative approach to recreation, parks, and leisure research.* State College, PA: Venture.

Hollander, M., and Wolfe, D. A. (1973). *Nonparametric statistical methods.* New York: Wiley.

Huck, S. W., Cormier, W. H., and Bounds, W. G. (1974). *Reading statistics and research.* New York: Harper & Row.

Hult, J. S., and Trekell, M. (Eds.). (1991). *A century of women's basketball.* Reston, VA: American Alliance for Health, Physical Education, Recreation and Dance.

Ibrahim, H. (1992). *Pioneers in leisure and recreation.* Reston: VA: American Alliance for Health, Physical Education, Recreation and Dance.

Isaac, S., and Michael, W. B. (1976). *Handbook in research and evaluation.* San Diego: EdITS.

Isaac, S., and Michael, W. B. (1981). *Handbook in research and evaluation.* San Diego: EdITS.

Isaac, S., and Michael, W. B. (1995). *Handbook in research and evaluation.* San Diego: EdITS.

Keppel, G. (1991). *Design and analysis: A researcher's handbook.* Englewood Cliffs, NJ: Prentice-Hall.

Kerlinger, F. N. (1973). *Foundations of behavioral research* (3d ed.). New York: Holt, Rinehart, & Winston.

Kerlinger, F. N. (1986). *Foundations of behavioral research* (3d ed.). New York: Holt, Rinehart & Winston.

Kirk, J., and Miller, M. (1986). *Reliability and validity in qualitative research.* Beverly Hills, CA: Sage.

Kirk, R. E. (1982). *Experimental design: Procedures for the behavioral sciences.* Monterey, CA: Brooks/Cole.

Lawson, H. (1989). From rookie to veteran: Workplace conditions in physical education and induction into the profession. In T. J. Templin and P. G. Shemps (Eds.), *Socialization into physical education: Learning to teach* (pp. 145–164). Indianapolis: Benchmark.

Leininger, M. (1985). Nature, rationale importance of qualitative research in nursing. In M. Leininger (Ed.), *Qualitative research methods in nursing.* Orlando, FL: Grune & Stratton.

Lincoln, Y., and Guba, E. (1985). *Naturalistic inquiry.* Beverly Hills, CA: Sage.

Locke, L. F., and Spirduso, W. W. (1976). *Proposals that work: A guide for planning research.* New York: Columbia University Teachers College Press.

Marascuilo, L. A., and McSweeney, M. (1977). *Nonparametric and distribution-free methods for the social sciences.* Monterey, CA: Brooks/Cole.

Marshall, C., and Rossman, G. (1989). *Designing qualitative research.* Newbury Park, CA: Sage.

Maxwell, S. E., and Delaney, H. D. (1990). *Designing experiments and analyzing data: A model comparison perspective.* Belmont, CA: Wadsworth.

McMillan, J. H., and Schumacher, S. (1984). *Research in education.* Boston: Little, Brown.

Merriam, S. (1988). *Case study research in education.* San Francisco: Jossey-Bass.

Miles, M., and Huberman, M. (1984). *Qualitative data analysis.* Beverly Hills, CA: Sage.

Nevins, A. (1938). *The gateway to history.* New York: McGraw-Hill.

Nie, N. H., et al. (1975). *Statistical package for the social sciences* (2d ed.). New York: McGraw-Hill.

Patton, M. (1980). *Qualitative evaluation methods.* Beverly Hills, CA: Sage.

Pedhazur, E. J. (1982). *Multiple regression in behavioral research: Explanation and prediction* (2d ed.). New York: Holt, Rinehart & Winston.

Pelegrino, D. A. (1979). *Research methods for recreation and leisure: A theoretical and practical guide.* Dubuque, IA: Wm. C. Brown.

Powney, J., and Watts, M. (1987). *Interviewing in educational research.* London: Routledge & Kegan Paul.

Pyrczak, F., and Bruce, R. R. (1992). *Writing empirical research reports: A basic guide for students of the social and behavioral sciences.* Los Angeles: Psyczak.

Reason, P., and Rowan, J. (Eds.). (1981). *Human inquiry: A sourcebook of new paradigm research.* New York: John Wiley & Sons.

Rubin, H. J. (1983). *Applied social research.* Columbus, OH: Charles E. Merrill.

Rubinson, L., and Neutens, J. J. (1987). *Research techniques for the health sciences.* New York: Macmillan.

Safrit, M. J., and Wood, T. M. (1989). *Measurement concepts in physical education and exercise science.* Champaign, IL: Human Kinetics.

Sarvela, P., and McDermott, R. J. (1993). *Health education evaluation and measurement: A practitioner's perspective.* Madison, WI: Brown & Benchmark.

SAS. (1985). *SAS users guide: Statistics.* Cary, NC: SAS Institute.

Sax, G. (1979). *Foundations of educational research* (2d ed.). Englewood Cliffs, NJ: Prentice-Hall.

Siegel, S. (1956). *Nonparametric statistics for the behavioral sciences.* New York: McGraw-Hill.

Siegel, S., and Castellan, N. J. (1988). *Nonparametric statistics for the behavioral sciences* (2d ed.). New York: McGraw-Hill.

Spradley, J. (1979). *The ethnographic interview.* Chicago: Holt, Rinehart & Winston.

SPSSX. (1986). *SPSSX user's guide.* Chicago: SPSS.

Stevens, J. (1986). *Applied multivariate statistics for the social sciences.* Hillsdale, NJ: Erlbaum.

Stunkard, A. J., Sorenson, T., and Schulsinger, F. (1983). Use of the Danish adoption register for the study of obesity and thinness. In S. S. Kety, L. P. Rowland, R. L. Sidman and S. W. Matthysee (Eds.), *Genetics of neurological and psychiatric disorders.* New York: Raven.

Sudman, S., and Bradburn, N. M. (1988). *Asking questions: A practical guide to questionnaire design.* San Francisco: Jossey-Bass.

Tabachnick, B. G., and Fidell, L. S. (1989). *Using multivariate statistics.* New York: Harper & Row.

Tatsuoka, M. M. (1988). *Multivariate analysis: Techniques for educational and psychological research.* New York: Wiley.

Thomas, J. R., and Nelson, J. K. (1985). *Introduction to research in health, physical education, recreation, and dance.* Champaign, IL: Human Kinetics.

Thorndike, R. M., Cunningham, G. K., Thorndike, R. L., and Hagen, E. P. (1991). *Measurement and evaluation in psychology and education.* New York: Macmillan.

Tuckman, B. W. (1978). *Conducting educational research* (2d ed.). New York: Harcourt Brace Jovanovich.

Tuckman, B. W. (1988). *Conducting educational research* (3d ed.). San Diego: Harcourt Brace Jovanovich.

Turabian, K. L. (1973). *A manual for writers of term papers, theses, and dissertations.* Chicago: University of Chicago Press.

Tutko, T. A., Lyon, L. P., and Ogilvie, B. C. (1969). *Athletic motivation inventory.* San Jose: Institute for the Study of Athletic Motivation, California State University.

Van Dalen, D. B. (1959). The historical method. In M. G. Scott (Ed.), *Research methods in health, physical education, and recreation* (pp. 465–481). Washington, DC: American Association for Health, Physical Education, and Recreation.

Van Dalen, D. B. (1964). *Understanding educational research.* New York: McGraw-Hill.

Van Dalen, D. B. (1979). *Understanding educational research: An introduction* (4th ed.). New York: McGraw-Hill.

Walker, H. M., and Lev, J. (1969). *Elementary statistical methods* (3d ed.). New York: Holt, Rinehart & Winston.

Weisberg, H. F., and Bowen, B. D. (1977). *An introduction to survey research and data analysis.* San Francisco: W. H. Freeman.

Wiersma, W. (1991). *Research methods in education* (5th ed.). Boston: Allyn & Bacon.

Winer, B. J., Brown, D. R., and Michels, K. N. (1991). *Statistical principles in experimental design* (3d ed.). New York: McGraw-Hill.

Wolcott, H. (1990). *Writing up qualitative research.* Newbury Park, CA: Sage.

Catalogs

Sage Publications. (1996). Publications Catalog. Sage Publications, Inc., P.O. Box 5084, Thousand Oaks, CA, 91359-9924.

Dissertations and Theses

Abo Abdo, H. E. (1981). *Kinematic and kinetic analysis of the soccer instep kick.* Doctoral dissertation, Indiana University, Bloomington.

Absher, R. R. (1978). *The history of the Indiana State Board of Health from 1922–1954.* Doctoral dissertation, Indiana University, Bloomington.

Baptista, R. C. (1962). *A history of intercollegiate soccer in the United States of America.* Doctoral dissertation, Indiana University, Bloomington.

Bishop, R. (1963). *The origin and development of adapted physical education in the United States.* Doctoral dissertation, Indiana University, Bloomington.

Clark, J. K. (1991). *Two curricular settings of a HIV education unit related to secondary school students' HIV knowledge and attitude.* Doctoral dissertation, Indiana University, Bloomington.

Collins, M. E. (1989). *Body figure perceptions and preferences among preadolescent children.* Doctoral dissertation, Indiana University, Bloomington.

Cotter, L. L. (1978). *Group cohesiveness and team success among women's intercollegiate basketball teams.* Doctoral dissertation, Indiana University, Bloomington.

Fratzke, M. R. (1973). *Discriminant analysis of intramural basketball officials.* Doctoral dissertation, Indiana University, Bloomington.

Frye, P. A. (1977). *Selected coefficients for estimating the reliability of multiple trail motor performance tests.* Doctoral dissertation, Indiana University, Bloomington.

Gaunt, S. J. (1979). *Factor structure of basketball playing ability.* Doctoral dissertation, Indiana University, Bloomington.

Grosshans, I. R. (1975). *Delbert Oberteuffer: His professional activities and contributions to the fields of health and physical education.* Doctoral dissertation, Indiana University, Bloomington.

Hashim, T. J. (1988). *A health knowledge test for male college freshmen in Saudi Arabia.* Doctoral dissertation, Indiana University, Bloomington.

Hendrick, J. (1981). *Biomechanical analysis of selected parameters in the field hockey drive.* Master degree thesis, Indiana University, Bloomington.

Henry, G. M. (1974). *The shooting accuracy of third grade students who practiced shooting at goals less than ten feet high.* Doctoral dissertation, Indiana University, Bloomington.

Holland, J. C. (1970). *Heart rates of Indiana high school basketball officials as measured by electrocardiographic radio telemetry.* Doctoral dissertation, Indiana University, Bloomington.

Ketlinski, R. C. (1973). *Teaching strategies and student achievement as related to learning concepts of skeletal muscular contraction.* Doctoral dissertation, Indiana University, Bloomington.

Kramer, W. D. (1970). *A computerized system for analyzing and evaluating performance data in physical education.* Doctoral dissertation, Indiana University, Bloomington.

Luedke, G. C. (1980). *Range of motion as the focus of teaching the overhand throwing pattern to children.* Doctoral dissertation, Indiana University, Bloomington.

Ogletree, R. J. (1991). *Selected factors related to help-seeking behavior in college women victims of sexual coercion.* Doctoral dissertation, Indiana University, Bloomington.

Peña, C. (1990). *Needs assessment of Indiana convention and visitor bureaus.* Master's thesis, Indiana University, Bloomington.

Piercy, I. (1978). *The extent of influence of Lloyd Bridges Sharp as identified in the lives and professional careers of selected educators and youth leaders.* Doctoral dissertation, University of Oregon, Eugene.

Scheibner, H. L. (1974). *A history of the evolution of health education as a specialized area of professional education in Indiana colleges and universities, 1816–1973.* Doctoral dissertation, Indiana University, Bloomington.

Sells, T. D. (1977). *Selected movement and anthropometric variables of football defensive tackles.* Doctoral dissertation, Indiana University, Bloomington.

Stoner, J. (1990). *George Warren Donaldson: His professional philosophy, influences and contributions to outdoor education.* Doctoral dissertation, Indiana University, Bloomington.

Umansky, W. (1976). *Prediction of preschool performance in selected areas from perinatal factors.* Doctoral dissertation, Indiana University, Bloomington.

Van Clief, E. W. (1982). *Influential physical education books of the twentieth century.* Doctoral dissertation, Indiana University, Bloomington.

Van Oteghen, S. L. (1973). *Two speeds of isokinetic exercise as related to the vertical jump performance of women.* Doctoral dissertation, Indiana University, Bloomington.

Visker, T. L. (1986). *Self-consciousness and physical self-efficacy in relationship to exercise adherence.* Doctoral dissertation, Indiana University, Bloomington.

Wasilak, J. M. (1988). *Training at various velocities on the biokinetic swim bench related to the three-dimensional pattern of the front crawl stroke.* Doctoral dissertation, Indiana University, Bloomington.

West, J. (1989). *Perceptions of self and physical activity in a culturally diverse physical education class.* Doctoral dissertation, University of Georgia, Athens.

Williams, L. D. (1976). *Julian Warner Smith: His life, professional career, and contributions.* Doctoral dissertation, East Texas State University, Commerce.

Nonprint Media

Andrews, J., and Drake, A. (Hosts). (1991). *Hanya: Portrait of a pioneer: The story of dancer/choreographer Hanya Holm* (Cassette Recording No. 243–28682). Reston, VA: American Alliance for Health, Physical Education, Recreation and Dance.

MYSTAT. (1994). Cambridge, MA: Course Technology.

Prusoczuk, K., and Baumgartner, T. A. (1986). TSCORE. Dubuque, IA: Wm. C. Brown.

Student SYSTAT. (1994). Cambridge, MA: Course Technology.

SYSTAT. (1992). Evanston, IL: SYSTAT.

Periodicals

Bain, L. (1985). A naturalistic study of students' responses to an exercise class. *Journal of Teaching in Physical Education, 5*(1), 2–12.

Bain, L., Wilson, T., and Chaikind, E. (1989). Participant perceptions of exercise programs for overweight women. *Research Quarterly for Exercise and Sport, 60*(2), 134–143.

Baumann, L. J., and Adair, E. G. (1992). The use of ethnographic interviewing to inform questionnaire construction. *Health Education Quarterly, 19*(1), 9–24.

Baumgartner, T. A. (1969). Stability of physical performance scores. *Research Quarterly, 40,* 257–261.

Baumgartner, T. A. (1978). Modified pull-up test. *Research Quarterly, 49,* 80–84.

Brennan, M. A. (1983). Dance creative measures: A reliability study. *Research Quarterly for Exercise and Sport, 54,* 293–295.

Caruthers, D., Fleming, W., and Willis, J. (1982). One hundred sixty years of rugby football (1823–1983). *National Intramural and Recreational Sports Association Journal, 7*(1), 2–5.

Chilcott, J. (1987). Where are you coming from and where are you going? The reporting of ethnographic research. *American Educational Research Journal, 24*(2), 199–218.

Cooper, J. M., and Andrews, E. W. (1975). Rhythm as a linguistic art: Signs, symbols, sounds and motions. *Quest, 23,* 68–74.

Dempsey, K. (1990). Women's life and leisure in an Australian rural community. *Leisure Studies, 9,* 35–44.

Dixey, R. (1987). It's a great feeling when you win: Women and bingo. *Leisure Studies, 6,* 199–214.

Eisner, E. (1981). On the differences between scientific and artistic approaches to qualitative research. *Educational Researcher, 10*(4), 5–9.

Ennis, C., and Chepyator-Thomson, J. (1990). Learning characteristics of field-dependent children within an analytical concept-based curriculum. *Journal of Teaching in Physical Education, 10,* 170–187.

Ennis, C., Ross, J., and Chen, A. (1992). The role of value orientations in curricular decision-making: A rationale for teacher's goals and expectations. *Research Quarterly for Exercise and Sport, 35*(4), 38–47.

Gaunt, S. (1987). Practical improvements in the Ross and Dill computer program for T-scores. *The GAHPERD Journal, 10*(3), 8–10.

Graham, C. (1991). The influence of teacher education on preservice development: Beyond a custodial orientation. *Quest, 43,* 1–19.

Green, K. N., East, W. B., and Hensley, L. D. (1987). A golf skills test battery for college males and females. *Research Quarterly for Exercise and Sport, 58,* 72–76.

Griffin, P. (1984). Girls participation pattern in a middle school team sport unit. *Journal of Teaching in Physical Education, 4,* 30–38.

Griffin, P. (1985). Boys participation styles in a middle school physical education sports unit. *Journal of Teaching in Physical Education, 4,* 100–110.

Henderson, K., and Bialeschki, M. (1987). A qualitative evaluation of a women's week experience. *Journal of Experiential Education, 10*(2), 25–28.

Howe, C. (1988). Using qualitative structured interviews in leisure research: Illustrations from one case study. *Journal of Leisure Research, 20*(4), 305–324.

Keller, K., Sliepcevich, E., Vitello, E., Lacey, E., and Wright, R. (1987). Assessing beliefs about and needs of senior citizens using the focus group interview: A qualitative approach. *Health Education, 18,* 44–49.

Krejcie, R. V., and Margan, D. W. (1970). Determining sample size for research activities. *Educational and Psychological Measurements, 30,* 607–610.

Lawson, H. (1983). Toward a model of socialization in physical education: The subjective warrant, recruitment, and teacher education (part 1). *Journal of Teaching in Physical Education, 2*(3), 3–16.

Lawson, H. (1986). Occupational socialization and the design of teacher education programs. *Journal of Teaching in Physical Education, 5*(2), 107–116.

Lincoln, Y., and Guba, E. (1990). Judging the quality of case study reports. *Qualitative Studies in Education, 3*(1), 53–59.

Locke, L. (1989). Qualitative research as a form of scientific inquiry in sport and physical education. *Research Quarterly for Exercise and Sport, 60*(1), 1–20.

Lumpkin, A. (1977). The growth of national women's tennis, 1904–1940. *Quest, 37,* 47–53.

Maatz-Majestic, E., and Tapp, M. (1992). College students' definitions of responsible alcohol use and perceived strategies for avoiding alcohol-related problems. *Research Quarterly for Exercise and Sport, 63*(1), A–40.

McClenaghan, B. A., and Williams, H. G. (1986). Design of an automated system to quantify dynamic stability. *Research Quarterly for Exercise and Sport, 57,* 78–81.

McLachlan, L. (1992). A model of constraints to family leisure: A study of families who have a child with Down's syndrome. *Research Quarterly for Exercise and Sport Supplement, 63*(1), A–50.

McLaughlin, J., Owen, S., Fors, S., and Levinson, R. (1992). The school child as health educator: Diffusion of hypertension information from sixth grade children to their parents. *Qualitative Studies in Education, 5*(2), 135–156.

McLaughlin, J., and Sliepcevich, F. (1985). The self-care behavior inventory: A model for behavioral instrument development. *Patient Education and Counseling, 7,* 289–301.

McLaughlin, J., and Zeeberg, I. (1993). Self-care and multiple sclerosis: A view from two cultures. *Social Science and Medicine, 37*(3), 315–329.

Mobley, T. A. (1980). Practitioner/researcher: A team. *Parks & Recreation, 15*(4), 40–43.

Morgan, D., and Laing, D. (1991). The diagnosis of Alzheimer's disease: Spouse's perspectives. *Qualitative Health Journal, 1*(3), 370–387.

Mull, S. S. (1991). The role of the health educator in development of self-esteem. *Journal of Health Education, 22*(6), 349–351.

Mullen, P. (1978). Cutting back after a heart attack: An overview. *Health Education Monographs, 6*(3), 295–311.

Reznik, J. W., and Stevenson, M. J. (1980). Elmer Dayton Mitchell: Father of intramurals. *NIRSA Journal, 4*(2), 14–16.

Rist, R. (1980). Blitzkrieg ethnography. *Educational Researcher, 9*(2), 8–10.

Robbins, M. P. (1966). A study of the validity of Delacato's theory of neurological organization. *Exceptional Children, 32* (April), 517–523.

Ross, D., and Dill, S. (1986). T-scores . . . calculate them the easy way. *Journal of Physical Education, Recreation, and Dance, 57*(5), 71–74.

Smith, M. (1987). Publishing qualitative research. *American Educational Research Journal, 24*(2), 178–183.

Steckler, A., Eng, E., and Goodman, R. (1991). Integrating qualitative and quantitative evaluation methods. *Hygie, 10,* 16–20.

Steckler, A., McLeroy, K., Goodman, R., McCormick, L., and Bird, S. (Eds.). (1992). Integrating qualitative and quantitative methods [Special edition]. *Health Education Quarterly, 19*(1).

Steckler, A., McLeroy, K., Goodman, R., Bird, S., and McCormick, L. (1992). Toward integrating qualitative and quantitative methods: An introduction. *Health Education Quarterly, 19*(1), 1–8.

Strong, C. (1981). Historical research: Does it apply to health education? *Health Education, 12*(4), 34–35.

Torabi, M. R. (1986). How to estimate practical significance in health education research. *Journal of School Health, 56*(6), 232–234.

Torabi, M. R. (1988). Factors affecting reliability coefficients of health attitude scales. *Journal of School Health, 58*(5), 186–189.

Torabi, M. R. (1990). The question of sample size. *Health Values, 14*(5), 53–56.

Torabi, M. R. (1991). Factors affecting response rate in mail survey questionnaires. *Health Values, 15*(5), 57–59.

Torabi, M. R. (1992). Significance of type II error and its calculation. *Health Values, 16*(5), 56–58.

Torabi, M. R. (1993). General standards for educational evaluations. *Health Values, 17*(4), 57–59.

Torabi, M. R., Bailey, W. J., and Massoumeh, M. J. (1993). Cigarette smoking as a predictor of alcohol and other drug use by children and adolescents: Evidence of the gateway drug effect. *Journal of School Health, 63*(7), 302–306.

Torabi, M. R., and Seffrin, J. R. (1986). A three component cancer attitude scale. *Journal of School Health, 56*(5), 170–174.

Torabi, M. R., and Seffrin, J. R. (1989). Evaluation of the effects of cancer education on knowledge, attitude, and behavior of university undergraduate students. *Journal of Cancer Education, 4*(1), 39–47.

Torabi, M. R., Seffrin, J. R., and Brashear, R. E. (1987). A statewide survey of hospital policy and practice concerning cigarette sales: A follow-up study. *Indiana Medicine, 80*(8), 756–758.

Torabi, M. R., and Yarber, W. (1992). Alternate forms of HIV prevention attitude scales for teenagers. *Aids Education and Prevention, 4*(2), 172–182.

Veenker, C. H. and Torabi, M. R. (1983). Multivariate analysis of dimensionality in health attitude structure. *Health Education.*

Wettan, R. G., and Willis, J. D. (1977). William Buckingham Curtis: The founding father of American amateur athletics, 1837–1900. *Quest, 37,* 28–37.

Wiggins, D. K. (1991). Prized performers, but frequently overlooked students: The involvement of black athletes in intercollegiate sports in predominantly white university campuses, 1890–1972. *Research Quarterly for Exercise and Sport, 62*(2), 164 -177.

Williamson, K. (1990). The ivory tower: Myth or reality? *Journal of Teaching in Physical Education, 9,* 95–105.

Wilson, S. (1977). The use of ethnographic techniques in educational research. *Review of Educational Research, 47,* 245–265.

Wolcott, H. (1980). How to look like an anthropologist without really being one. *Practicing Anthropology, 3*(2), 6–7, 56–59.

Presentations

Lincoln, Y. (1991, January). *Ethics and the new paradigm.* Presented at the Qualitative Methods in Education Conference, Athens, GA.

McLaughlin, J., and Owen, S. (1986, September). *Utilization of focus groups in school health evaluation: A case study.* Paper presented at American School Health Association Meeting, Denver, CO.

Reports

The University of Georgia. (1995). *Guidelines for appointment, promotion, and tenure.* Athens, GA: Author.

Indiana University Libraries. (1992). *ERIC, Sport Discus, Medline and PsycLIT on CD-ROM.* Bloomington, IN: Author.

Unpublished Manuscripts

Miller, D. E. (1990). *Challenge education programs related to the development of selected personality characteristics in psychologically troubled adolescents.* Unpublished research proposal, Indiana University, Bloomington.

Padilla, S. (1986). *Five options related to the improvement of smoking-damaged air quality in the military workplace.* Unpublished research proposal, Indiana University, Bloomington.

Pate, D. J. (1987). *Sea kayak touring and self-concept of persons with low level spinal cord injury.* Unpublished research proposal, Indiana University, Bloomington.

Seaman, J. (1970). *Example of an application of the research process: An abstract.* Unpublished manuscript, Indiana University, Bloomington.

Sun, D. C. (1988). *Fat loss in moderately obese women using two walking protocols.* Unpublished research proposal, Indiana University, Bloomington.

Welcher, C. L. (1991). *Shift rotation related to night nurse performance and frequency of medication errors in a hospital setting.* Unpublished research proposal, Indiana University, Bloomington.

Appendix A

Critical Values of t						

	LEVEL OF SIGNIFICANCE FOR ONE-TAILED TEST					
	.10	.05	.025	.01	.005	.0005
	LEVEL OF SIGNIFICANCE FOR TWO-TAILED TEST					
df	.20	.10	.05	.02	.01	.001
1	3.078	6.314	12.706	31.821	63.657	636.619
2	1.886	2.920	4.303	6.965	9.925	31.598
3	1.638	2.353	3.182	4.541	5.841	12.941
4	1.533	2.132	2.776	3.747	4.604	8.610
5	1.476	2.015	2.571	3.365	4.032	6.859
6	1.440	1.943	2.447	3.143	3.707	5.959
7	1.415	1.895	2.365	2.998	3.499	5.405
8	1.397	1.860	2.306	2.896	3.355	5.041
9	1.383	1.833	2.262	2.821	3.250	4.781
10	1.372	1.812	2.228	2.764	3.169	4.587
11	1.363	1.796	2.201	2.718	3.106	4.437
12	1.356	1.782	2.179	2.681	3.055	4.318
13	1.350	1.771	2.160	2.650	3.012	4.221
14	1.345	1.761	2.145	2.624	2.977	4.140
15	1.341	1.753	2.131	2.602	2.947	4.073
16	1.337	1.746	2.120	2.583	2.921	4.015
17	1.333	1.740	2.110	2.567	2.898	3.965
18	1.330	1.734	2.101	2.552	2.878	3.922
19	1.328	1.729	2.093	2.539	2.861	3.883
20	1.325	1.725	2.086	2.528	2.845	3.850
21	1.323	1.721	2.080	2.518	2.831	3.819
22	1.321	1.717	2.074	2.508	2.819	3.792
23	1.319	1.714	2.069	2.500	2.807	3.767
24	1.318	1.711	2.064	2.492	2.797	3.745
25	1.316	1.708	2.060	2.485	2.787	3.725

Critical Values of *t*—Concluded

	LEVEL OF SIGNIFICANCE FOR ONE-TAILED TEST					
	.10	.05	.025	.01	.005	.0005
	LEVEL OF SIGNIFICANCE FOR TWO-TAILED TEST					
DF	.20	.10	.05	.02	.01	.001
26	1.315	1.706	2.056	2.479	2.779	3.707
27	1.314	1.703	2.052	2.473	2.771	3.690
28	1.313	1.701	2.048	2.467	2.763	3.674
29	1.311	1.699	2.045	2.462	2.756	3.659
30	1.310	1.697	2.042	2.457	2.750	3.646
40	1.303	1.684	2.021	2.423	2.704	3.551
60	1.296	1.671	2.000	2.390	2.660	3.460
120	1.289	1.658	1.980	2.358	2.617	3.373
∞	1.282	1.645	1.960	2.326	2.576	3.291

Appendix A is taken from Table III of Fisher & Yates; STATISTICAL TABLES FOR BIOLOGICAL, AGRICULTURAL AND MEDICAL RESEARCH Published by Longman Group UK Ltd., 1974. Reprinted by permission of Addison Wesley Longman Ltd.

Appendix B

Critical Values of F
.05 level (light type) and .01 level (bold type) points for the distribution of F

DEGREES OF FREEDOM FOR DENOMINATOR

DEGREES OF FREEDOM FOR NUMERATOR

	1	2	3	4	5	6	7	8	9	10	11	12
1	161	200	216	225	230	234	237	239	241	242	243	244
	4052	**4999**	**5403**	**5625**	**5764**	**5859**	**5928**	**5981**	**6022**	**6056**	**6082**	**6106**
2	18.51	19.00	19.16	19.25	19.30	19.33	19.36	19.37	19.38	19.39	19.40	19.41
	98.49	**99.01**	**99.17**	**99.25**	**99.30**	**99.33**	**99.34**	**99.36**	**99.38**	**99.40**	**99.41**	**99.42**
3	10.13	9.55	9.28	9.12	9.01	8.94	8.88	8.84	8.81	8.78	8.76	8.74
	34.12	**30.81**	**29.46**	**28.71**	**28.24**	**27.91**	**27.67**	**27.49**	**27.34**	**27.23**	**27.13**	**27.05**
4	7.71	6.94	6.59	6.39	6.26	6.16	6.09	6.04	6.00	5.96	5.93	5.91
	21.20	**18.00**	**16.69**	**15.98**	**15.52**	**15.21**	**14.98**	**14.80**	**14.66**	**14.54**	**14.45**	**14.37**
5	6.61	5.79	5.41	5.19	5.05	4.95	4.88	4.82	4.78	4.74	4.70	4.68
	16.26	**13.27**	**12.06**	**11.39**	**10.97**	**10.67**	**10.45**	**10.27**	**10.15**	**10.05**	**9.96**	**9.89**
6	5.99	5.14	4.76	4.53	4.39	4.28	4.21	4.15	4.10	4.06	4.03	4.00
	13.74	**10.92**	**9.78**	**9.15**	**8.75**	**8.47**	**8.26**	**8.10**	**7.98**	**7.87**	**7.79**	**7.72**
7	5.59	4.74	4.35	4.12	3.97	3.87	3.79	3.73	3.68	3.63	3.60	3.57
	12.25	**9.55**	**8.45**	**7.85**	**7.46**	**7.19**	**7.00**	**6.84**	**6.71**	**6.62**	**6.54**	**6.47**
8	5.32	4.46	4.07	3.84	3.69	3.58	3.50	3.44	3.39	3.34	3.31	3.28
	11.26	**8.65**	**7.59**	**7.01**	**6.63**	**6.37**	**6.19**	**6.03**	**5.91**	**5.82**	**5.74**	**5.67**
9	5.12	4.26	3.86	3.63	3.48	3.37	3.29	3.23	3.18	3.13	3.10	3.07
	10.56	**8.02**	**6.99**	**6.42**	**6.06**	**5.80**	**5.62**	**5.47**	**5.35**	**5.26**	**5.18**	**5.11**
10	4.96	4.10	3.71	3.48	3.33	3.22	3.14	3.07	3.02	2.97	2.94	2.91
	10.04	**7.56**	**6.55**	**5.99**	**5.64**	**5.39**	**5.21**	**5.06**	**4.95**	**4.85**	**4.78**	**4.71**
11	4.84	3.98	3.59	3.36	3.20	3.09	3.01	2.95	2.90	2.86	2.82	2.79
	9.65	**7.20**	**6.22**	**5.67**	**5.32**	**5.07**	**4.88**	**4.74**	**4.63**	**4.54**	**4.46**	**4.40**
12	4.75	3.88	3.49	3.26	3.11	3.00	2.92	2.85	2.80	2.76	2.72	2.69
	9.33	**6.93**	**5.95**	**5.41**	**5.06**	**4.82**	**4.65**	**4.50**	**4.39**	**4.30**	**4.22**	**4.16**
13	4.67	3.80	3.41	3.18	3.02	2.92	2.84	2.77	2.72	2.67	2.63	2.60
	9.07	**6.70**	**5.74**	**5.20**	**4.86**	**4.62**	**4.44**	**4.30**	**4.19**	**4.10**	**4.02**	**3.96**
14	4.60	3.74	3.34	3.11	2.96	2.85	2.77	2.70	2.65	2.60	2.56	2.53
	8.86	**6.51**	**5.56**	**5.03**	**4.69**	**4.46**	**4.28**	**4.14**	**4.03**	**3.94**	**3.86**	**3.80**

From G. W. Snedecor and W. G. Cochran, *Statistical Methods,* 7th edition, Table of Critical Values of *F,* 1980. Copyright © 1980 Iowa State University Press, Ames, Iowa. Reprinted by permission.

14	16	20	24	30	40	50	75	100	200	500	∞
245	246	248	249	250	251	252	253	253	254	254	254
6142	**6169**	**6208**	**6234**	**6258**	**6286**	**6302**	**6323**	**6334**	**6352**	**6361**	**6366**
19.42	19.43	19.44	19.45	19.46	19.47	19.47	19.48	19.49	19.49	19.50	19.50
99.43	**99.44**	**99.45**	**99.46**	**99.47**	**99.48**	**99.48**	**99.49**	**99.49**	**99.49**	**99.50**	**99.50**
8.71	8.69	8.66	8.64	8.62	8.60	8.58	8.57	8.56	8.54	8.54	8.53
26.92	**26.83**	**26.69**	**26.60**	**26.50**	**26.41**	**26.35**	**26.27**	**26.23**	**26.18**	**26.14**	**26.12**
5.87	5.84	5.80	5.77	5.74	5.71	5.70	5.68	5.66	5.65	5.64	5.63
14.24	**14.15**	**14.02**	**13.93**	**13.83**	**13.74**	**13.69**	**13.61**	**13.57**	**13.52**	**13.48**	**13.46**
4.64	4.60	4.56	4.53	4.50	4.46	4.44	4.42	4.40	4.38	4.37	4.36
9.77	**9.68**	**9.55**	**9.47**	**9.38**	**9.29**	**9.24**	**9.17**	**9.13**	**9.07**	**9.04**	**9.02**
3.96	3.92	3.87	3.84	3.81	3.77	3.75	3.72	3.71	3.69	3.68	3.67
7.60	**7.52**	**7.39**	**7.31**	**7.23**	**7.14**	**7.09**	**7.02**	**6.99**	**6.94**	**6.90**	**6.88**
3.52	3.49	3.44	3.41	3.38	3.34	3.32	3.29	3.28	3.25	3.24	3.23
6.35	**6.27**	**6.15**	**6.07**	**5.98**	**5.90**	**5.85**	**5.78**	**5.75**	**5.70**	**5.67**	**5.65**
3.23	3.20	3.15	3.12	3.08	3.05	3.03	3.00	2.98	2.96	2.94	2.93
5.56	**5.48**	**5.36**	**5.28**	**5.20**	**5.11**	**5.06**	**5.00**	**4.96**	**4.91**	**4.88**	**4.88**
3.02	2.98	2.93	2.90	2.86	2.82	2.80	2.77	2.76	2.73	2.72	2.71
5.00	**4.92**	**4.80**	**4.73**	**4.64**	**4.56**	**4.51**	**4.45**	**4.41**	**4.36**	**4.33**	**4.31**
2.86	2.82	2.77	2.74	2.70	2.67	2.64	2.61	2.59	2.56	2.55	2.54
4.60	**4.52**	**4.41**	**4.33**	**4.25**	**4.17**	**4.12**	**4.05**	**4.01**	**3.96**	**3.93**	**3.91**
2.74	2.70	2.65	2.61	2.57	2.53	2.50	2.47	2.45	2.42	2.41	2.40
4.29	**4.21**	**4.10**	**4.02**	**3.94**	**3.86**	**3.80**	**3.74**	**3.70**	**3.66**	**3.62**	**3.60**
2.64	2.60	2.54	2.50	2.46	2.42	2.40	2.36	2.35	2.32	2.31	2.30
4.05	**3.98**	**3.86**	**3.78**	**3.70**	**3.61**	**3.56**	**3.49**	**3.46**	**3.41**	**3.38**	**3.36**
2.55	2.51	2.46	2.42	2.38	2.34	2.32	2.28	2.26	2.24	2.22	2.21
3.85	**3.78**	**3.67**	**3.59**	**3.51**	**3.42**	**3.37**	**3.30**	**3.27**	**3.21**	**3.18**	**3.16**
2.48	2.44	2.39	2.35	2.31	2.27	2.24	2.21	2.19	2.16	2.14	2.13
3.70	**3.62**	**3.51**	**3.43**	**3.34**	**3.26**	**3.21**	**3.14**	**3.11**	**3.06**	**3.02**	**3.00**

Critical Values of F—Continued

DEGREES OF FREEDOM FOR DENOMINATOR	DEGREES OF FREEDOM FOR NUMERATOR											
	1	2	3	4	5	6	7	8	9	10	11	12
15	4.54	3.68	3.29	3.06	2.90	2.79	2.70	2.64	2.59	2.55	2.51	2.48
	8.68	**6.36**	**5.42**	**4.89**	**4.56**	**4.32**	**4.14**	**4.00**	**3.89**	**3.80**	**3.73**	**3.67**
16	4.49	3.63	3.24	3.01	2.85	2.74	2.66	2.59	2.54	2.49	2.45	2.42
	8.53	**6.23**	**5.29**	**4.77**	**4.44**	**4.20**	**4.03**	**3.89**	**3.78**	**3.69**	**3.61**	**3.55**
17	4.45	3.59	3.20	2.96	2.81	2.70	2.62	2.55	2.50	2.45	2.41	2.38
	8.40	**6.11**	**5.18**	**4.67**	**4.34**	**4.10**	**3.93**	**3.79**	**3.68**	**3.59**	**3.52**	**3.45**
18	4.41	3.55	3.16	2.93	2.77	2.66	2.58	2.51	2.46	2.41	2.37	2.34
	8.28	**6.01**	**5.09**	**4.58**	**4.25**	**4.01**	**3.88**	**3.71**	**3.60**	**3.51**	**3.44**	**3.37**
19	4.38	3.52	3.13	2.90	2.74	2.63	2.55	2.48	2.43	2.38	2.34	2.31
	8.18	**5.93**	**5.01**	**4.50**	**4.17**	**3.94**	**3.77**	**3.63**	**3.52**	**3.43**	**3.36**	**3.30**
20	4.35	3.49	3.10	2.87	2.71	2.60	2.52	2.45	2.40	2.35	2.31	2.28
	8.10	**5.85**	**4.94**	**4.43**	**4.10**	**3.87**	**3.71**	**3.56**	**3.45**	**3.37**	**3.30**	**3.23**
21	4.32	3.47	3.07	2.84	2.68	2.57	2.49	2.42	2.37	2.32	2.28	2.25
	8.02	**5.78**	**4.87**	**4.37**	**4.04**	**3.81**	**3.65**	**3.51**	**3.40**	**3.31**	**3.24**	**3.17**
22	4.30	3.44	3.05	2.82	2.66	2.55	2.47	2.40	2.35	2.30	2.26	2.23
	7.94	**5.72**	**4.82**	**4.31**	**3.99**	**3.76**	**3.59**	**3.45**	**3.35**	**3.26**	**3.18**	**3.12**
23	4.28	3.42	3.03	2.80	2.64	2.53	2.45	2.38	2.32	2.28	2.24	2.20
	7.88	**5.66**	**4.76**	**4.26**	**3.94**	**3.71**	**3.54**	**3.41**	**3.30**	**3.21**	**3.14**	**3.07**
24	4.26	3.40	3.01	2.78	2.62	2.51	2.43	2.36	2.30	2.26	2.22	2.18
	7.82	**5.61**	**4.72**	**4.22**	**3.90**	**3.67**	**3.50**	**3.36**	**3.25**	**3.17**	**3.09**	**3.03**
25	4.24	3.38	2.99	2.76	2.60	2.49	2.41	2.34	2.28	2.24	2.20	2.16
	7.77	**5.57**	**4.68**	**4.18**	**3.86**	**3.63**	**3.46**	**3.32**	**3.21**	**3.13**	**3.05**	**2.99**
26	4.22	3.37	2.98	2.74	2.59	2.47	2.39	2.32	2.27	2.22	2.18	2.15
	7.72	**5.53**	**4.64**	**4.14**	**3.82**	**3.59**	**3.42**	**3.29**	**3.17**	**3.09**	**3.02**	**2.96**
27	4.21	3.35	2.96	2.73	2.57	2.46	2.37	2.30	2.25	2.20	2.16	2.13
	7.68	**5.49**	**4.60**	**4.11**	**3.79**	**3.56**	**3.39**	**3.26**	**3.14**	**3.06**	**2.98**	**2.93**
28	4.20	3.34	2.95	2.71	2.56	2.44	2.36	2.29	2.24	2.19	2.15	2.12
	7.64	**5.45**	**4.57**	**4.07**	**3.76**	**3.53**	**3.36**	**3.23**	**3.11**	**3.03**	**2.95**	**2.90**
29	4.18	3.33	2.93	2.70	2.54	2.43	2.35	2.28	2.22	2.18	2.14	2.10
	7.60	**5.42**	**4.54**	**4.04**	**3.73**	**3.50**	**3.33**	**3.20**	**3.08**	**3.00**	**2.92**	**2.87**
30	4.17	3.32	2.92	2.69	2.53	2.42	2.34	2.27	2.21	2.16	2.12	2.09
	7.56	**5.39**	**4.51**	**4.02**	**3.70**	**3.47**	**3.30**	**3.17**	**3.06**	**2.98**	**2.90**	**2.84**
32	4.15	3.30	2.90	2.67	2.51	2.40	2.32	2.25	2.19	2.14	2.10	2.07
	7.50	**5.34**	**4.46**	**3.97**	**3.66**	**3.42**	**3.25**	**3.12**	**3.01**	**2.94**	**2.86**	**2.80**
34	4.13	3.28	2.88	2.65	2.49	2.38	2.30	2.23	2.17	2.12	2.08	2.05
	7.44	**5.29**	**4.42**	**3.93**	**3.61**	**3.38**	**3.21**	**3.08**	**2.97**	**2.89**	**2.82**	**2.76**
36	4.11	3.26	2.86	2.63	2.48	2.36	2.28	2.21	2.15	2.10	2.06	2.03
	7.39	**5.25**	**4.38**	**3.89**	**3.58**	**3.35**	**3.18**	**3.04**	**2.94**	**2.86**	**2.78**	**2.72**

14	16	20	24	30	40	50	75	100	200	500	∞
2.43	2.39	2.33	2.29	2.25	2.21	2.18	2.15	2.12	2.10	2.08	2.07
3.56	**3.48**	**3.36**	**3.29**	**3.20**	**3.12**	**3.07**	**3.00**	**2.97**	**2.92**	**2.89**	**2.87**
2.37	2.33	2.28	2.24	2.20	2.16	2.13	2.09	2.07	2.04	2.02	2.01
3.45	**3.37**	**3.25**	**3.18**	**3.10**	**3.01**	**2.96**	**2.89**	**2.86**	**2.80**	**2.77**	**3.75**
2.33	2.29	2.23	2.19	2.15	2.11	2.08	2.04	2.02	1.99	1.97	1.96
3.35	**3.27**	**3.16**	**3.08**	**3.00**	**2.92**	**2.86**	**2.79**	**2.76**	**2.70**	**2.67**	**2.65**
2.29	2.25	2.19	2.15	2.11	2.07	2.04	2.00	1.98	1.95	1.93	1.92
3.27	**3.19**	**3.07**	**3.00**	**2.91**	**2.83**	**2.78**	**2.71**	**2.68**	**2.62**	**2.59**	**2.57**
2.26	2.21	2.15	2.11	2.07	2.02	2.00	1.96	1.94	1.91	1.90	1.88
3.19	**3.12**	**3.00**	**2.92**	**2.84**	**2.76**	**2.70**	**2.63**	**2.60**	**2.54**	**2.51**	**2.49**
2.23	2.18	2.12	2.08	2.04	1.99	1.96	1.92	1.90	1.87	1.85	1.84
3.13	**3.05**	**2.94**	**2.86**	**2.77**	**2.69**	**2.63**	**2.56**	**2.53**	**2.47**	**2.44**	**2.42**
2.20	2.15	2.09	2.05	2.00	1.96	1.93	1.89	1.87	1.84	1.82	1.81
3.07	**2.99**	**2.88**	**2.80**	**2.72**	**2.63**	**2.58**	**2.51**	**2.47**	**2.42**	**2.38**	**2.36**
2.18	2.13	2.07	2.03	1.98	1.93	1.91	1.87	1.84	1.81	1.80	1.78
3.02	**2.94**	**2.83**	**2.75**	**2.67**	**2.58**	**2.53**	**2.46**	**2.42**	**2.37**	**2.33**	**2.31**
2.14	2.10	2.04	2.00	1.96	1.91	1.88	1.84	1.82	1.79	1.77	1.76
2.97	**2.89**	**2.78**	**2.70**	**2.62**	**2.53**	**2.48**	**2.41**	**2.37**	**2.32**	**2.28**	**2.26**
2.13	2.09	2.02	1.98	1.94	1.89	1.86	1.82	1.80	1.76	1.74	1.73
2.93	**2.85**	**2.74**	**2.66**	**2.58**	**2.49**	**2.44**	**2.36**	**2.33**	**2.27**	**2.23**	**2.21**
2.11	2.06	2.00	1.96	1.92	1.87	1.84	1.80	1.77	1.74	1.72	1.71
2.89	**2.81**	**2.70**	**2.62**	**2.54**	**2.45**	**2.40**	**2.32**	**2.29**	**2.23**	**2.19**	**2.17**
2.10	2.05	1.99	1.95	1.90	1.85	1.82	1.78	1.76	1.72	1.70	1.69
2.86	**2.77**	**2.66**	**2.58**	**2.50**	**2.41**	**2.36**	**2.28**	**2.25**	**2.19**	**2.15**	**2.13**
2.08	2.03	1.97	1.93	1.88	1.84	1.80	1.76	1.74	1.71	1.68	1.67
2.83	**2.74**	**2.63**	**2.55**	**2.47**	**2.38**	**2.33**	**2.25**	**2.21**	**2.16**	**2.12**	**2.10**
2.06	2.02	1.96	1.91	1.87	1.81	1.78	1.75	1.72	1.69	1.67	1.65
2.80	**2.71**	**2.60**	**2.52**	**2.44**	**2.35**	**2.30**	**2.22**	**2.18**	**2.13**	**2.09**	**2.06**
2.05	2.00	1.94	1.90	1.85	1.80	1.77	1.73	1.71	1.68	1.65	1.64
2.77	**2.68**	**2.57**	**2.49**	**2.41**	**2.32**	**2.27**	**2.19**	**2.15**	**2.10**	**2.06**	**2.03**
2.04	1.99	1.93	1.89	1.84	1.79	1.76	1.72	1.69	1.66	1.64	1.62
2.74	**2.66**	**2.55**	**2.47**	**2.38**	**2.29**	**2.24**	**2.16**	**2.13**	**2.07**	**2.03**	**2.01**
2.02	1.97	1.91	1.86	1.82	1.76	1.74	1.69	1.67	1.64	1.61	1.59
2.70	**2.62**	**2.51**	**2.42**	**2.34**	**2.25**	**2.20**	**2.12**	**2.08**	**2.02**	**1.98**	**1.96**
2.00	1.95	1.89	1.84	1.80	1.74	1.71	1.67	1.64	1.61	1.59	1.57
2.66	**2.58**	**2.47**	**2.38**	**2.30**	**2.21**	**2.15**	**2.03**	**2.04**	**1.98**	**1.94**	**1.91**
1.98	1.93	1.87	1.82	1.78	1.72	1.69	1.65	1.62	1.59	1.56	1.55
2.62	**2.54**	**2.43**	**2.35**	**2.26**	**2.17**	**2.12**	**2.04**	**2.00**	**1.94**	**1.90**	**1.87**

Critical Values of F—Concluded

DEGREES OF FREEDOM FOR DENOMINATOR	DEGREES OF FREEDOM FOR NUMERATOR											
	1	2	3	4	5	6	7	8	9	10	11	12
38	4.10	3.25	2.85	2.62	2.46	2.35	2.26	2.19	2.14	2.09	2.05	2.02
	7.35	**5.21**	**4.34**	**3.86**	**3.54**	**3.32**	**3.15**	**3.02**	**2.91**	**2.82**	**2.75**	**2.69**
40	4.08	3.23	2.84	2.61	2.45	2.34	2.25	2.18	2.12	2.07	2.04	2.00
	7.31	**5.18**	**4.31**	**3.83**	**3.51**	**3.29**	**3.12**	**2.99**	**2.88**	**2.80**	**2.73**	**2.66**
42	4.07	3.22	2.83	2.59	2.44	2.32	2.24	2.17	2.11	2.06	2.02	1.99
	7.27	**5.15**	**4.29**	**3.80**	**3.49**	**3.26**	**3.10**	**2.96**	**2.86**	**2.77**	**2.70**	**2.64**
44	4.06	3.21	2.82	2.58	2.43	2.31	2.23	2.16	2.10	2.05	2.01	1.98
	7.24	**5.12**	**4.26**	**3.78**	**3.46**	**3.24**	**3.07**	**2.94**	**2.84**	**2.75**	**2.68**	**2.62**
46	4.05	3.20	2.81	2.57	2.42	2.30	2.22	2.14	2.09	2.04	2.00	1.97
	7.21	**5.10**	**4.24**	**3.76**	**3.44**	**3.22**	**3.05**	**2.92**	**2.82**	**2.73**	**2.66**	**2.60**
48	4.04	3.19	2.80	2.56	2.41	2.30	2.21	2.14	2.08	2.03	1.99	1.96
	7.19	**5.08**	**4.22**	**3.74**	**3.42**	**3.20**	**3.04**	**2.90**	**2.80**	**2.71**	**2.64**	**2.58**
50	4.03	3.18	2.79	2.56	2.40	2.29	2.20	2.13	2.07	2.02	1.98	1.95
	7.17	**5.06**	**4.20**	**3.72**	**3.41**	**3.18**	**3.02**	**2.88**	**2.78**	**2.70**	**2.62**	**2.56**
55	4.02	3.17	2.78	2.54	2.38	2.27	2.18	2.11	2.05	2.00	1.97	1.93
	7.12	**5.01**	**4.16**	**3.68**	**3.37**	**3.15**	**2.98**	**2.85**	**2.75**	**2.66**	**2.59**	**2.53**
60	4.00	3.15	2.76	2.52	2.37	2.25	2.17	2.10	2.04	1.99	1.95	1.92
	7.08	**4.98**	**4.13**	**3.65**	**3.34**	**3.12**	**2.95**	**2.82**	**2.72**	**2.63**	**2.56**	**2.50**
65	3.99	3.14	2.75	2.51	2.36	2.24	2.15	2.08	2.02	1.98	1.94	1.90
	7.04	**4.95**	**4.10**	**3.62**	**3.31**	**3.09**	**2.93**	**2.79**	**2.70**	**2.61**	**2.54**	**2.47**
70	3.98	3.13	2.74	2.50	2.35	2.23	2.14	2.07	2.01	1.97	1.93	1.89
	7.01	**4.92**	**4.08**	**3.60**	**3.29**	**3.07**	**2.91**	**2.77**	**2.67**	**2.59**	**2.51**	**2.45**
80	3.96	3.11	2.72	2.48	2.33	2.21	2.12	2.05	1.99	1.95	1.91	1.88
	6.96	**4.88**	**4.04**	**3.56**	**3.25**	**3.04**	**2.87**	**2.74**	**2.64**	**2.55**	**2.46**	**2.41**
100	3.94	3.09	2.70	2.46	2.30	2.19	2.10	2.03	1.97	1.92	1.88	1.85
	6.90	**4.82**	**3.98**	**3.51**	**3.20**	**2.99**	**2.82**	**2.69**	**2.59**	**2.51**	**2.43**	**2.36**
125	3.92	3.07	2.68	2.44	2.29	2.17	2.08	2.01	1.95	1.90	1.86	1.83
	6.84	**4.78**	**3.94**	**3.47**	**3.17**	**2.95**	**2.79**	**2.65**	**2.56**	**2.47**	**2.40**	**2.33**
150	3.91	3.06	2.67	2.43	2.27	2.16	2.07	2.00	1.94	1.89	1.85	1.82
	6.81	**4.75**	**3.91**	**3.44**	**3.14**	**2.92**	**2.76**	**2.62**	**2.53**	**2.44**	**2.37**	**2.30**
200	3.89	3.04	2.65	2.41	2.26	2.14	2.05	1.98	1.92	1.87	1.83	1.80
	6.76	**4.71**	**3.88**	**3.41**	**3.11**	**2.90**	**2.73**	**2.60**	**2.50**	**2.41**	**2.34**	**2.28**
400	3.86	3.02	2.62	2.39	2.23	2.12	2.03	1.96	1.90	1.85	1.81	1.78
	6.70	**4.66**	**3.83**	**3.36**	**3.06**	**2.85**	**2.69**	**2.55**	**2.46**	**2.37**	**2.29**	**2.23**
1000	3.85	3.00	2.61	2.38	2.22	2.10	2.02	1.95	1.89	1.84	1.80	1.76
	6.66	**4.62**	**3.80**	**3.34**	**3.04**	**2.82**	**2.66**	**2.53**	**2.43**	**2.34**	**2.26**	**2.20**
∞	3.84	2.99	2.60	2.37	2.21	2.09	2.01	1.94	1.88	1.83	1.79	1.75
	6.64	**4.60**	**3.78**	**3.32**	**3.02**	**2.80**	**2.64**	**2.51**	**2.41**	**2.32**	**2.24**	**2.18**

14	16	20	24	30	40	50	75	100	200	500	∞
1.96	1.92	1.85	1.80	1.76	1.71	1.67	1.63	1.60	1.57	1.54	1.53
2.59	**2.51**	**2.40**	**2.32**	**2.22**	**2.14**	**2.08**	**2.00**	**1.97**	**1.90**	**1.86**	**1.84**
1.95	1.90	1.84	1.79	1.74	1.69	1.66	1.61	1.59	1.55	1.53	1.51
2.56	**2.49**	**2.37**	**2.29**	**2.20**	**2.11**	**2.05**	**1.97**	**1.94**	**1.88**	**1.84**	**1.81**
1.94	1.89	1.82	1.78	1.73	1.68	1.64	1.60	1.57	1.54	1.51	1.49
2.54	**2.46**	**2.35**	**2.26**	**2.17**	**2.08**	**2.02**	**1.94**	**1.91**	**1.85**	**1.80**	**1.78**
1.92	1.88	1.81	1.76	1.72	1.66	1.63	1.58	1.56	1.52	1.50	1.48
2.52	**2.44**	**2.32**	**2.24**	**2.15**	**2.06**	**2.00**	**1.92**	**1.88**	**1.82**	**1.78**	**1.75**
1.91	1.87	1.80	1.75	1.71	1.65	1.62	1.57	1.54	1.51	1.48	1.46
2.50	**2.42**	**2.30**	**2.22**	**2.13**	**2.04**	**1.98**	**1.90**	**1.86**	**1.80**	**1.76**	**1.72**
1.90	1.86	1.79	1.74	1.70	1.64	1.61	1.56	1.53	1.50	1.47	1.45
2.48	**2.40**	**2.28**	**2.20**	**2.11**	**2.02**	**1.96**	**1.88**	**1.84**	**1.78**	**1.73**	**1.70**
1.90	1.85	1.78	1.74	1.69	1.63	1.60	1.55	1.52	1.48	1.46	1.44
2.46	**2.39**	**2.26**	**2.18**	**2.10**	**2.00**	**1.94**	**1.86**	**1.82**	**1.76**	**1.71**	**1.68**
1.88	1.83	1.76	1.72	1.67	1.61	1.58	1.52	1.50	1.46	1.43	1.41
2.43	**2.35**	**2.23**	**2.15**	**2.06**	**1.96**	**1.90**	**1.82**	**1.78**	**1.71**	**1.66**	**1.64**
1.86	1.81	1.75	1.70	1.65	1.59	1.56	1.50	1.48	1.44	1.41	1.39
2.40	**2.32**	**2.20**	**2.12**	**2.03**	**1.93**	**1.87**	**1.79**	**1.74**	**1.68**	**1.63**	**1.60**
1.85	1.80	1.73	1.68	1.63	1.57	1.54	1.49	1.46	1.42	1.39	1.37
2.37	**2.30**	**2.18**	**2.09**	**2.00**	**1.90**	**1.84**	**1.76**	**1.71**	**1.64**	**1.60**	**1.56**
1.84	1.79	1.72	1.67	1.62	1.56	1.53	1.47	1.45	1.40	1.37	1.35
2.35	**2.28**	**2.15**	**2.07**	**1.98**	**1.88**	**1.82**	**1.74**	**1.69**	**1.62**	**1.56**	**1.53**
1.82	1.77	1.70	1.65	1.60	1.54	1.51	1.45	1.42	1.38	1.35	1.32
2.32	**2.24**	**2.11**	**2.03**	**1.94**	**1.84**	**1.78**	**1.70**	**1.65**	**1.57**	**1.52**	**1.49**
1.79	1.75	1.68	1.63	1.57	1.51	1.48	1.42	1.39	1.34	1.30	1.28
2.26	**2.19**	**2.06**	**1.98**	**1.89**	**1.79**	**1.73**	**1.64**	**1.59**	**1.51**	**1.46**	**1.43**
1.77	1.72	1.65	1.60	1.55	1.49	1.45	1.39	1.36	1.31	1.27	1.25
2.23	**2.15**	**2.03**	**1.94**	**1.85**	**1.75**	**1.68**	**1.59**	**1.54**	**1.46**	**1.40**	**1.37**
1.76	1.71	1.64	1.59	1.54	1.47	1.44	1.37	1.34	1.29	1.25	1.22
2.20	**2.12**	**2.00**	**1.91**	**1.83**	**1.72**	**1.66**	**1.56**	**1.51**	**1.43**	**1.37**	**1.33**
1.74	1.69	1.62	1.57	1.52	1.45	1.42	1.35	1.32	1.26	1.22	1.19
2.17	**2.09**	**1.97**	**1.88**	**1.79**	**1.69**	**1.62**	**1.53**	**1.48**	**1.39**	**1.33**	**1.28**
1.72	1.67	1.60	1.54	1.49	1.42	1.38	1.32	1.28	1.22	1.16	1.13
2.12	**2.04**	**1.92**	**1.84**	**1.74**	**1.64**	**1.57**	**1.47**	**1.42**	**1.32**	**1.24**	**1.19**
1.70	1.65	1.58	1.53	1.47	1.41	1.36	1.30	1.26	1.19	1.13	1.08
2.09	**2.01**	**1.89**	**1.81**	**1.71**	**1.61**	**1.54**	**1.44**	**1.38**	**1.28**	**1.19**	**1.11**
1.69	1.64	1.57	1.52	1.46	1.40	1.35	1.28	1.24	1.17	1.11	1.00
2.07	**1.99**	**1.87**	**1.79**	**1.69**	**1.59**	**1.52**	**1.41**	**1.36**	**1.25**	**1.15**	**1.00**

Appendix C

Appendix C is taken from Table IV of Fisher & Yates; STATISTICAL TABLES FOR BIOLOGICAL, AGRICULTURAL AND MEDICAL RESEARCH Published by Longman Group UK Ltd., 1974. Reprinted by permission of Addison Wesley Longman Ltd.

Critical Values of CHI-SQUARE

PROBABILITY UNDER H_0 THAT $X^2 \geq$ CHI-SQUARE

df	.99	.98	.95	.90	.80	.70	.50	.30	.20	.10	.05	.02	.01	.001
1	.00016	.00063	.0039	.016	.064	.15	.46	1.07	1.64	2.71	3.84	5.41	6.64	10.83
2	.02	.04	.10	.21	.45	.71	1.39	2.41	3.22	4.60	5.99	7.82	9.21	13.82
3	.12	.18	.35	.58	1.00	1.42	2.37	3.66	4.64	6.25	7.82	9.84	11.34	16.27
4	.30	.43	.71	1.06	1.65	2.20	3.36	4.88	5.99	7.78	9.49	11.67	13.28	18.46
5	.55	.75	1.14	1.61	2.34	3.00	4.35	6.06	7.29	9.24	11.07	13.39	15.09	20.52
6	.87	1.18	1.64	2.20	3.07	3.83	5.35	7.23	8.56	10.64	12.59	15.03	16.81	22.46
7	1.24	1.56	2.17	2.83	3.82	4.67	6.35	8.38	9.80	12.02	14.07	16.62	18.48	24.32
8	1.65	2.03	2.73	3.49	4.59	5.53	7.34	9.52	11.03	13.36	15.51	18.17	20.09	26.12
9	2.09	2.53	3.32	4.17	5.38	6.39	8.34	10.66	12.24	14.68	16.92	19.68	21.67	27.88
10	2.56	3.06	3.94	4.86	6.18	7.27	9.34	11.78	13.44	15.99	18.31	21.16	23.21	29.59
11	3.05	3.61	4.58	5.58	6.99	8.15	10.34	12.90	14.63	17.28	19.68	22.62	24.72	31.26
12	3.57	4.18	5.23	6.30	7.81	9.03	11.34	14.01	15.81	18.55	21.03	24.05	26.22	32.91
13	4.11	4.76	5.89	7.04	8.63	9.93	12.34	15.12	16.98	19.81	22.36	25.47	27.69	34.53
14	4.66	5.37	6.57	7.79	9.47	10.82	13.34	16.22	18.15	21.06	23.68	26.87	29.14	36.12
15	5.23	5.98	7.26	8.55	10.31	11.72	14.34	17.32	19.31	22.81	25.00	28.26	30.58	37.70
16	5.81	6.61	7.96	9.31	11.15	12.62	15.34	18.42	20.46	23.54	26.30	29.83	32.00	39.29
17	6.41	7.26	8.67	10.08	12.00	13.53	16.34	19.51	21.62	24.77	27.59	31.00	33.41	40.75
18	7.02	7.91	9.39	10.86	12.86	14.44	17.34	20.60	22.76	25.99	28.87	32.35	34.80	42.31
19	7.63	8.57	10.12	11.65	13.72	15.35	18.34	21.69	23.90	27.20	30.14	33.69	36.19	43.82
20	8.26	9.24	10.85	12.44	14.58	16.27	19.34	22.78	25.04	28.41	31.41	35.02	37.57	45.82
21	8.90	9.92	11.59	13.24	15.44	17.18	20.34	23.86	26.17	29.62	32.67	36.34	38.93	46.80
22	9.54	10.60	12.34	14.04	16.31	18.10	21.34	24.94	27.30	30.81	33.92	37.66	40.29	48.27
23	10.20	11.29	13.09	14.85	17.19	19.02	22.34	26.02	28.43	32.01	35.17	38.97	41.64	49.73
24	10.86	11.99	13.85	15.66	18.06	19.94	23.34	27.10	29.55	33.20	36.42	40.27	42.98	51.18
25	11.52	12.70	14.61	16.47	18.94	20.87	24.34	28.17	30.68	34.38	37.65	41.57	44.31	52.62
26	12.20	13.41	15.38	17.29	19.82	21.79	25.34	29.25	31.80	35.58	38.88	42.86	45.64	54.05
27	12.88	14.12	16.15	18.11	20.70	22.72	26.34	30.32	32.91	36.74	40.11	44.14	46.96	55.48
28	13.56	14.85	16.93	18.94	21.59	23.65	27.34	31.39	34.03	37.92	41.34	45.42	48.28	56.89
29	14.26	15.57	17.71	19.77	22.48	24.58	28.34	32.46	35.14	39.09	42.56	46.69	49.59	58.30
30	14.95	16.31	18.49	20.60	23.36	25.51	29.34	33.53	36.25	40.26	43.77	47.96	50.89	59.70

Index

Abdo, Abo, H.E., 267
Absher, R.R., 161
Abstract
    elements of, 284
    research report, 261, 268–69
Acceptance page, research report, 261, 263
Achtert, W.S., 251
Acknowledgments page, research report, 261, 264
Action research, elements of, 13–14, 17, 134
Affective measures, types of, 79
After-the-fact research, 134
Alpha level, 222
    alternate alpha level, 227–28
    meaning of, 220
    and type II error, 228
American Alliance for Health, Physical Education, Recreation, and Dance (AAHPERD) Fitness Tests Opinionnaire, 146–49
American Psychological Association (APA)
    ethical guidelines, 24
    research report format guide, 261
Analysis of covariance (ANCOVA), 124–25, 244
    uses of, 244
Analysis of variance (ANOVA), 229–41
    mean square (MS) value, 229
    one-way ANOVA, 229–32
    random blocks ANOVA, 234–35

Analysis of variance (ANOVA)—Cont.
    repeated measures ANOVA, 232–34
    sum of squares (SS), 229, 230
    two-way ANOVA, 235–41
Andrews, E.W., 21
Andrews, J., 160
A posteriori comparisons, 243
Appendixes, research report, 278
Applied research, nature of, 13
Arkin, H., 105
Ary, D., 105
Assumptions, research proposal, 44–45
Attribute variables, 75

Babbie, E., 136, 137, 150
Baiely, W.J., 20
Bain, L., 174, 179
Ballou, S.V., 261
Baptista, R.C., 160
Basic research, nature of, 12–13
Baumgartner, T.A., 89, 90, 91, 116, 128, 133, 168, 169, 196, 206
Becker, H., 179
Bell-shaped curve, 202
Best, J.W., 8, 11, 17, 75, 76, 78, 80, 82, 85, 91, 104, 134, 150, 152
Beta, 228
Bialeschki, M., 188
Bibliographic Index of Health Education Periodicals (BIHEP), 51
Biklen, S., 181, 185
Biographical research, 157–59
Bird, S., 175, 188

Bishop, R., 160
Block designs, 123
Blommers, P.J., 218–19
Blumer, H., 177
BMDP, 251
Body of report, research report, 261, 269–78
Bogdan, R., 181, 185
Bookwalter, C.W., 46, 48
Bookwalter, K.W., 46, 48
Borg, W.R., 137
Bounds, W.G., 125, 244
Bowan, J., 179
Bowen, B.D., 150
Bradburn, N.M., 135
Brennan, M.A., 169
Brown, D.R., 124, 125, 238, 241, 243, 244
Burgess, R.G., 175

Campbell, D., 115, 118, 122, 124
Campbell, D.T., 122
Campbell, W.G., 261
Caruthers, D., 160
Case studies, elements of, 15, 132
Castellan, N.J., 244
Causal comparative/ex post facto approach, elements of, 16
Cell, 232
Central tendency error, 126
Central tendency measures, 203–4
Chaikind, E., 179
Checklists, 86
Chen, A., 176

Chepyator-Thomson, J., 188

Chilcott, J., 186

Chi-square test
one-way chi-square test, 245–47
table for, 318
two-way chi-square test, 247–49

Clark, J.K., 262, 263

Closed-ended questionnaire, 85–86

Closed-ended questions, questionnaires, 138–39, 141

Cluster sampling, 101

Coefficient of determination, 212

Cognitive measures, types of, 78

Cohen, J., 253

Cohen, P., 253

Collins, M.E., 32, 41, 50, 91, 268, 269, 284

Colton, R.R., 105

Completion items, questionnaires, 138

Computer analysis
MYSTAT program, 197
SYSTAT program, 197–98, 200, 202, 207, 209, 214, 222, 223–24, 231, 249
of test scores, 196–98

Computer program development, creative activity, 168

Computer search
database systems, 60
library catalogs, 47–48
steps in, 61

Conceptual literature, 33

Conclusions
in research report, 275, 280
in scientific method, 8, 10–11

Confirmability, in qualitative studies, 186

Contingency table, two-way chi-square test, 247–49

Continuous scores, 195

Continuous variables, 72

Control and experimental research, 122–25
block designs, 123
counter-balanced design, 123–24
matched pairs, 123
physical manipulation, 122–23
selective manipulation, 123
statistical methods, 124–25

Cook, T.D., 122, 173, 174, 175

Cooper, J.M., 21

Core variable, 178

Cormier, W.H., 125, 244

Correlation, 210–14
correlation coefficient, 210–13
meaning of, 251

Correlational research, elements of, 16, 132–33

Correlation coefficient, 210–13
accuracy issues, 213–14
interpretation of, 212–13
negativity of, 212
rank order correlation coefficient, 212
rank order of, 211
testing of, 253–54

Cotter, L.L., 38, 40, 41

Council of Biology Editors, 261

Counter-balanced design, 123–24

Covariates, 124–25, 244

Creative activity, 165–71
computer program development, 168
documentation, 169–70
elements of, 165–66
fine arts department example, 167–68
for graduate students, 170–71
in health and human performance (HHP), 166–67
procedure development, 168–69
standards, 169

Credibility, in qualitative studies, 185

Criterion-referenced standards, 133–34

Critical region, 222

Critical theory, qualitative research, 179

Critical value, 222

Cross-sectional research, 132

Cross-validation, 252

Cunningham, G.K., 128

Curvilinear relationship, 213

Data analysis
computers in, 196–98
descriptive statistics, 196–214
in experimental research, 114
inductive analysis, 174–75
in qualitative research, 184–85
research report, 270, 274–75
in scientific method, 8, 9
of scores, 195–214
steps in, 193

Data collection
plan in research proposal, 62
in qualitative research, 180–81
research report section, 270

Data collection—*Cont.*
in scientific method, 8, 9

Data collection instruments, 89–93
development of, 92–93
objectivity of, 89
reliability of, 89–90
revision of instrument, 91–92
selection of, 90–91
validity, 90

Data collection methods, 76–89
criteria for selection of, 88–89
measurement methods, 78–85
observation, 76, 77
questioning methods, 85–88

Day, R.A., 261

Dayton, C.M., 125, 241

Deductive reasoning, process of, 6, 7

Definition of terms, research proposal, 45–46

Degrees of freedom, 222, 228, 230, 232, 233

Delaney, H.D., 238, 241

Deliberate sampling, 101

Delimitations, research proposal, 42–43

Delphi technique, 88

Dempsey, K., 179

Denzin, N., 177, 184

Dependability, in qualitative studies, 186

Dependent variables, 72–73

Descriptive research, 130–50
action research, 134
case studies, 132
correlational research, 132–33
cross-sectional research, 132
elements of, 15, 69, 130–31
ex post facto research, 134
longitudinal research, 131–32
normative research, 133–34
observational research, 134
surveys, 131, 135–50

Descriptive statistics, 193, 202–14
correlation, 210–14
descriptive values, 202
mean, 204
median, 204
mode, 203
percentile ranks/percentiles, 206–7
range, 205
standard deviation, 205
standard scores, 207
uses of, 193

Descriptive statistics—*Cont.*
  variability measures, 204–6
  variance, 205–6
Descriptive values, data analysis, 202
Design of experiment, 114, 118–21
  pre-experimental design, 119
  quasi-experimental design, 120
  true experimental design, 119–20
Developmental research, elements of, 15, 131–32
Dill, S., 168
Dillman, D.A., 150
Direct Access to Reference Information (DATRIX), 60
Directional statement, of research hypothesis, 18
Direct observation, 77, 181
Discrete scores, 195
Discrete variables, 71
Distributed questionnaire, 138
Dixey, R., 179
Document analysis, qualitative research, 183
Documentation, creative activity, 169–70
Double-blind study, 127
  post hoc error, 127
Drake, A., 160

East, W.B., 169
Education Resources Information Center (ERIC), 60
Eisner, E., 186
Empiricism, meaning of, 12
Eng, E., 188
Ennis, C., 188
Error and experimental research, 125–27
  central tendency error, 126
  experimenter bias effect, 126–27
  halo effect, 126
  Hawthorne effect, 125
  John Henry effect, 126
  overrater error, 126
  placebo effect, 125–26
  subject-researcher interaction effect, 127
  underrater error, 126
Ethics and research, 22–27
  APA guidelines, 24
  Informed Consent Statement, 23–24, 26–27
  privacy/confidentiality, 23–24

Ethics and research—*Cont.*
  Protection of Human Subjects Form, 22–23, 24–25
Ethnographic research, as qualitative approach, 175
Expected frequency, 245–46
Experimental research, 110–28
  control methods in, 122–25
  designs, 119
  elements of, 16, 69
  error sources in, 125–27
  hypothesis in, 112
  measurement in, 128
  pre-experimental design, 119
  quasi-experimental design, 120
  steps in, 111–14
  true experimental design, 119–20
  validity, 114–18
  variables in, 111–12, 113
Experimental setting, and validity, 118
Experimenter bias effect, 126–27
Experiment-wise error rate, 243
Ex post facto research, elements of, 16, 134
External criticism, historical research, 155
External validity
  meaning of, 115, 122
  threats to, 117–18
Extraneous variables, 74–75

Factorial design, 236
Feminist theory, qualitative research, 179
Ferguson, G.A., 195, 213, 214, 218, 229, 235, 243, 244, 253
Fidell, L.S., 251
Field notes
  nature of, 181
  reflective field notes, 181
Field research, as qualitative research, 175
Fine arts, creative activity in, 167–68
Fishbowl technique, in sampling, 98
Fleming, W., 160
Focus groups, 183
Fors, S., 183, 188
Fox, D.J., 30, 31, 33, 70, 76, 77, 78, 80, 82, 85, 101, 152, 153
F ratio, 231–32
Fratzke, M.R., 31
Frequency polygon, 201–2

Friedman two-way ANOVA, 245
Frye, P.A., 40
F statistic, 229, 230–31
F table, 231, 312–17
F test, 229, 243

Gaunt, S.J., 31, 168
Geertz, C., 177, 181
Gibaldi, J., 251
Glaser, B., 178
Goetz, J., 175, 176, 185, 186
Good, C.V., 5
Goodman, R., 172–73, 175, 188
Goodness of fit, one-way chi-square test, 245–47
Gorden, R., 182
Graham, C., 179
Graphs, 200–202
  curvilinear relationship, 213
  frequency polygon, 201–2
  histogram, 202
  leptokurtic curve, 202
  linear relationship in, 213
  normal curve, 202
  platykurtic curve, 202
  positively/negatively skewed curve, 202
  of prediction equation, 252
  scattergram, 209
Green, K.N., 169
Green, L., 128
Griffin, P., 174
Grosshans, I.R., 158, 161
Grounded theory, qualitative research, 178–79
Guba, E., 175, 185, 186

Hagen, E.P., 128
Halo effect, 126
  rating scales, 82
Handrick, J., 39, 50, 265
Harrington, W., 174
Harris, R.J., 251
Hashim, T.J., 38
Hawthorne effect, 125
Health and human performance (HHP)
  creative activity in, 166–67
  historical research in, 157, 159–61
  purpose of research in, 20–22
  qualitative research in, 173–74, 187–88

Henderson, K.A., 137, 173, 176, 179, 185, 186, 188
Hensley, L.D., 169
Histogram, 202
Historical research, 151–53, 157
    biographical research, 157–59
    elements of, 14, 69, 151–52
    external criticism of, 155
    format for, 161–63
    in health and human performance (HHP), 159–61
    hypotheses in, 159
    internal criticism of, 156
    interpretation of, 153
    oral history, 156–57
    primary data sources, 153–54
    problems related to, 152–53
    secondary data sources, 154–55
History, and internal validity, 115–16, 117
Holland, J.C., 31, 104
Hollander, M., 244
Howe, C., 188
Huberman, M., 184
Huck, S.W., 125, 244
Hult, J.S., 160
Hypotheses
    in experimental research, 112
    in historical research, 159
    research hypothesis, 17–20
    research proposal, 45
    in scientific method, 8, 9–10
    time for use of, 70
Hypothesis-testing method, 219–21
    accepting/rejecting null hypothesis, 220–21
    alternate hypotheses, uses of, 227–29
    null hypothesis in, 219, 220–21
    probability level selection, 220
    research hypothesis, 219
    statement of hypothesis, 219
    statistical hypothesis, 219
    statistical table, use of, 220

Imperfect induction, meaning of, 7
Implementations section, research report, 275, 281
Independent variables, 72–73, 111–12
Indexes
    library research, 51–52
    listing of, 51–52
Indiana University Libraries Bulletin, 60
Indirect observation, 77

Induction
    process of, 6–7
    types of, 7
Inductive analysis, in qualitative research, 174–75
Inferential statistics, 217–54
    analysis of covariance (ANCOVA), 124–25, 244
    analysis of variance (ANOVA), 229–41
    assumptions related to statistical tests, 241
    hypothesis-testing method, 219–21
    inference in, 218–19
    multivariate tests, 249, 251
    one-group t test, 221–22
    one-way chi-square test, 245–47
    prediction-regression analysis, 251–53
    two dependent groups t test, 224–27
    two-group comparisons, 243
    two independent groups t test, 223–24
    two-way chi-square test, 247–49
    type I and type II errors, 228–29
    univariate tests, 249
    uses of, 193, 218
Informed Consent Statement, 23–24, 26–27
Internal consistency reliability, 89–90
Internal criticism, historical research, 156
Internal validity
    meaning of, 114–15, 122
    threats to, 115–17
Internet, 47
Interpretation, 177
Interval scores, 195–96
Intervening variables, 73–74
Interview guide, 86–87
Interviews
    focus groups, 183
    interviewer methods in, 182–83
    interview schedule, 181–82
    personal interviews, 136–37
    phone interviews, 136
    qualitative research, 181–83
    semistructured interviews, 136
    structured interviews, 136, 181
    unstructured interviews, 136, 181–82
Introduction
    of research proposal, 39–40
    of research report, 269

Inventory method, 79–80
Isaac, S., 14, 82, 111, 115, 134, 137, 149, 166, 289, 290

Jackson, A.S., 89, 90, 91, 116, 128, 133, 169, 196, 206
Jacobs, L.C., 105
John Henry effect, 126
Journal articles. *See* Published articles
Justification for study, research proposal, 41–42

Kahn, J.V., 134, 150
Keller, K., 183
Keppel, G., 124, 125, 238, 241, 244
Kerlinger, F.N., 82
Key informants, 181
Kirk, J., 186
Kirk, R.E., 241
Kramer, W.D., 168
Krejcie, R.V., 105
Kruskal-Wallis one–way ANOVA, 245

Lacey, E., 183
Laing, D., 178
LeCompte, M., 175, 176, 185, 186
Leninger, M., 174
Leptokurtic curve, 202
Levinson, R., 183, 188
Lev, J., 214
Lewis, F.M., 128
Library, classification systems used, 47
Likert scale, 84–85
Limitations, research proposal, 43–44
Lincoln, Y., 175, 185, 186, 187
Linear relationship, 213
Line of best fit, 209
List of figures, research report, 261, 267
List of tables, research report, 261, 266
Literary Digest presidential election sample, 103
Literature review, 49–51
    classification of readings, 49–50
    research proposal, 49–51
    summary for, 50–51
    time factors, 47
Literature search, 46–48, 51–61
    computer search, 60–61
    of conceptual literature, 33
    and critical reading, 48
    indexes for, 51–52
    library classification systems, 47
    note-taking in, 48–49

Literature search—*Cont.*
periodicals, 53–60
of related literature, 33
reviews, 52–53
and working bibliography, 47
Locke, L.F., 172, 261
Longitudinal research, 131–32
Luedke, G.C., 45
Lumpkin, A., 160
Lyon, L.P., 79

Maatz-Majestic, E., 188
Marascuilo, L.A., 244
Margan, D.W., 105
Marshall, C., 180, 186
Massoumeh, M.J., 20
Matched pairs, 123
Matched pairs design, 224, 225–26
Maxwell, C., 238, 241
McClenaghan, B.A., 169
McCormick, L., 175, 188
McDermott, R.J., 128
McLachlan, L., 178
McLaughlin, J., 180, 183, 188, 189
McLeroy, K., 175, 188
McMillan, J.H., 150
McSweeney, M., 244
Mean, 204
Mean square (MS) value, 229
Measurement methods, 78–85
affective measures, 79
cognitive measures, 78
inventory method, 79–80
physical measures, 78
projective technique, 80
scaling methods, 80–85
sociometric method, 80
Median, 204
Medline, 60
Member checks, 185
Merriam, S., 175
Michael, W.B., 14, 82, 111, 115, 134, 137, 149, 166, 289, 290
Michels, K.N., 124, 125, 238, 241, 243, 244
Miles, M., 184
Miller, M., 186
Mobley, T.A., 5
Mode, 203
Morgan, D., 178
Mullen, P., 178
Mull, S.S., 33

Multiple-choice questions, questionnaires, 138–39
Multiple comparisons, 243
Multiple prediction, 252–53
Multistage sampling, 101
Multivariate tests, 249, 251
types of, 251
uses of, 193
MYSTAT program, 197

Naturalistic inquiry, and qualitative research, 173
Negatively skewed curve, 202
Nelson, J.K., 100, 165
Nevins, A., 157
Nominal scores, 196
Nondirectional statement, of research hypothesis, 18
Nonlinear regression, 253
Nonparametric statistics, uses of, 193, 244–45
Nonparticipant observers, 181
Nonprobability samples, 102
Nonsignificant statistical test, 221
Normal curve, 202
Normative research, 133–34
Norm-referenced standards, 133
Note-taking, library research, 48–49
Null hypothesis, 19–20, 219, 220–21
acceptance of, 220–21
meaning of, 19
rejection of, 220
and type II error, 228

Objectivity, in data collection instrument, 89
Observation, 76, 77
direct observation, 77, 181
field notes in, 181
indirect observation, 77
nonparticipant observers, 181
participant observation, 77, 181
in various research methods, 76
Observational research, 134
Observed frequency, 245–46
Ogilvie, B.C., 79
Ogletree, R.J., 46, 266
One-group *t* test, 221–22
One-tailed statistical test, 228
One-way ANOVA, 229–32
Kruskal-Wallis one-way ANOVA, 245
steps in, 231–32

One-way chi-square test, 245–47
expected and observed frequencies, 245–46
steps in, 246–47
Open-ended questionnaire, 86
Open-ended questions, 138
Oral history, historical research, 156–57
Ordinal scores, 196
Outline, of research problem, 35–37
Overrater error, 126
Owen, S., 183, 188

Padilla, S., 41
Paired-comparison scale, 84
Parameters, 193
Parametric statistics, uses of, 193, 244
Participant observation, 77, 181
Pate, D.J., 45
Patton, M., 177
Pearson, Karl, 210
Pedhazur, E.J., 253
Pelegrino, D.A., 21
Peña, C., 38
Percentile ranks, 206–7
Percentiles, 206–7
Per-comparison error rate, 243
Perfect induction, meaning of, 7
Periodicals, listing for HHP field, 53–60
Phenomenology, qualitative research, 177–78
Phone interviews, 136
Photographs, in qualitative research, 183
Physical Education Index, 51
Physical manipulation, of variables, 122–23
Physical measures, types of, 78
Piercy, I., 159
Placebo, meaning of, 126
Placebo effect, 125–26
Platykurtic curve, 202
Polynomial regression, 253
Population, 96–97
meaning of, 96
parameters, 193
and sampling, 96–97
Positively skewed curve, 202
Post hoc error, 127
Prediction, meaning of, 251
Prediction-regression analysis, 251–53
multiple prediction, 252–53
simple prediction, 252
Pre-experimental design, 119

Primary data sources, historical research, 153–54

Privacy/confidentiality, of research subjects, 23–24

Probes, in interviews, 182

Problem identification, in scientific method, 7–8, 9

Problem statement, research proposal, 39–40

Procedure development, creative activity, 168–69

Procedures section, research proposal, 62–66

Projective technique, 80

Proposal. *See* Research proposal

Protection of Human Subjects Form, 22–23, 24–25

Prusoczuk, K., 168

PsycLIT, 60

Published articles
   critiquing article, 289–90
   elements of, 285
   parts of, 286–87
   pre-writing activities, 286
   proofreading of, 287
   submitted to journals, 288–89
   thesis/dissertation for, 285

Purpose statement, research proposal, 40–41

Qualitative research, 172–89
   compared to quantitative research, 175–76
   critical theory, 179
   data analysis, 184–85
   data collection in, 180–81
   direct observation, 181
   document analysis, 183
   elements of, 174–75
   ethnographic research as, 175
   feminist theory, 179
   field research as, 175
   grounded theory, 178–79
   in health and human performance (HHP), 173–74, 187–88
   interview, 181–83
   and naturalistic inquiry, 173
   phenomenology, 177–78
   photos/videos, use of, 183
   reader's approach to, 186–87
   reseach idea in, 180
   research question in, 180

Qualitative research—*Cont.*
   research report, 185
   supporting quantitative data, 184
   symbolic interaction, 177
   triangulation in, 184
   trustworthiness of data, 185–86
   uses/applications of, 187–89

Qualitative variables, 71

Quantitative research, compared to qualitative research, 175–76

Quantitative variables, 71

Quasi-experimental design, 120

Questioning methods, 85–88
   checklists, 86
   Delphi technique, 88
   structured interview, 86–87
   structured questionnaire, 85–86
   unstructured interview, 87–88
   unstructured questionnaire, 86

Questionnaires, 137–50
   administration of, 137–38
   analysis of data from, 143–44
   distributed questionnaire, 138
   distribution of, 142–43
   example of, 146–49
   format for, 140–41, 144–46
   questions, types of, 138–39
   reliability, 140
   return of completed questionnaires, 143–44
   validity, 139

Random blocks ANOVA, 234–35
   steps in, 239–41

Random Numbers program, 100

Random sample, 97–99
   collection methods for, 98
   research subjects, 75
   and validity, 117, 118

Range, 205

Rank order correlation coefficient, 211

Rank order scales, 82

Rating scales, 80–82
   halo effect, 82
   Likert scale, 84–85
   paired-comparison scale, 84
   rank order scales, 82
   semantic differential scale, 82

Ratio scores, 195

Razeveih, A., 105

Reader's Guide to Periodical Literature, 51

Real difference, 219

Reason, P., 179

Reasoning
   deductive, 5–6
   inductive, 6–7

Recommendations, research report, 275, 281–82

References, research report, 278, 283

Reflective field notes, 181

Regression
   meaning of, 251
   nonlinear regression, 253
   polynomial regression, 253
   prediction-regression analysis, 251–53

Regression line, 209

Reichardt, C.S., 173, 174, 175

Related literature, 33

Reliability
   in data collection instrument, 89–90
   internal consistency reliability, 89–90
   questionnaires, 140
   stability reliability, 90

Repeated measures ANOVA, 232–34
   steps in, 233–34

Repeated measures design, 224–25, 226–27

Reports. *See* Research report

Representative sample, 97

Research
   applied research, 13
   basic research, 12–13
   ethical issues, 22–27

Research approach
   intent of study, 70
   time frame of interest in, 69

Research classifications
   action approach, 13–14, 17
   case and field approach, 15, 132
   causal comparative/ex post facto approach, 16
   correlational approach, 16
   creative activity, 165–71
   descriptive approach, 15, 130–50
   developmental approach, 15
   experimental approach, 16, 110–28
   historical approach, 14, 151–63
   qualitative research, 172–89

Research hypothesis, 17–20, 219
   characteristics of, 17–18
   directional/nondirectional statement of, 18
   and null hypothesis, 19–20

Research process
 criteria for research problem, 33–35
 data collection instruments, 89–93
 data collection methods, 76–89
 hypotheses statement, 70
 literature consulted in, 33
 outline of problem, 35–37
 problem definition, 33
 problem selection, 31–32
 research approach, 69–70
 research proposal, 37–66
 steps in, 30–31
 and variables, 71–76
Research proposal, 37–66
 assumptions, 44–45
 data collection plan, 62
 definition of terms, 45–46
 delimitations, 42–43
 hypotheses, 45
 introduction, 39–40
 justification for study, 41–42
 limitations, 43–44
 literature review, 49–51
 literature search, 46–47, 48, 51–61
 problem statement, 39–40
 procedures section, 62–66
 purpose statement, 40–41
 title of, 38
 working bibliography, 47
Research report, 114
 abstract, 261, 268–69
 acceptance page, 261, 263
 acknowledgments page, 261, 264
 appendixes, 278
 body of report, 261, 269–78
 checklist for, 291–93
 conclusions, 275, 280
 data analysis, 270, 274–75
 data collection procedures, 270
 data reporting tables, examples of,
  272–74
 discussion of findings, example of,
  276–77
 in experimental research, 114
 format for, 261
 implementations section, 275, 281
 introduction, 269
 list of figures, 261, 267
 list of tables, 261, 266
 opening paragraph, example of, 270
 in qualitative research, 185
 recommendations, 275, 281–82

Research report—*Cont.*
 references, 278, 283
 research problem/hypotheses,
  example of, 271
 review of related literature, 269–70
 summary, 275, 279
 table of contents, 261, 265
 title page, 261, 262
Research subjects, selection of.
 See Sampling
Reviews
 library research, 52–53
 listing of, 52–53
Reznik, J.W., 160
Rho, 211
Rist, R., 175
Robbins, M.P., 8, 9
Ross, D., 168
Ross, J., 176
Rossman, G., 180, 186
Rubin, H.J., 137, 150
Rubinson, L., 22, 88, 150, 155

Safrit, M.J., 253
Sage Publications, 135
Sample, meaning of, 96
Sampling
 appropriateness of sample, 104–5
 cluster sampling, 101
 deliberate sampling, 101
 multistage sampling, 101
 nonprobability samples, 102
 and population, 96–97
 random selection, 97–99
 sample size, 102–5
 simple random sample, 97–99
 stratified random sampling, 99–100
 systematic sampling, 100
Sampling error, 218–19
Sampling units, 101
Sarvela, P., 128
SAS, 197, 244, 251
Sax, G., 6, 100
Scaling methods, 80–85
 rating scales, 80–82
Scattergram, 209
Scheibner, H.L., 161
Schulsinger, F., 92
Schumacher, S., 150
Scientific method, 7–11
 application of, 8–10
 steps in, 7–8

Scores, 195–202
 analysis of. *See* Descriptive statistics
 computer analysis of, 196–98
 continuous scores, 195
 discrete scores, 195
 graphing of, 200–202
 interval scores, 195–96
 nominal scores, 196
 ordinal scores, 196
 ratio scores, 195
 simple frequency distributions,
  198–200
 standard scores, 207
Seaman, J., 8, 9
Secondary data sources, historical
  research, 154–55
Selective manipulation, of variables, 123
Sells, T.D., 271, 274
Semantic differential scale, 82
Semistructured interviews, 136
Siegel, S., 244
Significance, of statistical test, 220–21
Silverman, Stephen, 100
Simple effects test, 239–40
Simple frequency distributions, 198–200
Simple prediction, 252
Single-blind study, 127
Sliepcevich, E., 183, 189
Slope, 252
Smith, M., 186
Sociometric method, 80
Sorenson, T., 92
Spearman's rho, 211
Spirduso, W.W., 261
Sport Discus, 60
Spradley, J., 182, 185
SPSS, 197, 253
SPSSX, 244, 251
Stability reliability, 90
Standard deviation, 205
Standard error of prediction, 252
Standards, creative activity, 169
Standard scores, 207
Stanley, J., 115, 118, 122, 124
Statistical hypothesis, 219
Statistical power, 229
Statistical regression, and internal
  validity, 116–17
Statistics, 124–25, 203–6
 descriptive statistics, 193, 202–14
 inferential statistics, 193, 217–54
 multivariate statistics, 193

Statistics—*Cont.*
    nonparametric statistics, 193, 244–45
    parametric statistics, 193, 244
    selection of method, 254
    univariate statistics, 193
    See also Descriptive statistics;
        Inferential statistics
Steckler, A., 172–73, 175, 188
Stevens, J., 251
Stevenson, M.J., 160
Stoner, J., 160
Stratified random sampling, 99–100
Strauss, A., 178
Structured interviews, 86–87, 136, 181
Structured questionnaire, 85–86
Stunkard, A.J., 92
Sudman, S., 135
Summary, research report, 275, 279
Sum of squares (SS), 229, 230
Sun, D.C., 39, 42, 44
Surveys, 131, 135–50
    personal interviews, 136–37
    phone interviews, 136
    pre-research planning, 135
    questionnaires, 137–50
Syllogism, nature of, 6
Symbolic interaction, qualitative
    research, 177
SYSTAT program, 197–98, 200, 202,
    207, 209, 214, 222, 223–24, 231, 249
Systematic sampling, 100

Tabachnick, B.G., 251
Table of contents, research report, 261,
    265
Table of random numbers, in sampling,
    98–99
Tables for Statisticians, 105
Takane, Y., 195, 213, 214, 218, 229, 235,
    243, 244, 253
Tapp, M., 188
Tatsuoka, M.M., 251
Testing
    and external validity, 117–18
    and internal validity, 116
Theory
    meaning of, 11
    and research, 11–12
Thesis/dissertation
    abstract, 284
    compared to research report, 284
Thick description, 180–81

Thomas, J.R., 100, 165
Thorndike, R.L., 128
Thorndike, R.M., 128
Time frame of interest, for research
    project, 69
Title page
    of research proposal, 38
    of research report, 261, 262
Torabi, M.R., 20
Transferability, in qualitative studies,
    185–86
Triangulation, 184
True experimental design, 119–20
Truth, sources of evidence, 5–6
t scores, 207
t table, 310–11
t tests
    one-group *t* test, 221–22
    two dependent groups *t* test, 224–27
    two independent groups *t* test, 223–24
Tuckman, B.W., 150
Turabian, K.L., 261
Tutko, T.A., 79
Two-dimensional ANOVA, 236
Two-group comparisons, 243
Two independent groups *t* test, 223–24
    matched pairs design, 224, 225–26
    repeated measures design, 224–25,
        226–27
Two-tailed statistical test, 228
Two-way ANOVA, 235–41
    factorial design, 236
    Friedman two-way ANOVA, 245
    simple effects test, 239–40
    steps in, 239–41
    two-dimensional ANOVA, 236
Two-way chi-square test, 247–49
    steps in, 249
Type I errors, 228–29
Type II errors, 228–29
Typologies, 174

Underrater error, 126
Univariate statistics, uses of, 193
Univariate tests, 249
Unstructured interviews, 87–88, 136, 181
Unstructured questionnaire, 86

Validity
    in data collection instrument, 90
    in experimental research, 114–18
    external validity, 115, 122

Validity—*Cont.*
    internal validity, 114–15, 122
    questionnaires, 139
    threats to, 115–18
Van Clief, E.W., 88
Van Dalen, D.B., 115, 134, 154, 158
Van Oteghen, S.L., 50
Variability measures, 204–6
Variables, 71–76
    attribute variables, 75
    classification/identification of, 113
    continuous variables, 72
    control, methods for, 75–76, 122–25
    dependent variables, 72–73, 111–12
    discrete variables, 71
    extraneous variables, 74–75
    independent variables, 72–73, 111–12
    intervening variables, 73–74
    qualitative variables, 71
    quantitative variables, 71
Variance, 205–6
Variate, 124–25, 244
Videos, in qualitative research, 183
Visker, T.L., 38, 40, 270, 272, 273,
    279–82
Vitello, E., 183

Walker, H.M., 214
Weisberg, H.F., 150
Welcher, C.L., 42
West, J., 177
Wettan, R.G., 160
Wiersma, W., 134, 137, 149
Wiggins, D.K., 160
Williams, H.G., 169
Williamson, K., 178
Willis, J., 160
Willis, J.D., 160
Wilson, S., 177
Wilson, T., 179
Winer, B.J., 124, 125, 238, 241, 243, 244
Wolcott, H., 175, 186
Wolfe, D.A., 244
Wood, T.M., 253
Working bibliography, 47
    research proposal, 47
Wright, R., 183

Y-intercept, 252

Zeeberg, I., 180
Z scores, 207, 208